MEDICAL RADIOLOGY
Diagnostic Imaging

Editors:
A. L. Baert, Leuven
K. Sartor, Heidelberg

J. Golzarian · S. Sun · M. J. Sharafuddin (Eds.)

Vascular Embolotherapy

A Comprehensive Approach

Volume 1
General Principles, Chest, Abdomen, and Great Vessels

With Contributions by

H. T. Abada · D. M. Coldwell · M. D. Darcy · L. Defreyne · A. Fauconnier · J. Golzarian
D. Hunter · P. Lacombe · A. Laurent · L. Machan · H. Mimura · T. A. Nicholson · J. P. Pelage
J. S. Pollak · M. K. Razavi · J. A. Reekers · A. C. Roberts · G. T. Rosen · M. J. Sharafuddin
G. P. Siskin · S. Sun · K. Takahashi · J. C. van den Berg · D. Valenti · R. I. White, Jr.
J. J. Wong

Foreword by
A. L. Baert

With 171 Figures in 414 Separate Illustrations, 43 in Color and 33 Tables

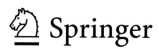 Springer

Jafar Golzarian, MD
Professor of Radiology, Department of Radiology
University of Iowa Hospitals and Clinics
Carver College of Medicine
200 Hawkins Drive
Iowa City, IA 52242
USA

Shiliang Sun, MD
Associate Professor of Radiology
University of Iowa Hospitals and Clinics
Carver College of Medicine
200 Hawkins Drive
Iowa City, IA 52242
USA

Melhelm J. Sharafuddin, MD
Departments of Radiology and Surgery
University of Iowa Hospitals and Clinics
Carver College of Medicine
200 Hawkins Drive
Iowa City, IA 52242
USA

Medical Radiology · Diagnostic Imaging and Radiation Oncology
Series Editors: A. L. Baert · L. W. Brady · H.-P. Heilmann · M. Molls · K. Sartor

Continuation of Handbuch der medizinischen Radiologie
Encyclopedia of Medical Radiology

Library of Congress Control Number: 2004117986

ISBN 3-540-21361-9 Springer Berlin Heidelberg New York
ISBN 978-3-540-21361-1 Springer Berlin Heidelberg New York

Springer is part of Springer Science+Business Media

http//www.springer.com
© Springer-Verlag Berlin Heidelberg 2006
Printed in Germany

Medical Editor: Dr. Ute Heilmann, Heidelberg
Desk Editor: Ursula N. Davis, Heidelberg
Production Editor: Kurt Teichmann, Mauer
Cover-Design and Typesetting: Verlagsservice Teichmann, Mauer

*T*o my parents
a wellspring of love and support without limit.
I owe you everything.

*T*o my wonderful wife, *Elham*
and my children *Sina* and *Sadra*

Dr. Golzarian

*T*o my wife, *Shuzhen*, and daughter, *Yue*
for their selfless support
Dr. Sun

*T*o my wife *Lucy*, and children *Jacob* and *Evan*
Dr. Sharafuddin

*T*o all our teachers

Foreword

Percutaneous image-guided treatment is now well recognized as an effective minimally invasive treatment modality in modern medicine. Its field of application is growing every year due to the availability of more and more sophisticated materials, tools and devices, but also because of the technical progress in reduction of the dose of ionizing irradiation incurred by both patient and radiologist during fluoroscopy.

Vascular embolotherapy is now one of the main forms of endovascular percutaneous treatment of diseases of the vascular system.

The editors of the two volumes of "Vascular Embolotherapy: a Comprehensive Approach", J. Golzarian, S. Sun and M.J. Sharafuddin, leading experts in the field, were successful in obtaining the collaboration of many other internationally renowned interventional radiologists. I am particularly indebted to Professor Golzarian for his original concept for these books and his relentless efforts to complete the project in good time.

I would like to congratulate the editors and authors on producing these well-written, superbly illustrated and exhaustive volumes covering all aspects of vascular embolotherapy. The readers will find comprehensive up-to-date information as a source of knowledge and as a guideline for their daily clinical work.

These two outstanding books will certainly meet with high interest from interventional radiologists and vascular surgeons. They – and therefore their patients – will greatly benefit from its contents. Also referring physicians may find these books very useful to learn more about the indications, possibilities and limitations of modern vascular embolotherapy

I am confident that these two volumes will encounter the same success with readers as the previous books in this series.

Leuven   ALBERT L. BAERT

Preface

Therapeutic embolization has now become a major part of modern interventional practice, and its applications have become an integral component of the modern multimodality management paradigms in trauma, gastrointestinal hemorrhage and oncology, and the endovascular therapy of vascular malformations and aneurysms. The past decade has also marked the emergence of several new indications for therapeutic embolization, such as uterine fibroid embolization, and the widespread acceptance of embolization therapy as an effective non-operative management modality for major hepatic, splenic and renal injuries that once posed tremendous challenge to the trauma surgeon. Embolization therapy has also become an integral facet of the modern oncology center, offering solid-organ chemoembolization, preoperative devascularization, hepatic growth stimulation prior to resection, and direct gene therapy delivery.

Despite this remarkable growth, there are currently few references available to summarize this major field in vascular interventional therapy. The purpose of our two-volume book was to organize and present the current state of the art of embolotherapy in a comprehensive yet manageable manner. Our goal was to provide a user-friendly, well-illustrated, and easy-to-browse resource to enable both experts and novices in this field to quickly derive high-yield clinically relevant information when needed. In addition to standard applications of embolotherapy, we have also included a number of closely related applications that have become intimately associated with the field of therapeutic embolization, such as stent-graft placement and radiofrequency ablation. The two volumes constitute the combined experience of many of the leading experts in the field and have been generously supplemented with helpful tables, illustrations and detailed imaging material. We have also striven to include insightful discussions and a "cookbook" segment in each topic to provide a quick outline of procedural preparation and technique. We have included a chapter on monitoring and resuscitation of the hemorrhaging patient that should be a "must-read" for the interventionist who is not well versed in surgical critical care. Readers will also find important coverage of pathophysiology and of diagnostic clinical as well as imaging workup.

We hope this reference will meet the needs of physicians providing therapeutic embolization, whether they are trainees, recent graduates or even well-established interventionists who wish to refresh their memory or learn the opinion of some of the field's renowned experts before embarking on a difficult case or trying a new technique or approach.

Iowa City

Jafar Golzarian
Shiliang Sun
Melhem J. Sharafuddin

Contents

General Principles

1 Embolotherapy: Basic Principles and Applications

Melhem J. Sharafuddin, Shiliang Sun, and Jafar Golzarian

CONTENTS

1.1 Introduction

Embolotherapy is defined as the percutaneous endovascular use of one or more of a variety of agents or materials to accomplish vascular occlusion. The number of applications of embolotherapy continues to expand. This text provides a brief overview of the current applications of embolotherapy, current embolic techniques and some related general principles.

Embolotherapy initially evolved as a minimally invasive means for arresting uncontrolled hemorrhage in a number of clinical scenarios including upper gastrointestinal (UGI) bleeding resulting from ulcerative disease, malignancy, pancreatitis

M. J. Sharafuddin, MD
Departments of Radiology and Surgery, University of Iowa Hospitals and Clinics, 200 Hawkins Drive, Iowa City, IA 52242, USA
S. Sun, MD
Associate Professor of Radiology, University of Iowa Hospitals and Clinics, 200 Hawkins Drive, Iowa City, IA 52242, USA
J. Golzarian, MD
Professor of Radiology, Director, Vascular and Interventional Radiology, University of Iowa Hospitals and Clinics, 200 Hawkins Drive, 3957 JPP, Iowa City, IA 52242, USA

and hemobilia [1–9]. Its efficacy was also described in lower gastrointestinal (LGI) hemorrhage due to tumors, diverticular disease, angiodysplasia [7, 10–14]. Embolotherapy was also determined to be a valuable tool in the management of obstetric and gynecologic bleeding due to peripartum complications, and in benign and malignant gynecologic tumors [15, 16]. Bronchial artery embolization is also a well recognized and often the only effective modality for the management of severe hemoptysis in a variety of inflammatory lung conditions [17, 18]. It has also been described in spontaneous retroperitoneal hemorrhage, as well as retroperitoneal and intraperitoneal hemorrhage due to vascular tumors [19].

Perhaps one of the most well recognized applications of embolotherapy is traumatic hemorrhage, especially from pelvic fractures, and appendicular musculoskeletal injuries [20–23]. In recent years, embolotherapy has also become increasingly recognized as an excellent modality for the non-operative management of solid organ trauma, including the liver [24–28], spleen [26, 29–32] and kidneys [26, 33–35]. Embolization is also the leading modality in the management of iatrogenic solid organ and vascular injuries, especially those cause by percutaneous biopsy and laparoscopy [36]. Transjugular embolization in conjunction with TIPS [37], as well as direct percutaneous transhepatic embolization [38, 39] of bleeding portosystemic varices are also effective approaches in the management of UGI and LGI hemorrhage due to portal venous hypertension.

With the current advances in technology allowing more accurate and controlled deployment of embolic agents, embolotherapy has now become the procedure of choice for the management of visceral and solid organ aneurysms [40–42]. In addition, embolotherapy has now arguably become the primary facet in the management of vascular malformations of all varieties, in the central nervous system and head and neck [43, 44], pulmonary circulation [45–48], viscera, trunk and extremities [49–54].

Embolotherapy is also an effective means for the management of symptomatic male varicocele [55], vasogenic impotence, and priapism [56, 57]. Embolotherapy is also the main effective modality for the management of the pelvic venous congestion syndrome in women [58].

Embolotherapy has recently gained acclaim as valid tissue ablation and devascularization modality. Portal vein embolization is becoming an increasingly well recognized tool for organ flow redistribution, to allow increased regeneration prior to planned hepatic resection [59–61]. It is also a promising modality to enhance vector expression in gene transfer therapy aimed at the hepatocyte [62]. Preoperative embolization of vascular skeletal metastases or vascular solid organ tumors was also recognized as a useful application in the early days of Embolotherapy [63–65]. Ablation of dysfunctioning organs using various embolization techniques and regimens has also been well described for management of hypertension or protein wasting in end-stage renal disease [66, 67], hypersplenism, and immune disorders of the spleen [30, 68–70], and recently in Graves' disease of the thyroid [71]. The evolution of uterine fibroid embolization has established the role of embolotherapy as a viable alternative to hysterectomy, and undoubtedly revolutionized the management options in this very common disorder [72–74]. Chemoembolization has also become a key component of the modern multimodality treatment paradigms of primary and metastatic hepatic tumors [75–77].

The advance of endovascular therapy for aortoiliac aneurysmal disease has also brought about yet another flourishing application of embolotherapy. Embolization of the internal iliac artery plays an important adjunct initial modality to allow endovascular treatment of aortic aneurysms with extension into the common iliac arteries [78–80]. It also plays an crucial role in the secondary management of complications related to endoleaks [81–84].

1.2
The Ideal Vascular Occlusion Technique

The ideal vascular occlusion technique is one that allows accurate guidance and delivery to the target with low risk of injury to normal structures. This characteristic is a function of various specific attributes: (1) radiopacity, radio-opaque markers or ability to mix into radiopaque suspension, (2) simplicity of the delivery technique, (3) reliability of delivery mechanism, (4) ability to reach distal vascular beds,

(5) amenability to trouble shooting/salvage in case of complications or device malfunction (for example ability to easily retrieve and preferably also redeploy the device in case of misplacement; (6) efficacy or the ability to result in rapid occlusion for a duration appropriate to the desired application; (7) being adaptable to allow selective occlusion of various vessel types and sizes; (8) biocompatible components, and (9) cost competitiveness.

1.2.1
Classification of Intravascular Embolic Agents

Numerous devices or materials have been used to accomplish effective vascular occlusion and their specific details are beyond the scope of this brief summary. A broad classification and examples are listed in Table 1.1. Broadly speaking, embolic materials can be classified into different categories based on their physical and biological properties. It is important to note that the level of occlusion, which is primarily determined by the size of the agent, can also be affected by the occurrence of secondary clumping of individual particles. Embolic materials and devices are now available that can allow the occlusion of anywhere from a large vessel to a distal arteriolar or capillary level. The majority of non-neurovascular embolization procedures are currently performed with coils, Gelfoam, particles, and liquid sclerosants. There has also been increased interest in solidifying liquid mixtures and tissue glues. Mechanical embolic agents function by causing a direct mechanical obstruction of the lumen as well as providing a matrix for thrombus formation ultimately resulting in occlusion. Certain agents can also incite an inflammatory reaction in and around the vessel, which further accentuates the occlusive effect. Liquid sclerosant agents such as absolute alcohol cause direct destruction and denaturation of endothelial proteins.

Of all the attributes and features of an embolic agent, the main factors influencing its selection in a specific application relate to the desired level of occlusion in the vascular tree and the desired permanency of occlusion. For example, when dealing with traumatic or degenerative hemorrhagic conditions, small particulate and liquid agents should be avoided as they can reach the capillary level resulting in significant non-target ischemia and infarction. On the other hand, such agents may be perfectly appropriate in conditions where hemorrhage is caused by a hypervascular tumor.

Table 1.1. Broad classification of intravascular embolic agents

Proximal mechanical:
- Coils:
  o Conventional Gianturco coils (0.035 inch) [110]
  o Microcoils (0.014–0.018 inch) [111]
  o Conventional Guglielmi detachable coil (GDC) [112, 113]
  o New 3D GDC [114]
  o Radioactive coils (Platinum coils implanted with radioactive 32P) [115]
  o Biodegradable coils [116, 117]
  o Mechanism of detachment:
    ▪ Simple wire pusher
    ▪ Electrically detachable (GDC) [118]
    ▪ Mechanically detachable [104, 119]
- Gelfoam: Level of occlusion depends on size and preparation (torpedoes, pledgets, slurry, powder)
- Detachable balloons [120]
- Shape memory polymers[121]
- Cast forming materials:
  o N-butyl 2-cyanoacrylate [122, 123]
  o Ethylene-vinyl alcohol copolymer/dimethyl sulfoxide/micronized tantalum mixture (Onyx)

Distal mechanical: small particulate agents:
- Standard polyvinyl alcohol (PVA): nonuniform size, aggregating
- Round PVA: calibrated uniform size, aggregating
- Trisacryl gelatin microspheres (Embosphere): calibrated, flexible, non-aggregating
- Embogold: radiopaque microspheres
- Yttrium-90 glass radioactive microspheres (TheraSphere) [124]

Liquid sclerosing liquids:
- Absolute ethanol [51, 52]
- Ethibloc: biodegradable fibrosing agent [125]
- Hypertonic dextrose
- Boiling contrast
- Providone iodine
- Sodium tetradecyl sulfate (Sotradecol)

Chemoembolization mixtures

Miscellaneous techniques:
- Stent-assisted and balloon-assisted coil remodeling technique (in wide neck aneurysms) [126–129]
- Direct fibrin adhesive injection during balloon inflation across neck [130]
- Covered stents [131, 132]
- Direct thrombin injection into aneurysms: [133, 134]
- Flow directed balloon catheterization [135]

1.3
Essential Elements for Success in Successful Embolotherapy

Embolotherapy is a delicate balance between safety and efficacy. Therefore, all involved parties (including the interventionist, referring physician and the patient or patient's family) need to be in agreement about expectations and risks before proceeding. The following criteria must always be satisfied: (1) clinical appropriateness of embolization, (2) proper pre-procedural imaging studies and/or angiographic localization of the bleeding abnormality or target vessel(s), (3) accurate determination of target vessel size, (4) accurate assessment of the status of collateral circulation, (5) appropriateness of embolic agent choice, (6) availability of modern angiographic equipment and a full array of diagnostic and interventional devices and supplies, and (7) technically skilled and experienced operator including knowledge of trouble shooting techniques.

1.3.1
Complications of Embolotherapy

The complications of embolotherapy are well described, but vary in their manifestations depending on the affected end-organ [85, 86]. By nature, success depends on complete abolishment of vascular supply, be it normal or abnormal vasculature. This can often be accomplished but not without a risk of compromise to adjacent normal tissue. Moreover, aggressive pursuit of difficult vascular territories poses a risk for non-target embolization.

Embolotherapy is associated with the usual iodinated contrast related risk of nephrotoxicity and access related hemorrhagic and thromboembolic complications. However, the most significant complication of embolization is non-target embolization. It occurs when normal vessels are unintentionally occluded due to a technical failure of a device of or if the embolic material or device refluxes out of the embolized vessel into the parent vessel. Non-target embolization can affect the systemic arterial system, and can take the form of pulmonary embolization when working in the venous system or when the embolic material passes through an AV fistula. Many post embolization complications are the results of inadequate technique, incomplete or suboptimal diagnostic angiography or inadequate evaluation of the vascular supply and collaterals before embolization. Adhering to meticulous technique and attention to details are crucial during the embolotherapy to minimize non-target embolization. Significant complications following embolotherapy can occur as a result of the use of an inappropriate embolic agent. Liquid sclerosant agents and small particles such as very small PVA or Gelfoam powder should be used very carefully as they can cause occlusion to the capillary level with significant tissue infarction.

Complex embolization procedures require prolonged fluoroscopic exposure to the skin especially when using the same projection under magnification and without proper collimation [87]. The operator needs to be cognizant of that risk and needs to reduce radiation exposure by using pulse fluoroscopy, minimizing magnification and periodically varying the angle of fluoroscopy beam.

A spectrum of end-organ ischemic complications can occur with embolotherapy. Bowel infarction can complicate splanchnic embolization targeting bleeding or could result from inadvertent non-target embolization from an upstream source [88]. Gallbladder infarction or bile duct necrosis can complicate hepatic artery embolization or chemoembolization [89, 90]. Splenic abscess and overwhelming sepsis can occurs following splenic embolization [91]. Skin necrosis and nerve injury have been reported as a result of ethanol embolization of vascular malformations [53, 54]. Buttock muscular necrosis, buttock claudication and sexual dysfunction can occur as a result of internal iliac branch embolization, especially when distal or bilateral [92–95].

The "post-embolization syndrome" comprises a constellation of symptoms including pain, fever, nausea, vomiting, and leukocytosis due to ischemia or infarction of the embolized organ [85]. The post-embolization syndrome *per se* is almost expected sequelae of the procedure and should not be considered a complication. It is much more common with a solid organ embolization and when sclerosant agents are used. Shock and cardiovascular collapse have also been rarely described during embolization with absolute alcohol [51].

1.4
Guidelines and Techniques to Prevent and Manage Complications

In order to minimize the risk of complications during embolotherapy, experience, thorough knowledge of relevant vascular anatomy, proper planning and execution using a well stocked modern inventory and availability of high quality fluoroscopy and digital subtraction angiograms cannot be overemphasized. In addition, safeguards have been recommended to reduce the risk of complications during embolization, such as ultraselective technique and the avoidance of pressor drugs [96]. The importance of correction of coagulopathy prior to embolotherapy cannot be overemphasized, with a number of studies demonstrating high failure rates noted in coagulopathic patients [97]. Conversely, in high risk embolization procedures not associated with active hemorrhage, heparinization or treatment with glycoprotein IIb/IIIa blockers have been shown to reduce thromboembolic complications [98]. When occlusion at a consistent level in the vascular tree is desired, some authors advocate using newer particulate agents such as Embosphere over conventional PVA; the inhomogeneity of PVA particle and their tendency to clumping may contribute to more proximal occlusion and lack of efficacy is cases where distal occlusion is desired [99]. Although Embosphere is reported to allow for more accurate and consistent occlusion at the desired level in patients undergoing uterine fibroid embolization (UFE) [100], the clinical outcome after UFE is not different between non-spherical PVA compared to Embosphere [101].

Familiarity with a variety of specific trouble shooting techniques is an important prerequisite to success in embolotherapy. When embolizing a large vessel, coil stability is essential. A study of the effect of sizing on stability suggests that a certain degree of oversizing is essential to minimize the risk of dislodgement. However, this should be weighed against the negative effect of an elongated and incompletely formed coil on hemostasis. An oversizing ratio of around 15% has been suggested in arteries, although in veins more oversizing is required [102]. Some authors recommended the use of tightly packed nested coils to enhance hemostatic efficacy [103]. Newer detachable coil designs allow testing of stability before detaching the coil and may be preferred in high risk situations [104]. Occlusion balloons in high flow situation or when using liquid agents are very useful to prevent non-target embolization. Of all trouble shooting techniques, the ability to quickly retrieve misplaced or migrated coils is a crucial skill [105, 106].

Finally, the injection technique of embolic particles is of paramount importance. Flow-directed injection of the particles respects the physiology of the circulation. Forceful injection can result not only in vessels damage or reflux but also in some situation, may provoke the opening of the normal vascular anastomosis with subsequent non-target embolization.

1.4.1
Guidelines and Principles in Selected Clinical Scenarios

1.4.1.1
Upper GI Bleeding

The most common etiology of UGI bleeding requiring angiographic intervention is from ulcers nonresponsive to endoscopic maneuvers [1, 4]. Gelfoam has been the favored material in the setting of upper GI bleeding. Oftentimes embolization of the left gastric or gastroduodenal artery is required. If a bleeding source is identified, a combination of gel foam slurry followed by larger pledgets can be used. However, if superselective catheterization of the bleeding vessel is performed, coil embolization is the technique of choice. If there is an associated pseudo aneurysm, embolization should be performed on both sides of the pseudo aneurysm with coils ("coil-sandwich" technique). Special care should be taken if the patient has a history of prior gastric or esophageal surgery. If collateral supply is compromised, a superselective embolization technique should be performed if at all possible. Duodenal embolization is technically challenging because of the dual blood supply to the duodenum from the celiac axis and superior mesenteric artery.

Antegrade obliteration of the superior duodenal branches via the gastroduodenal artery is often insufficient alone, as the bleeding points can be quickly pressurized via the rich anastomotic connections from the inferior pancreaticoduodenal arcade. In such cases, a "coil-sandwich" technique or alternatively direct obliteration of the bleeding segment or pseudoaneurysm by nested coils or a casting agent may be needed to prevent recurrence.

When no bleeding site is identified angiographically, some have advocated empiric embolization of either the left gastric artery of gastroduodenal artery. However, in our opinion this should be reserved as a last resort option. Aggressive non-selective embolization in UGI bleeding can cause infarction, pancreatitis, or severe gastroduodenal tissue ischemia and friability, which can markedly limit or complicate subsequent surgical options. When contemplating empiric embolization of the left gastric artery, care must be taken to exclude the possibility of replaced left hepatic artery completely originating from the left gastric artery [107].

Hemobilia is a subset of UGI bleeding that is particularly difficult to manage by conventional means. Embolotherapy is a valuable modality is the management of hemobilia resulting from trauma, iatrogenic injury or tumors [8].

1.4.1.2
Lower GI Bleeding

Recent evidence suggests an important role for embolotherapy in the management of lower GI bleeding. A variety of agents including Gelfoam, and coils have all been described. Proximal embolization should be avoided, and selective micro catheter catheterization and micro coil embolization, ideally at the level of the arcade or vasa recta is preferred. Selective embolization may be technically challenging in vasoconstricted shocky vessels or if vasospasm develops from repeated instrumentations. Pretreatment with a calcium channel blocker or intraarterial administration of a vasodilator may be beneficial. The use of vasopressin or other vasoconstrictors should be avoided following embolization because of the risk of intestinal infarction with this combination. Likewise, careful follow-up of the patient's symptoms and abdominal examination are crucial; should ischemic complications be suspected exploratory surgery should be performed to rule out infarction.

1.4.1.3
Hemoptysis/Bronchial Artery Embolization

Bronchial artery embolization is the therapeutic modality of choice for severe hemoptysis in chronic inflammatory conditions of the lungs such as cystic fibrosis, and bronchiectasis. The traditional teaching is to perform unilateral embolization of the involved side. Bronchoscopy is helpful to localize the site of bleeding. Curiously, the patient can also accurately localize the side of bleeding. It is important to realize that one must not rely on the demonstration of active extravasation from the bronchial artery to justify the bronchial artery embolization. Hypervascularity and/or enlargement of the bronchial arteries are sufficient to proceed with embolization. Particulate agents, such as PVA, are the embolic agent of choice although some investigators recommend the addition of Gelfoam plug into the proximal bronchial artery. Coils should not be used. One challenging aspect of bronchial embolization is the need to avoid unintended embolization of a spinal artery that can sometimes arise from the bronchial artery.

Cookbook: (Materials)

A. General Principles and Safeguards in Embolotherapy:

1. Appropriateness: Discuss indications, risk/benefits with referring physician, patient/family.

2. Establish clear procedure goals, priorities, acceptable endpoints, and alternative approaches. For example, in an unstable patient, procedural speed is paramount, and non-selective embolization should be preferred over a lengthy selective embolization of difficult to reach bleeding site(s).

3. Recognize high-risk situations for ischemic complications during embolization:
   - Multiple-vessel embolization
   - Altered collateral circulation: previous embolization, trauma/iatrogenic injury, atherosclerosis, shock, and pharmacological alteration (vasopressor therapy)

4. Procedure planning:
   - Ensure availability of equipment and resources: Adequate fluoroscopy/DSA, availability of catheters, guidewires, large inventory of coils and embolic materials.
   - Vascular access approach: retrograde versus antegrade, ipsilateral versus contralateral.
   - Choice of embolic material/method is paramount and must be based on the target vascular territory and the desired effect. Ability to reach distal vascular beds. For example, emergent non-selective embolization of a large vascular territory is best accomplished with a potentially temporary occlusive agent such as Gelfoam.
   - Be comfortable with a number of trouble shooting/salvage techniques in case of complications/malfunction. For example, snaring or forceps retrieval a misplaced coil, deployment of a coil stuck in a catheter with a saline flush using a TB syringe [108].
   - Go over available anatomic studies (CT, angiogram, scintigram). Active bleeding on the scintigram, enlarging hematoma, hematoma with a hematocrit level, and active contrast swirling or blush on contrast-enhanced helical CT are all helpful signs for localizing active bleeding.
   - Avoid particulate agents if significant AV shunting is noted on the angiogram.
   - Be familiar with the normal and collateral vascular supply of target territory, and the variant vascular anatomy especially if previously injured or compromised by trauma or prior embolization procedures. For example, when treating bleeding from a well-collateralized territory such as soft musculoskeletal tissue, liver, spleen, and the upper GI, using particles >500 μm is unlikely to cause significant ischemia. On the other hand, even proximal coil embolization of the superior gluteal artery territory following severe crush injury to the buttocks may result in muscular necrosis.
   - Correct coagulopathy. Uncorrected coagulopathy is a significant cause of failure.

5. Start with a nonselective regional angiogram, before proceeding to more selective injections, with the uncommon exception of circumstances the bleeding vessel is identified before the procedure (via imaging or endoscopy).

6. After completion of the primary embolization procedure, it is important to check other potential collateral pathways. For example, profunda femoris and contralateral internal iliac arteries are injected following embolization of an internal iliac bleeding source.

7. Avoid "burning bridges". For example, placement of proximal coils for a multifocal small vascular bleed will preclude a subsequent attempt to correct recurrent bleeding supplied from collateral anastomoses.

8. Safety tips during embolization:
   - Maintain fluoroscopic monitoring (use pulse-fluoroscopy).
   - If possible attempt to use an opacified embolic agent/mixture, for example n-butyl cyanoacrylate can be mixed with Ethiodol [109].
   - Carefully estimate volume of embolic material quantity to be used (excess leads to overflow reflux).
   - Beware of causes of reflux of embolic material which can cause non-target embolization:
     - Excess of embolic material quantity
     - Stagnation from prior embolic injections
     - Excessively forceful injection
   - Use frequent contrast injections to check residual flow rate/volume needed to fill the target territory without reflux.

- Beware of signs of imminent backflow: stasis/near-stasis, obstruction of segmental branches.
- Maintain tactile feedback during embolic material injection or coils deployment and void forceful contrast injections.
- During embolization through occlusion balloon (always aspirate before balloon deflation).

B) Specific Trauma Embolotherapy Guidelines:
- Embolize early when requested by the trauma service.
- To avoid delays, have a reliable plan in place to provide prompt coverage in case of trauma bleeding emergencies.
- Ensure procedural speed in unstable patient: non-selective embolization is preferred over lengthy selective embolization of multiple bleeding sites.
- Realize that arterial embolization alone may not be sufficient in the following scenarios:
  - Uncorrected coagulopathy
  - Concomitant venous/bone marrow hemorrhage (major venous injury, unstable pelvic fracture with marrow bleeding)
- In patients with severe unstable pelvic bony injuries it is important pelvic fixation be first attempted (pelvic binder or external fixator)
- Be cognizant of the fact that complications attributed to the embolization procedure may in fact be due to the trauma itself. For example, impotence/incontinence may be the result of sacral plexus injury in iliosacral fractures, and muscle necrosis could be the result of crush injury in blunt trauma.

1.5
Trauma

Interventional angiographic techniques now play a key role in the modern approach to traumatic hemorrhagic injuries. Indications for angiographic exploration in a trauma victim include: (a) musculoskeletal injury, associated with hemodynamic instability and not responding to stabilization (pelvic binder/traction); (b) wide-impact blunt trauma; (c) penetrating trauma, especially with a trans-axial wound-tract, or when more than one anatomic region is involved; (d) difficult operative access to a suspected injury;

(e) presence of an overwhelming contraindication to surgery, as in massive extraperitoneal hemorrhage from pelvic ring disruption; (f) continued bleeding following initial surgery, especially damage control laparotomy where visceral injuries were packed.

With pelvic trauma, the goal is to rapidly and temporarily reduce the pressure head with cessation of bleeding. Therefore, Gelfoam is the preferred agent initially, although coils can also be used. Prolonged attempts at subselective catheterization of bleeding sites are counter productive, and there should be no hesitation in embolizing the entire internal iliac artery, especially when multifocal bleeding from various branches of the internal iliac artery is present. The goal is to rapidly stabilize the patient before they become hypothermic and coagulopathic and the embolization should be performed in an expeditious manner.

1.6
Conclusion

Embolization therapy has become a major arm of modern interventional therapy. Its applications have become fundamental cores in the multimodality treatment paradigms in trauma, oncology, and endovascular therapy of vascular malformations and aneurysms. Knowledge of different techniques, materials and vascular anatomy and variants is essential to obtain good clinical outcome and minimize complications.

References

1. Defreyne L, Vanlangenhove P, De Vos M, et al. (2001) Embolization as a first approach with endoscopically unmanageable acute nonvariceal gastrointestinal hemorrhage. Radiology 218:739–748
2. Lang EK (1992) Transcatheter embolization in management of hemorrhage from duodenal ulcer: long-term results and complications. Radiology 182:703–707
3. Lang EV, Picus D, Marx MV, Hicks ME (1990) Massive arterial hemorrhage from the stomach and lower esophagus: impact of embolotherapy on survival. Radiology 177:249–252
4. Lang EV, Picus D, Marx MV, Hicks ME, Friedland GW (1992) Massive upper gastrointestinal hemorrhage with normal findings on arteriography: value of prophylactic embolization of the left gastric artery. AJR Am J Roentgenol 158:547–549
5. Golzarian J, Nicaise N, Deviere J, et al. (1997) Transcatheter embolization of pseudoaneurysms complicating pancreatitis. Cardiovasc Intervent Radiol 20:435–440

6. Gambiez LP, Ernst OJ, Merlier OA, Porte HL, Chambon JP, Quandalle PA (1997) Arterial embolization for bleeding pseudocysts complicating chronic pancreatitis. Arch Surg 132:1016–1021

7. Gomes AS, Lois JF, McCoy RD (1986) Angiographic treatment of gastrointestinal hemorrhage: comparison of vasopressin infusion and embolization. AJR Am J Roentgenol 146: 1031–1037

8. Moodley J, Singh B, Lalloo S, Pershad S, Robbs JV (2001) Non-operative management of haemobilia. Br J Surg 88:1073–1076

9. Savader SJ, Trerotola SO, Merine DS, Venbrux AC, Osterman FA (1992) Hemobilia after percutaneous transhepatic biliary drainage: treatment with transcatheter embolotherapy. J Vasc Intervent Radiol 3:345–352

10. Gordon RL, Ahl KL, Kerlan RK, et al. (1997) Selective arterial embolization for the control of lower gastrointestinal bleeding. Am J Surg 174: 24–28

11. Funaki B, Kostelic JK, Lorenz J, et al. (2001) Superselective microcoil embolization of colonic hemorrhage. AJR Am J Roentgenol 177:829–836

12. Kerns SR (1994) How safe is the use of platinum microcoils for embolization of small mesenteric arteries in patients with gastrointestinal bleeding? AJR Am J Roentgenol 162:1497

13. Peck DJ, McLoughlin RF, Hughson MN, Rankin RN (1998) Percutaneous embolotherapy of lower gastrointestinal hemorrhage.[see comment]. J Vasc Intervent Radiol 9:747–751

14. Zuckerman DA, Bocchini TP, Birnbaum EH (1993) Massive hemorrhage in the lower gastrointestinal tract in adults: diagnostic imaging and intervention. AJR Am J Roentgenol 161:703–711

15. Pelage JP, Soyer P, Repiquet D, et al. (1999) Secondary postpartum hemorrhage: treatment with selective arterial embolization. Radiology 212:385–389

16. Yamashita Y, Harada M, Yamamoto H, et al. (1994) Transcatheter arterial embolization of obstetric and gynaecological bleeding: efficacy and clinical outcome. Br J Radiol 67:530–534

17. Mal H, Rullon I, Mellot F, et al. (1999) Immediate and long-term results of bronchial artery embolization for life-threatening hemoptysis [see comment]. Chest 115:996–1001

18. Uflacker R, Kaemmerer A, Picon PD, et al. (1985) Bronchial artery embolization in the management of hemoptysis: technical aspects and long-term results. Radiology 157:637–644

19. Sharafuddin MJ, Andresen KJ, Sun S, Lang E, Stecker MS, Wibbenmeyer LA (2001) Spontaneous extraperitoneal hemorrhage with hemodynamic collapse in patients undergoing anticoagulation: management with selective arterial embolization. J Vasc Intervent Radiol 12:1231–1234

20. Agolini SF, Shah K, Jaffe J, Newcomb J, Rhodes M, Reed JF, 3rd (1997) Arterial embolization is a rapid and effective technique for controlling pelvic fracture hemorrhage [see comment]. J Trauma 43:395–399

21. Ben-Menachem Y, Coldwell DM, Young JW, Burgess AR (1991) Hemorrhage associated with pelvic fractures: causes, diagnosis, and emergent management. AJR Am J Roentgenol 157:1005–1014

22. Fisher RG, Ben-Menachem Y (1987) Interventional radiology in appendicular skeletal trauma. Radiol Clin North Am 25:1203–1209

23. Velmahos GC, Toutouzas KG, Vassiliu P, et al. (2002) A prospective study on the safety and efficacy of angiographic embolization for pelvic and visceral injuries. J Trauma 53:303–308

24. Ciraulo DL, Luk S, Palter M, et al. (1998) Selective hepatic arterial embolization of grade IV and V blunt hepatic injuries: an extension of resuscitation in the nonoperative management of traumatic hepatic injuries. J Trauma 45:353–358

25. Denton JR, Moore EE, Coldwell DM (1997) Multimodality treatment for grade V hepatic injuries: perihepatic packing, arterial embolization, and venous stenting. J Trauma 42:964–967; discussion 967–968

26. Hagiwara A, Murata A, Matsuda T, Matsuda H, Shimazaki S (2004) The usefulness of transcatheter arterial embolization for patients with blunt polytrauma showing transient response to fluid resuscitation. J Trauma 57:271–276

27. Mohr AM, Lavery RF, Barone A, et al. (2003) Angiographic embolization for liver injuries: low mortality, high morbidity. J Trauma 55:1077–1081

28. Schwartz RA, Teitelbaum GP, Katz MD, Pentecost MJ (1993) Effectiveness of transcatheter embolization in the control of hepatic vascular injuries. J Vasc Intervent Radiol 4:359–365

29. Sekikawa Z, Takebayashi S, Kurihara H, et al. (2004) Factors affecting clinical outcome of patients who undergo transcatheter arterial embolisation in splenic injury. Br J Radiol 77:308–311

30. Sakai T, Shiraki K, Inoue H, et al. (2002) Complications of partial splenic embolization in cirrhotic patients. Dig Dis Sci 47:388–391

31. Dent D, Alsabrook G, Erickson BA, et al. (2004) Blunt splenic injuries: high nonoperative management rate can be achieved with selective embolization. J Trauma 56:1063–1067

32. Liu PP, Lee WC, Cheng YF, et al. (2004) Use of splenic artery embolization as an adjunct to nonsurgical management of blunt splenic injury. J Trauma 56:768–772

33. Hagiwara A, Sakaki S, Goto H, et al. (2001) The role of interventional radiology in the management of blunt renal injury: a practical protocol. J Trauma 51:526–531

34. Dinkel HP, Danuser H, Triller J (2002) Blunt renal trauma: minimally invasive management with microcatheter embolization experience in nine patients. Radiology 223:723–730

35. Fisher RG, Ben-Menachem Y, Whigham C (1989) Stab wounds of the renal artery branches: angiographic diagnosis and treatment by embolization. AJR Am J Roentgenol 152:1231–1235

36. Perini S, Gordon RL, LaBerge JM, et al. (1998) Transcatheter embolization of biopsy-related vascular injury in the transplant kidney: immediate and long-term outcome. J Vasc Intervent Radiol 9:1011–1019

37. Hidajat N, Stobbe H, Hosten N, et al. (2002) Transjugular intrahepatic portosystemic shunt and transjugular embolization of bleeding rectal varices in portal hypertension. AJR. Am J Roentgenol 178:362–363

38. L'Hermine C, Chastanet P, Delemazure O, Bonniere PL, Durieu JP, Paris JC (1989) Percutaneous transhepatic embolization of gastroesophageal varices: results in 400 patients. AJR. Am J Roentgenol 152:755–760

39. Shimamura T, Nakajima Y, Une Y, et al. (1997) Efficacy and safety of preoperative percutaneous transhepatic portal embolization with absolute ethanol: a clinical study. Surgery 121:135–141

40. Reber PU, Baer HU, Patel AG, Wildi S, Triller J, Buchler MW (1998) Superselective microcoil embolization: treatment of choice in high-risk patients with extrahepatic pseudoaneurysms of the hepatic arteries. J Am Coll Surg 186:325–330

41. Routh WD, Keller FS, Gross GM (1990) Transcatheter thrombosis of a leaking saccular aneurysm of the main renal artery with preservation of renal blood flow. AJR Am J Roentgenol 154:1097–1099

42. Kasirajan K, Greenberg RK, Clair D, Ouriel K (2001) Endovascular management of visceral artery aneurysm. J Endovasc Ther 8:150–155

43. Soderman M, Andersson T, Karlsson B, Wallace MC, Edner G (2003) Management of patients with brain arteriovenous malformations. Eur J Radiol 46:195–205

44. Sreevathsa MR, Lalitha RM, Prasad K (2003) Arteriovenous malformations of the head and neck: experience with magnetic resonance angiography and therapeutic embolisation. Br J Oral Maxillofac Surg 41:75–77

45. White RI, Jr. (1996) Pulmonary arteriovenous malformations and hereditary hemorrhagic telangiectasia: embolotherapy using balloons and coils [comment]. Arch Intern Med 156:2627–2628

46. Dinkel H-P, Triller J (2002) Pulmonary arteriovenous malformations: embolotherapy with superselective coaxial catheter placement and filling of venous sac with Guglielmi detachable coils. Radiology 223:709–714

47. Mager JJ, Overtoom TT, Blauw H, Lammers JW, Westermann CJ (2004) Embolotherapy of pulmonary arteriovenous malformations: long-term results in 112 patients. J Vasc Intervent Radiol 15:451–456

48. Prasad V, Chan RP, Faughnan ME (2004) Embolotherapy of pulmonary arteriovenous malformations: efficacy of platinum versus stainless steel coils. J Vasc Intervent Radiol 15(2 Pt 1):153–160

49. Tan KT, Simons ME, Rajan DK, Terbrugge K (2004) Peripheral high-flow arteriovenous vascular malformations: a single-center experience. J Vasc Intervent Radiol 15:1071–1080

50. Rockman CB, Rosen RJ, Jacobowitz GR, et al. (2003) Transcatheter embolization of extremity vascular malformations: the long-term success of multiple interventions. Ann Vasc Surg 17:417–423

51. Yakes WF, Haas DK, Parker SH, et al. (1989) Symptomatic vascular malformations: ethanol embolotherapy. Radiology 170(3 Pt 2):1059–1066

52. Fan X, Zhang Z, Zhang C, et al. (2002) Direct-puncture embolization of intraosseous arteriovenous malformation of jaws. J Oral Maxillofac Surg 60:890–896

53. Dickey KW, Pollak JS, Meier GH, 3rd, Denny DF, White RI, Jr. (1995) Management of large high-flow arteriovenous malformations of the shoulder and upper extremity with transcatheter embolotherapy. J Vasc Intervent Radiol 6:765–773

54. Yakes WF, Luethke JM, Merland JJ, et al. (1990) Ethanol embolization of arteriovenous fistulas: a primary mode of therapy. J Vasc Intervent Radiol 1:89–96

55. Shlansky-Goldberg RD, VanArsdalen KN, Rutter CM, et al. (1997) Percutaneous varicocele embolization versus surgical ligation for the treatment of infertility: changes in seminal parameters and pregnancy outcomes. J Vasc Intervent Radiol 8:759–767

56. Fernandez Arjona M, Oteros R, Zarca M, Diaz Fernandez J, Cortes I (2001) Percutaneous embolization for erectile dysfunction due to venous leakage: prognostic factors for a good therapeutic result. Eur Urol 39:15–19

57. Kawakami M, Minagawa T, Inoue H, et al. (2003) Successful treatment of arterial priapism with radiologic selective transcatheter embolization of the internal pudendal artery. Urology 61:645

58. Maleux G, Stockx L, Wilms G, Marchal G (2000) Ovarian vein embolization for the treatment of pelvic congestion syndrome: long-term technical and clinical results. J Vasc Intervent Radiol 11:859–864

59. Farges O, Belghiti J, Kianmanesh R, et al. (2003) Portal vein embolization before right hepatectomy: prospective clinical trial. Ann Surg 237:208–217

60. Abdalla EK, Hicks ME, Vauthey JN (2001) Portal vein embolization: rationale, technique and future prospects [see comment]. Br J Surg 88:165–175

61. Madoff DC, Hicks ME, Abdalla EK, Morris JS, Vauthey JN (2003) Portal vein embolization with polyvinyl alcohol particles and coils in preparation for major liver resection for hepatobiliary malignancy: safety and effectiveness-study in 26 patients. Radiology 227:251–260

62. Duncan JR, Hicks ME, Cai SR, Brunt EM, Ponder KP (1999) Embolization of portal vein branches induces hepatocyte replication in swine: a potential step in hepatic gene therapy. Radiology 210:467–477

63. Prabhu VC, Bilsky MH, Jambhekar K, et al. (2003) Results of preoperative embolization for metastatic spinal neoplasms. J Neurosurg Spine 98:156–164

64. Sun S, Lang EV (1998) Bone metastases from renal cell carcinoma: preoperative embolization. J Vasc Intervent Radiol 9:263–269

65. Soulen MC, Faykus MH, Jr., Shlansky-Goldberg RD, Wein AJ, Cope C (1994) Elective embolization for prevention of hemorrhage from renal angiomyolipomas. J Vasc Intervent Radiol 5:587–591

66. De Baere T, Lagrange C, Kuoch V, Morice P, Court B, Roche A (2000) Transcatheter ethanol renal ablation in 20 patients with persistent urine leaks: an alternative to surgical nephrectomy. J Urol 164:1148–1152

67. Keller FS, Coyle M, Rosch J, Dotter CT (1986) Percutaneous renal ablation in patients with end-stage renal disease: alternative to surgical nephrectomy. Radiology 159:447–451

68. Jones DV, Jr., Lawrence DD, Patt YZ (1995) Percutaneous transcatheter arterial embolization for hypersplenism. Ann Intern Med 123:810–811

69. Kimura F, Itoh H, Ambiru S, et al. (2002) Long-term results of initial and repeated partial splenic embolization for the treatment of chronic idiopathic thrombocytopenic purpura. AJR Am J Roentgenol 179:1323–1326

70. Kumpe DA, Rumack CM, Pretorius DH, Stoecker TJ, Stellin GP (1985) Partial splenic embolization in children with hypersplenism. Radiology 155:357–362

71. Xiao H, Zhuang W, Wang S, et al. (2002) Arterial embolization: a novel approach to thyroid ablative therapy for Graves' disease. J Clin Endocrinol Metabol 87:3583–3589

72. Lefebvre GG, Vilos G, Asch M, Society of Obstetricians and Gynaecologists of C, Canadian Association of R, Canadian

Interventional Radiology A (2004) Uterine fibroid embolization (UFE). J Obstet Gynaecol Can 26:899–911

73. Spies JB, Cooper JM, Worthington-Kirsch R, Lipman JC, Mills BB, Benenati JF (2004) Outcome of uterine embolization and hysterectomy for leiomyomas: results of a multicenter study. Am J Obstet Gynecol 191: 22–31

74. Hovsepian DM, Siskin GP, Bonn J, et al. (2004) Quality improvement guidelines for uterine artery embolization for symptomatic leiomyomata [see comment]. Cardiovasc Intervent Radiol 27:307–313

75. Llovet JM, Bruix J (2003) Systematic review of randomized trials for unresectable hepatocellular carcinoma: chemoembolization improves survival. Hepatology 37:429–442

76. Lee KH, Sung KB, Lee DY, Park SJ, Kim KW, Yu JS (2002) Transcatheter arterial chemoembolization for hepatocellular carcinoma: anatomic and hemodynamic considerations in the hepatic artery and portal vein. Radiographics 22:1077–1091

77. Dodd GD, 3rd, Soulen MC, Kane RA, et al. (2000) Minimally invasive treatment of malignant hepatic tumors: at the threshold of a major breakthrough. Radiographics 20:9–27

78. Lin PH, Bush RL, Chaikof EL, et al. (2002) A prospective evaluation of hypogastric artery embolization in endovascular aortoiliac aneurysm repair. J Vasc Surg 36:500–506

79. Engelke C, Elford J, Morgan RA, Belli AM (2002) Internal iliac artery embolization with bilateral occlusion before endovascular aortoiliac aneurysm repair – clinical outcome of simultaneous and sequential intervention. J Vasc Intervent Radiol 13:667–676

80. Schoder M, Zaunbauer L, Holzenbein T, et al. (2001) Internal iliac artery embolization before endovascular repair of abdominal aortic aneurysms: frequency, efficacy, and clinical results. AJR Am J Roentgenol 177:599–605

81. Golzarian J, Struyven J, Abada HT, et al. (1997) Endovascular aortic stent-grafts: transcatheter embolization of persistent perigraft leaks. Radiology 202:731–734

82. Sheehan MK, Barbato J, Compton CN, Zajko A, Rhee R, Makaroun MS (2004) Effectiveness of coiling in the treatment of endoleaks after endovascular repair. J Vasc Surg 40:430–434

83. Rhee SJ, Ohki T, Veith FJ, Kurvers H (2003) Current status of management of type II endoleaks after endovascular repair of abdominal aortic aneurysms. Ann Vasc Surg 17:335–344

84. Baum RA, Cope C, Fairman RM, Carpenter JP (2001) Translumbar embolization of type 2 endoleaks after endovascular repair of abdominal aortic aneurysms. J Vasc Intervent Radiol 12:111–116

85. Hemingway AP, Allison DJ (1988) Complications of embolization: analysis of 410 procedures. Radiology 166:669–672

86. Rosenwasser RH, Berenstein A, Nelson PK, Setton A, Jafar JJ, Marotta T (1993) Safety of embolic materials [comment]. J Neurosurg 79:153–155

87. O'Dea TJ, Geise RA, Ritenour ER (1999) The potential for radiation-induced skin damage in interventional neuroradiological procedures: a review of 522 cases using automated dosimetry. Med Phys 26:2027–2033

88. Hemingway AP, Allison DJ (1998) Colonic embolisation: useful but caution required [comment]. Gut 43:4–5

89. Takayasu K, Moriyama N, Muramatsu Y, et al. (1985) Gallbladder infarction after hepatic artery embolization. AJR Am J Roentgenol 144:135–138

90. Makuuchi M, Sukigara M, Mori T, et al. (1985) Bile duct necrosis: complication of transcatheter hepatic arterial embolization. Radiology 156:331–334

91. Back LM, Bagwell CE, Greenbaum BH, Marchildon MB (1987) Hazards of splenic embolization. Clinical Pediatrics 26:292–295

92. Ramirez JI, Velmahos GC, Best CR, Chan LS, Demetriades D (2004) Male sexual function after bilateral internal iliac artery embolization for pelvic fracture. J Trauma 56:734–739

93. Su WT, Stone DH, Lamparello PJ, Rockman CB (2004) Gluteal compartment syndrome following elective unilateral internal iliac artery embolization before endovascular abdominal aortic aneurysm repair. J Vasc Surg 39:672–675

94. Kritpracha B, Pigott JP, Price CI, Russell TE, Corbey MJ, Beebe HG (2003) Distal internal iliac artery embolization: a procedure to avoid. J Vasc Surg 37:943–348

95. Cynamon J, Prabhaker P, Twersky T (2001) Techniques for hypogastric artery embolization. Tech Vasc Intervent Radiol 4:236–242

96. Guy GE, Shetty PC, Sharma RP, Burke MW, Burke TH (1992) Acute lower gastrointestinal hemorrhage: treatment by superselective embolization with polyvinyl alcohol particles. AJR Am J Roentgenol 159:521–526

97. Encarnacion CE, Kadir S, Beam CA, Payne CS (1992) Gastrointestinal bleeding: treatment with gastrointestinal arterial embolization. Radiology 183:505–508

98. Qureshi AI, Luft AR, Sharma M, Guterman LR, Hopkins LN (2000) Prevention and treatment of thromboembolic and ischemic complications associated with endovascular procedures: Part I–Pathophysiological and pharmacological features. Neurosurgery 46:1344–1359

99. Repa I, Moradian GP, Dehner LP, et al. (1989) Mortalities associated with use of a commercial suspension of polyvinyl alcohol. Radiology 170:395–399

100. Chua GC, Wilsher M, Young MP, Manyonda I, Morgan R, Belli AM (2005) Comparison of particle penetration with non-spherical polyvinyl alcohol versus trisacryl gelatin microspheres in women undergoing premyomectomy uterine artery embolization. Clin Radiol 60:116–122

101. Spies JB, Allison S, Flick P, et al. (2004) Polyvinyl alcohol particles and tris-acryl gelatin microspheres for uterine artery embolization for leiomyomas: results of a randomized comparative study. J Vasc Interv Radiol 15:793–800

102. Nancarrow PA, Fellows KE, Lock JE (1987) Stability of coil emboli: an in vitro study. Cardiovasc Intervent Radiol 10:226–229

103. Butto F, Hunter DW, Castaneda-Zuniga W, Amplatz K (1986) Coil-in-coil technique for vascular embolization. Radiology 161:554–555

104. Coley SC, Jackson JE (1998) Endovascular occlusion with a new mechanical detachable coil. AJR Am J Roentgenol 171:1075–1079

105. Gabelmann A, Kramer S, Gorich J (2001) Percutaneous retrieval of lost or misplaced intravascular objects. AJR Am J Roentgenol 176:1509–1513

106. Huggon IC, Qureshi SA, Reidy J, Dos Anjos R, Baker EJ, Tynan M (1994) Percutaneous transcatheter retrieval of misplaced therapeutic embolisation devices. Br Heart J 72:470–475

107. Brown KT, Friedman WN, Marks RA, Saddekni S (1989) Gastric and hepatic infarction following embolization of

the left gastric artery: case report. Radiology 172:731–732

108. Tarazov PG, Gapchenko EM, Dmitrieva IA, Ryzhkov VK (1992) Coil embolization using a saline flush technique [comment]. Br J Radiol 65:1055–1056

109. Sadato A, Wakhloo AK, Hopkins LN (2000) Effects of a mixture of a low concentration of n-butylcyanoacrylate and ethiodol on tissue reactions and the permanence of arterial occlusion after embolization. Neurosurgery 47:1197–1203

110. Lund G, Rysavy J, Kotula F, Castaneda-Zuniga WR, Amplatz K (1985) Detachable steel spring coils for vessel occlusion. Radiology 155:530

111. Kaufman SL, Martin LG, Zuckerman AM, Koch SR, Silverstein MI, Barton JW (1992) Peripheral transcatheter embolization with platinum microcoils. Radiology 184:369–372

112. Guglielmi G, Vinuela F, Dion J, Duckwiler G (1991) Electrothrombosis of saccular aneurysms via endovascular approach. Part 2: Preliminary clinical experience [see comment]. J Neurosurg 75:8–14

113. Guglielmi G, Vinuela F, Sepetka I, Macellari V (1991) Electrothrombosis of saccular aneurysms via endovascular approach. Part 1: Electrochemical basis, technique, and experimental results. J Neurosurg 75:1–7

114. Guglielmi G (1999) Treatment of an intracranial aneurysm using a new three-dimensional-shape Guglielmi detachable coil: technical case report [comment]. Neurosurgery 45:959–961

115. Raymond J, Roy D, Leblanc P, et al. (2003) Endovascular treatment of intracranial aneurysms with radioactive coils: initial clinical experience. Stroke 34:2801–2806

116. Abrahams JM, Forman MS, Grady MS, Diamond SL (2001) Biodegradable polyglycolide endovascular coils promote wall thickening and drug delivery in a rat aneurysm model. Neurosurgery 49:1187–1193

117. Ino T, Kishiro M, Ito H (1996) New occluding spring coil made from atelocollagen. Lancet 347:1187

118. Rao VR, Mandalam RK, Joseph S, et al. (1990) Embolization of large saccular aneurysms with Gianturco coils. Radiology 175:407–410

119. Murphy KJ, Houdart E, Szopinski KT, et al. (2001) Mechanical detachable platinum coil: report of the European phase II clinical trial in 60 patients. Radiology 219:541–544

120. Wholey MH (1977) The technology of balloon catheters in interventional angiography. Radiology 125:671–676

121. Echigo S, Matsuda T, Kamiya T, et al. (1990) Development of a new transvenous patent ductus arteriosus occlusion technique using a shape memory polymer. ASAIO Transactions 36:Jul–Sep

122. Huang F, Kuo YL, Ko SF, Ng SH, Lui CC, Jeng SF (2003) Percutaneous puncture and pre-operative cyanoacrylate obliteration of a traumatic false aneurysm of an angular artery branch [see comment]. Br J Radiol 76:746–749

123. Ishimaru H, Murakami T, Matsuoka Y, et al. (2004) N-butyl 2-cyanoacrylate injection via pancreatic collaterals to occlude splenic artery distal to large splenic aneurysm after proximal coil embolization. AJR Am J Roentgenol 182:213–215

124. Salem R, Lewandowski R, Roberts C, et al. (2004) Use of yttrium-90 glass microspheres (TheraSphere) for the treatment of unresectable hepatocellular carcinoma in patients with portal vein thrombosis. J Vasc Interv Radiol 15:335–345

125. Niechajev I, Clodius L (1990) Histologic investigation of vascular malformations of the face after transarterial embolization with ethibloc and other agents. Plast Reconstr Surg 86:664–671

126. Phatouros CC, Sasaki TY, Higashida RT, et al. (2000) Stent-supported coil embolization: the treatment of fusiform and wide-neck aneurysms and pseudoaneurysms. Neurosurgery 47:107–113

127. Benitez RP, Silva MT, Klem J, Veznedaroglu E, Rosenwasser RH (2004) Endovascular occlusion of wide-necked aneurysms with a new intracranial microstent (Neuroform) and detachable coils. Neurosurgery 54:1359–1367

128. Lefkowitz MA, Gobin YP, Akiba Y, et al. (1999) Balloon-assisted Guglielmi detachable coiling of wide-necked aneurysma: Part II – clinical results. Neurosurgery 45:531–537

129. Malek AM, Halbach VV, Phatouros CC, et al. (2000) Balloon-assisted technique for endovascular coil embolization of geometrically difficult intracranial aneurysms. Neurosurgery 46:1397–1406

130. Matson MB, Morgan RA, Belli AM (2001) Percutaneous treatment of pseudoaneurysms using fibrin adhesive. Br J Radiol 74:690–694

131. Althaus SJ, Keskey TS, Harker CP, Coldwell DM (1996) Percutaneous placement of self-expanding stent for acute traumatic arterial injury. J Trauma 41:145–148

132. Haas PC, Angelini P, Leachman DR, Krajcer Z (2000) Percutaneous treatment of life-threatening congenital arteriovenous malformations with the Wallgraft endoprosthesis. J Endovasc Ther 7:333–339

133. Cope C, Zeit R (1986) Coagulation of aneurysms by direct percutaneous thrombin injection. AJR Am J Roentgenol 147:383–387

134. Gale SS, Scissons RP, Jones L, Salles-Cunha SX (2001) Femoral pseudoaneurysm thrombinjection [see comment]. Am J Surg 181:379–383

135. Mazer M, Smith CW, Martin VN (1985) Distal splenic artery embolization with a flow-directed balloon catheter. Radiology 1541:245

2 Embolization Tools

Jafar Golzarian, Gary P. Siskin, Melhem Sharafuddin, Hidefumi Mimura, and Douglas M. Coldwell

CONTENTS

J. Golzarian, MD
Professor of Radiology, Director, Vascular and Interventional Radiology, University of Iowa, Department of Radiology, 200 Hawkins Drive, 3957 JPP, Iowa City, IA 52242, USA
G. P. Siskin, MD
Associate Professor of Radiology and Obstetrics and Gynecology, Department of Radiology, Albany Medical College, 47 New Scotland Avenue, MC-113, Albany, NY 12208-3479, USA
M. J. Sharafuddin, MD
Departments of Radiology and Surgery, 3JPP, University of Iowa Hospitals and Clinics, 200 Hawkins Drive, Iowa City, IA 52242-1077, USA
H. Mimura, MD
Associate Professor of Radiology, University of Iowa Hospitals and Clinics, Department of Radiology, 200 Hawkins Dr, 3957 JPP, Iowa City, IA 52242, USA
D. M. Coldwell, MD
Professor of Radiology, University of Texas Southwestern Medical Center, 5323 Harry Hines Blvd, Dallas, TX 75390-8834, USA

2.1 Introduction

Embolotherapy is a major aspect of Interventional Radiology and, as such, there are an increasing number of indications, ongoing research, and new developments. Numerous materials have been used for embolization and, recently, many new embolic agents, and devices have been developed. In this chapter we review the most common materials used in daily practice of most interventional radiologists. In this two-volume textbook, each chapter discusses separately the optimal embolic materials related to the corresponding clinical indications. We will also refer the readers to Chap. 10.6 in volume I, and Chap. 17 in Volume II, discussing future development in embolic materials.

2.2 Embolic Agents

The key decision in the performance of any embolization procedure is the choice of agent. Based on their physical and chemical properties, embolic agents can induce mechanical occlusion of the vessels; provoke the formation of thrombus by inflammatory reactions or destroy the endothelium leading to thrombosis. In this section, we will discuss the particulate agents, liquid agents and metallic embolic materials.

2.2.1 Particulate Agents

Particulate embolic agents are typically used for the embolization of tumor and tumor-related symptoms in addition to the treatment of certain hemorrhagic conditions. In general, these agents are administered from a selective position within the arterial vasculature of the target organ and are subsequently flow-directed towards the abnormal area being treated. This differs from coils and other mechanical agents which are administered directly into the abnormal blood vessels and are expected to cause their effect while they remain where they are administered. Particulate agents tend to be classified as either absorbable or non-absorbable. This tends to pertain to the agent itself and not necessarily to the occlusion induced by the agent.

2.2.1.1
Polyvinyl Alcohol Particles

Polyvinyl alcohol, which interventionalists know as the most commonly used particulate embolic agent, is also well known for its use in a variety of domestic and industrial products (Fig. 2.1). In particular, it has historically been used in cements, packaging materials, water-resistant adhesives (such as the backing of postage stamps), cosmetics, and household sponges. In 1949, GRINDLAY and CLAGGETT [1] established the biocompatibility of PVA by using it as filling material after pneumonectomy. Since then, it has been used as a skin substitute in burn patients [2], for support in patients with rectal prolapse [3], and for closure of a variety of congenital heart defects [4].

The preparation of polyvinyl alcohol for use as an embolic agent first involves its conversion into absorbable foam that is subsequently compressed [5]. Once the compressed foam is dried, it retains its compressed shape but when placed into solution, it resumes its original shape [5]. The particles themselves are prepared by rasping or blending a compressed block of polyvinyl alcohol or punching out polyvinyl alcohol plugs [5-7]. The irregularly shaped particles that are formed from this process are passed through sieves with sequentially smaller holes to separate them into various size ranges. One potential problem with this method is the axes of the particles may be oriented in such a way that large particles may be able to pass through small holes depending on the orientation of the individual particles as they pass through the sieves [6]. Some early reported problems with PVA were directly related to the variability in size of early particle preparations, before changes were made in the manufacturing process to ensure size uniformity [8].

TADAVARTHY et al. reported the first use of PVA as an embolic agent in patients with cervical carcinoma, hemangiosarcoma of the liver, hemangioendothelioma of the neck and forehead, and an arte-

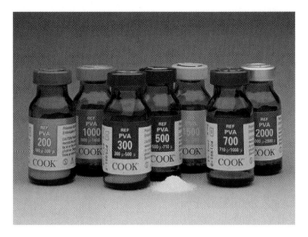

Fig. 2.1. PVA particles of different sizes. (Courtesy of Cook inc.)

riovenous malformation of the spine [5, 9]. Since then, PVA has been successfully used to embolize vessels in patients with a variety of disorders including head and neck arteriovenous malformations and tumors [10], lower gastrointestinal bleeding [11], bone metastases from renal cell carcinoma [12], hemoptysis caused by cystic fibrosis [13], priapism [14], and hemorrhage caused by pelvic neoplasms and arteriovenous malformations [15, 16]. Today, PVA is perhaps best known for its role in uterine fibroid embolization [17-20] and hepatic chemoembolization procedures [21-23].

One potential advantage of particulate agents in general is the potential to occlude a target vessel at a desired point along the course of that vessel (proximal or distal) by selecting a particle size that corresponds to that diameter. Generally, the use of small particles will result in a more distal occlusion and larger particles result in a more proximal embolization. However, this is less reliable with irregularly shaped PVA particles than with newer, spherical embolic agents. The tendency of irregularly shaped PVA to clump together due to the surface electrostatic charge often makes the effective size of this agent larger than that of the individual particles, which may lead to an embolization that is more proximal than intended [24]. Dilution and slow infusion of particles during the embolization procedures may be technical factors that can reduce the tendency for particulate aggregation, which may subsequently lead to a more distal embolization [24].

Several studies have described the histologic effects of PVA particles on embolized blood vessels. Initially, PVA particles do not occupy the entire lumen of the embolized vessel [25, 26]. Instead, they tend to adhere to the vessel wall, perhaps due to the irregular configuration of the particles, leading to slow flow in the vessel [27]. Slow flow ultimately leads to inflammatory and foreign body reactions, which results in platelet aggregation and thrombus formation within the intraluminal lattice of the PVA particles. These inflammatory changes can last for as long as 28 months after embolization [13]. These changes can result in thrombosis and focal angionecrosis of the vessel wall [8, 28–33]. Angionecrosis tends to be localized to the points where particles directly contact the vessel wall and can potentially lead to perivascular extravasation of particles [13, 30]. However, this finding has not been consistently observed [8].

PVA has been described as a non-absorbable or permanent embolic agent because it is not biodegradable. DAVIDSON and TERBRUGGE described the appearance of intravascular PVA in a specimen that was resected 8 years after embolization of a facial vascular malformation [31]. In this patient, particle fragments were found and the only change in particle morphology was slight calcification. However, PVA particles are not consistently found in specimens obtained after embolization [32], either due to distal particle migration [8, 29] or to the use of H and E staining during the preparation of pathologic slides; polyvinyl alcohol particles are best seen with the Verhoeff-van Gieson stain [33].

While the permanence of PVA as an embolic agent is well established, it is also clear that the occlusion caused by PVA particles is not permanent. Some reports cite occlusions lasting for at least several months [5, 13, 28]. More persistent occlusions will occur with the organization of thrombus, disappearance of inflammatory infiltrate, and ingrowth of connective tissue into the particles, all of which can lead to extensive fibrotic changes [13, 28, 29]. Luminal recanalization after PVA embolization has also been reported [13, 16, 31, 34, 35]. Proposed mechanisms for recanalization have included angioneogenesis and capillary regrowth caused by vascular proliferation inside the organized thrombus [8, 13] and resorption of the thrombus found between clumps of PVA in the lumen of an embolized vessel after the resolution of inflammation [8, 25, 30]. Recanalization does seem to occur in the portion of the vessel lumen previously containing thrombus and not in the portion containing polyvinyl alcohol particles [30].

To date, there have been no complications reported that have related directly to intravascular polyvinyl alcohol. That is not to say that there have not been complications seen after embolization procedures utilizing polyvinyl alcohol as the embolic agent. These complications, however, relate more to the effects of occluding blood vessels in the target organ vasculature than to the embolic agent used. As described earlier, the inclusion of small particles in early preparations of PVA increased the risk for inadvertent end-organ injury. Specific complications have included facial nerve palsy after external carotid artery embolization [36], paralysis after bronchial artery embolization [37], bladder or muscle necrosis and paralysis after pelvic embolization [38, 39], premature ovarian failure after fibroid embolization [40], and two infant deaths after the embolization of hepatic arteriovenous malformations [41]. Both of the deaths were attributed to pulmonary hypertension, presumably caused by particles passing through the malformation and into the pulmonary artery circulation. In response to these reports, manufacturing techniques were modified to minimize the number of particles smaller than the sizes specified for a given preparation of polyvinyl alcohol [6, 41].

2.2.1.1.1
How To Use PVA

PVA particles are available in different sizes from 50 to 1200 μ. They are distributed dry or in solution. To be used, they have to be mixed in a solution of contrast and saline. The proportion of contrast varies related to the concentration of iodine. We usually use a solution containing 40% contrast (Visipaque 300). Practically, the mixtures should provoke a suspension of the particles in the solution to prevent flocculation (Fig. 2.2). To obtain a uniform suspension, different methods are utilized. First, the particles are placed in a sterile bowl and mixed with contrast and saline. A 10- or 20-cc syringe is used to aspirate the solution and will serve as a reservoir. It is connected to the middle hub of a stopcock and a 3- or 5-ml syringe connected to the end-hub is used to aspirate back and forth to mix the particles (Fig. 2.3). Another way is to use a 3-ml non-lower lock syringe. After aspirating the solution, the syringe is rotated continuously during the slow injection of the particle. This rotation can prevent precipitation of the particles. As stated previously, the use of high dilution of the particles is essential to prevent catheter occlusion or clumping that may result in a proximal embolization (Fig. 2.4). We routinely dilute the particles in a 40-cc solution of contrast and saline. After the first syringe is used,

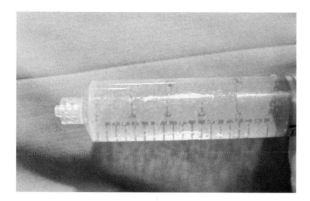

Fig. 2.2. PVA suspension

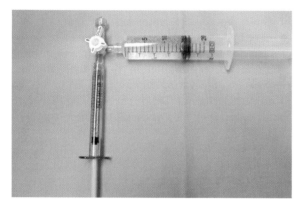

Fig. 2.3. A 20-cc syringe used as a reservoir connected to a three-way stopcock. The PVA solution is aspirated with the 3-cc syringe and injected to the catheter

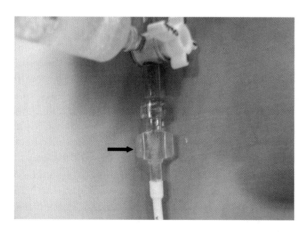

Fig. 2.4. The *arrow* demonstrates the agglomeration of the PVA particles occluding the catheter

we usually add another 10-cc solution to the bowl to obtain a better dilution. Sometimes this dilution continues up to a final solution of 70–80 ml for a vial of 1 ml PVA particles.

2.2.1.2
Spherical Embolic Agents

The recent interest in embolization procedures has led to the development of a new class of particulate agent, the spherical embolic agent. The movement towards a spherical configuration has its basis largely in the previously mentioned disadvantages of irregularly shaped PVA particles as an embolic agent. These include the size variability in particle preparations, the tendency for PVA particles to aggregate potentially leading to more a proximal embolization than intended, and anecdotal reports citing difficulty in injecting these particles through microcatheter. Any agent that addressed these difficulties with irregular PVA and resulted in an effective embolization along with a successful clinical outcome could be expected to become quickly accepted within the interventional radiology community which has been the case with spherical agents.

2.2.1.2.1
Trisacryl Gelatin Microspheres

In 1996, Laurent et al. reported on the development of a new, non-resorbable embolization agent with a spherical configuration [42]. These spheres were made from a trisacryl polymer matrix impregnated with gelatin that is hydrophilic, biocompatible and nontoxic (Fig. 2.5) [42]. The trisacryl polymer has been used for many years as a base material for chromatography media used to purify biopharmaceuticals. The presence of denatured collagen on the sphere surface supports cellular adhesion onto the material [42, 43]. Even in this initial publication, the ability of these spheres to address the disadvantages of irregularly shaped PVA particles were highlighted. In particular, these spheres can be more effectively separated by size with a sieving process than irregularly shaped PVA since they only have one dimension [42]. This leads to a narrow range of sphere sizes within a given preparation of spheres (± 20 to ± 100 µ). In addition, these investigators describe the ability of these spheres to be administered easily through most microcatheters [42]. Finally, they were shown to have no tendency to form aggregates, which theoretically would minimize the chance for an embolic occlusion to be more proximal than intended. It has been suggested that the hydrophilic interaction of these spheres with fluids and a positive surface charge, both contribute to the reduced formation of particle aggregates

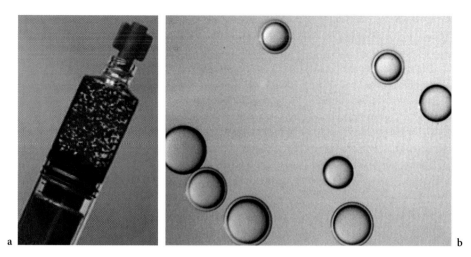

Fig. 2.5a,b. Trisacryl gelatin microspheres or embospheres (courtesy of Biosphere Medical). **a** Trisacryl gelatin microspheres in suspension. **b** Microscopic images demonstrating the spheres

[42, 44, 45]. In its original form, these spheres are clear, which make them somewhat difficult to see during the process of preparing them for us. Trisacryl gelatin microspheres stained with elemental gold are also available (EmboGold, Biosphere Medical Inc., Rockland, MA) for easier visualization of the spheres during preparation.

The initial clinical experience with trisacryl gelatin microspheres was reported by BEAUJEUX et al. in 105 patients with tumors or arteriovenous malformations in the head, neck or spine [46]. From this experience, it was learned that the precise calibration of these spheres enables interventionalists to have good control over the desired site of occlusion by appropriate size selection. In addition, the embolization were clinically effective, demonstrating that complete devascularization of the target pathology was often not possible but may not have been necessary to meet the goals of the embolization procedure [46].

To date, the use of trisacryl gelatin microspheres (Embospheres, Biosphere Medical, Rockland, MA) in several different clinical applications has been reported. BENDSZUS et al. demonstrated that trisacryl gelatin microspheres are effective in the preoperative evaluation of meningiomas, producing significantly less blood loss at surgery than irregularly shaped PVA particles [47]. YOON has described its use in bronchial artery embolization for hemoptysis [48]. These spheres have also been utilized effectively in the treatment of uterine fibroids [49–52]. PELAGE et al. have suggested that a limited approach be utilized with this application in an effort to reduce the extent of tissue

necrosis associated with this procedure [49]. They have advocated this limited approach given the ability of these microspheres to precisely target certain vessels. The flow-directed nature of microspheres makes it likely that the embolic material is first directed into the hypervascular pathology being targeted for embolization. A more limited approach can therefore potentially limit the effects of the embolization to the target tissue and minimize unintended embolization of the normal tissue surrounding the target pathology.

As described, the ability to target the level of occlusion with spherical agents such as trisacryl gelatin microspheres is one of the most appealing aspects of this class of agent. In animal studies, DERDEYN et al. demonstrated that for a given vessel and particle size, trisacryl gelatin microspheres penetrate significantly deeper into the blood vessel than PVA particles [44]. If one selects spheres that are the same size as PVA particles, the spheres will travel more distal in the vasculature of the target organ. Therefore, if an interventionalist is seeking to occlude a vessel at a similar point in the vessel to PVA particles, larger spheres will need to be selected, which was confirmed early on by BEAUJEUX et al. [46]. The ability to achieve a controlled arterial occlusion was highlighted by PELAGE et al. in their work studying uterine artery embolization in sheep. They found that the proximal aggregates formed by PVA particles cause the actual level of occlusion to be both proximal and distal and to correlate poorly with the size of the PVA particles [53]. Conversely, they found a significant correlation between the level of arterial occlusion and the diameter of the trisacryl gelatin microspheres used for embolization [45]. Therefore, large diameter spheres can be used if a proximal embolization is desired while small diameter spheres are recommended if a distal embolization is indicated. These findings were confirmed in humans by LAURENT et al. [54], who appropriately called for additional research focusing on the optimal size spherical agent required for particular types of pathology since without this knowledge, the ability to size match the spheres with the target vessel cannot be fully utilized.

Histologically, the initial work of LAURENT et al. and BEAUJEUX et al. found that these spheres provoke a moderate giant cell and polymorphonuclear inflammatory cell reaction [42, 46]. SISKIN et al. found that at 7 days, the response to the trisacryl gelatin microspheres consisted of macrophages and occasional lymphocytes and increased over time. When gold-colored microspheres were evaluated, the response consisted almost exclusively of lymphocytes, with occasional giant cells noted [35].

There have been complications reported in association with the use of trisacryl gelatin microspheres. DE BLOK et al. reported a case of fatal sepsis after uterine artery embolization performed with this agent. In this case, diffuse necrosis of the vaginal wall and cervix was found, attributed to distal penetration of spheres measuring 500–700 μ in diameter [55]. These authors agree with PELAGE et al. that a more limited approach to embolization should be utilized when using this agent. BROWN reported three deaths in patients with hepatocellular carcinoma embolized with 40- to 120 μ microspheres [56]. All three patients died after demonstrating progressive, irreversible hypoxemia. Two of the patients had autopsy confirmation of microspheres in small pulmonary arteries. Signs felt to place patients at risk for this event included tumor extending high into the dome of the liver, a large adrenal metastasis with tumor thrombus extending into the inferior vena cava, and presence of a systemic draining vein [56]. BROWN et al. theorized that the small size of these spheres was likely responsible for this complication and that patients embolized with either larger spheres due to their size or PVA particles due to their tendency to aggregate are likely protected from this potential complication. RICHARD et al. reported on a series of patients with non-infective endometritis after uterine artery embolization performed with gold-colored trisacryl microspheres [57]. While it is not known if these clinical findings could be attributed to the elemental gold in these microspheres, the

manufacturer has recommended that only the non-colored microspheres be used for uterine fibroid embolization at the present time.

2.2.1.2.1.1
How To Use Embospheres

The particles are loaded in a syringe or in a vial. When loaded, the syringe containing the particles is connected to a three-way stopcock. Another 5-cc syringe with contrast material is also connected. The contrast is aspirated and after 3–5 min a uniform suspension is obtained. The solution can be injected easily and slowly. There is no need to perform the back and forth aspiration like for PVA particles. This maneuver is not recommended since it might damage the spheres. In our experience, there is still some clumping with these particles so we usually use a 10- or 20-cc contrast solution to have a bigger dilution.

2.2.1.2.2
Polyvinyl Alcohol Microspheres

Recently, microspheres consisting of polyvinyl alcohol have been released and approved for use to treat hypervascular tumors (Fig. 2.6). These spheres were developed to address the shortcomings of PVA particles, similar to the trisacryl gelatin microspheres. Histologically, PVA-based microspheres are associated with a milder inflammatory response than both PVA particles and trisacryl gelatin microspheres [35]. The acute cellular response to embolization with PVA microspheres consists exclusively of Neutrophils. At 7 and 28 days after embolization, the inflammatory response consists of macrophages and occasional lymphocytes, which is different than the macrophages and giant cells seen after embolization with PVA particles. SISKIN et al. have presented their preliminary success with PVA microspheres for uterine fibroid embolization. However, there are increasing concerns on the results of uterine artery embolization for fibroids using PVA microspheres. Recent reports (abstracts) demonstrate a higher rate of partial devascularization of fibroids with these particles (see the Chap. 10.5). LAURENT et al. have also demonstrated that Contour SE particles are highly compressible [58]. This compressibility is associated to a change of the spherical shape of the particles becoming more oval. The failures may be explained by the higher compressibility of the particles and early proximal occlusion resulting to insufficient embolization.

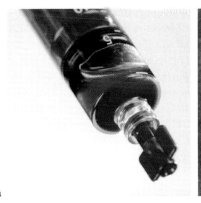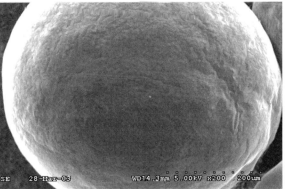

a

b

Fig. 2.6a,b. Spherical PVA (Beadblock hydrogel spheres; courtesy of Terumo). **a** Suspension of the BeadBlock particles. **b** Microscopic image showing the sphere

2.2.1.3
Gelfoam

Gelfoam, a water-insoluble hemostatic material prepared from purified skin gelatin (a non-antigenic carbohydrate), is frequently used as a biodegradable, absorbable embolic agent [59]. CORRELL and WISE [60] were the first to report the hemostatic properties of Gelfoam and its potential for use during surgery. It has been reported that in this setting, Gelfoam promotes hemostasis by hastening the supporting thrombus development [61]. In 1964, Gelfoam was first used as an intravascular agent for occluding a traumatic carotid cavernous fistula [62]. Since then, Gelfoam has been successfully used as an embolic agent for a variety of indications including renal cell carcinoma before resection [63], bone cancers [64], gastrointestinal bleeding [65], hemobilia [66], and arterial injury caused by trauma [67]. In 1979, HEASTON et al. [68] described the first use of Gelfoam in the pelvis for postpartum hemorrhage after bilateral hypogastric artery ligation. Since then, postpartum hemorrhage [69–71], postoperative hemorrhage [72], arteriovenous fistulas [73], cervical ectopic pregnancies [74], and bleeding caused by pelvic malignancies [75] and uterine fibroids [76–79], have all been effectively treated with Gelfoam embolization of the uterine or internal iliac arteries. Pelvic embolization remains one of the most common indications for the use of Gelfoam as an embolic agent, primarily because of support in the medical literature demonstrating fertility preservation after embolization [70–72, 77, 80, 81].

Histologically, Gelfoam initiates an acute full-thickness necrotizing arteritis of the arterial wall, with local edema and interruption of the elastic interna [63, 82]. Within 6 days after Gelfoam administration, acute inflammatory and foreign body, giant cell reactions have been observed [83]. These reactions induce thrombus formation, the residue of which can be found for several months [84]. However, LIGHT and PRENTICE [83] noted that the cellular reaction initiated by Gelfoam abated by day 30 and no Gelfoam or thrombus was seen at day 45, which served as the basis for the premise that Gelfoam is a temporary embolic agent. Studies have revealed that the resorption time for Gelfoam typically occurs within 7–21 days of embolization [84, 85]. However, when used for surgical hemostasis, unabsorbed gelatin sponges have been found in wounds 2–12 months after implantation [86].

Classically, the occlusion caused by a Gelfoam embolization has been considered "temporary" in that flow becomes reestablished to a treated vessel over time. The literature, however, provides support for both a temporary and permanent occlusion after Gelfoam embolization. In animals, the time to recanalization after a Gelfoam embolization has ranged from 3 weeks to 4 months [84, 85, 87]. BRACKEN et al. [63] found arterial recanalization in two patients who underwent embolization for renal cell carcinoma after 5 and 6 months. However, persistent occlusion after Gelfoam embolization has also been observed [63, 88]. JANDER and RUSSINOVICH [88] found that the permanence of Gelfoam occlusion might be related to the amount of Gelfoam used, stating that if a bleeding vessel was densely packed with Gelfoam, the occlusion would be permanent. It has also been suggested that an aggressive inflammatory reaction caused by introduction of Gelfoam into the vasculature may cause fibrotic and other changes in the vessel wall that result in a more permanent occlusion.

Ischemic and infectious complications have been reported when using Gelfoam as an embolic agent. Ischemic complications associated with the use of Gelfoam in the pelvis include buttock ischemia [68], lower limb paresis [38], and bladder gangrene [89]. These complications have been attributed to the small size of the embolic agent used, prompting recommendations that Gelfoam powder not be used in the nonmalignant setting [90]. Infectious complications, including at least three pelvic abscesses, have been reported after pelvic embolization with Gelfoam [72, 91, 92]. In addition, hepatic infections resulting in abscess formation have been reported when using Gelfoam during hepatic arterial chemoembolization procedures [93]. These infections may be caused by the potential for Gelfoam to retain enough air bubbles to support aerobic organisms [86]. Because of this potential, early surgical articles recommended using as little Gelfoam as possible, avoiding prolonged exposure of Gelfoam to con-

taminated air, and thoroughly compressing the Gelfoam so that large air bubbles are eliminated and not introduced into a patient [86].

Gelfoam is currently available in two forms: a powder containing particles ranging in diameter from 40 to 60 μ or a sheet from which sections of various sizes can be cut [59]. Gelfoam, like PVA, is not radiopaque and is typically mixed with contrast before injection. The small size of the particles in Gelfoam powder increases the risk for ischemia caused by distal artery occlusion [38]. The pledgets cut from a sheet of Gelfoam are typically larger and result in a more proximal artery occlusion than Gelfoam powder [59]. An additional technique is to create Gelfoam slurry by mixing pledgets between two syringes via a three-way stopcock. This method will decrease the size of the injected Gelfoam and allow a more distal delivery than that achieved with pledgets. There are different ways to cut the Gelfoam sheet. One way is to use a blade and cut a thin layer of the Gelfoam. Then this layer is cut longitudinally and transversally to small pieces using scissors (Fig. 2.7). Other possibility is to

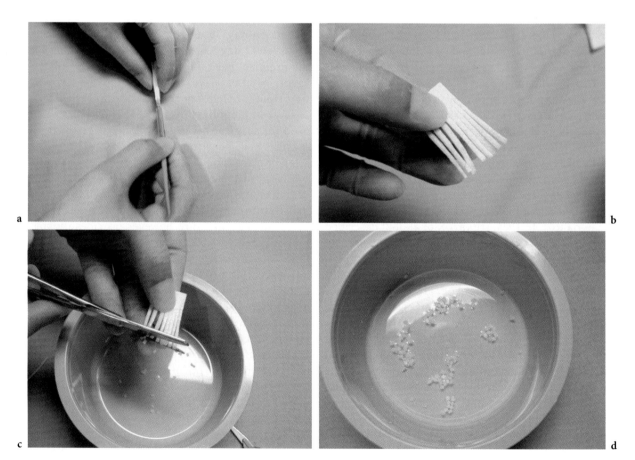

a
b
c
d

Fig. 2.7a–d. Gelfoam. **a** First cut the Gelfoam pledget longitudinally with blade. **b** The pledget is then cut to size vertically using scissors. **c** Each fragment is then cut to small cubes. **d** The particles are soaked in contrast and ready to be used

scratch the Gelfoam sheet carefully with the blade to obtain small size fragments (Fig. 2.8). The sizes of particles will be much less homogenous than the previous approach. However, forceful mixing of the particles with contrast can make it possible to obtain a jelly-form solution that can be injected easily. Finally, Gelfoam can be cut to long and tiny fragments also called 'torpedo'. Torpedo fragments are usually used for obtaining a proximal vessel occlusion in major arteries or as a complementary embolization to prevent from rebleeding (Fig. 2.9).

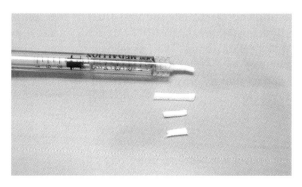

Fig. 2.9. Gelfoam "torpedo"

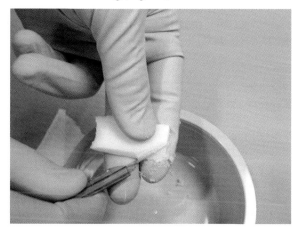

Fig. 2.8. Gelfoam slurry. The Gelfoam pledget is shaved with the blade at a 45° angle. The slurry is mixed with the contrast. After several back and fro aspirations, a jelly-like solution is obtained

2.2.1.4
Other Resorbable Agents

2.2.1.4.1
Oxycel/Surgicel

Oxycel (Becton Dickinson, Franklin Lakes, NJ) is composed of fibrillar absorbable oxidized regenerated cellulose. The basic functional unit of oxidized cellulose is the anhydroglucuronic acid. It is most commonly used as a local hemostatic agent in open surgical procedures by acting as a matrix for normal blood coagulation. It absorbs up to ten times its weight in blood. Oxycel is available in various forms and preparations: pads, strips, cotton, and powder. Although it was primarily used as a local hemostatic agents in open surgery to control oozing from raw tissues, its use in endovascular procedures has also been described both experimentally and clinically [94, 95].

As with Gelfoam, the main occlusion segments were recanalized by 4 months and no trace of either Oxycel remained, nor tissue reaction against either material [94]. Oxycel is highly effective in applications where temporary occlusion is desired such as trauma and pre-operative vascular reduction [96, 97]. Depending on the application and desired effect, Oxycel may be delivered as slurry suspended in a radiopaque mixture or in autologous blood through an angiographic catheter, or can be injected in its powdered form through a microcatheter [96–99].

2.2.1.4.2
Avitene

The agent is composed of a microfibrillar collagen preparation supplied in the form of a powder. It has been shown to be an effective particulate embolic agent in a number of experimental studies and clinical reports. In arteries embolized with Avitene suspended in saline moderate recanalization occurred by 2 weeks and total recanalization by 2 months. Arteries embolized with Avitene suspended in sodium Sotradecol remained occluded at 2 months with the longer occlusion duration attributed to increased inflammatory changes induced by Sotradecol [100]. It is a useful agent for tumor necrosis and organ ablation [101]. The agent is delivered through a microcatheter.

2.2.2
Liquid Agents

Sclerosants permanently destroy the vascular endothelium through different mechanisms depending on the type of agents: chemical (iodine or alcohol); osmotic effect (salicylates or hypertonic saline); detergents (morrhuate sodium, Sotradecol, polidocanol, and diatrizoate sodium) [102]. If injected in the artery, they can pass the capillary level allowing distal embolization. Their usage is thus much more challenging. They are mostly used in organ ablation such as tumors, veins or arteriovenous malformations (AVM).

2.2.2.1
Ethanol or Absolute Alcohol

Absolute alcohol is a very effective embolization agent. It destroys the walls of the blood vessels by inciting a strong inflammatory reaction and causes an instant precipitation of endothelial cells proteins and rapid thrombosis. Ethanol can result in transmural vessel necrosis, and diffusion into the surrounding tissue. It can be used intravascular or through direct puncture of the lesion. Because of its lack of radio-opacity, inflow occlusion with the use of balloon catheters is important to prevent from untargeted embolization. If inflow occlusion is not possible in case of AVMs, then outflow occlusion can be achieved with the use of orthopedic tourniquets, blood pressure cuffs or manual compression depending on the location of the lesion. Contrast is injected into the vessel in order to measure the volume of alcohol. In case of AVM, contrast is injected to the nidus during inflow occlusion until the draining veins are seen. This reflects the volume of alcohol needed to fill the nidus without spilling into the draining veins. Alcohol needs to be retained for several minutes within the lesion then drawn up. The balloon is then deflated and contrast injection should be repeated to evaluate the degree of vessel occlusion. In AVM embolization, the injection should be continued till the nidus is thrombosed.

If the inflow occlusion is not possible, alcohol can be mixed to Ethiodol in an 8:2 or 7:3 ratios in order to become more radiopaque [103]. This mixture makes it possible not only to see the flow, but it also increases the distribution and embolic effect of alcohol [104].

It is important to consider the risk of necrosis of neighboring tissues and of the skin when using alcohol by a percutaneous or endovascular route. The risk of systemic toxicity increases in doses above 1 ml/kg or if a volume greater than 60 ml is used. Complications can be as high as 15% of patients treated with absolute alcohol (range: 7.5%–23%) [105]. Severe complications such as cardiac arrest and pulmonary embolism have been reported [106,

107]. The mechanism remains unknown and may include pulmonary vasospasm, pulmonary embolism, and direct cardiotoxicity. Patients must be monitored closely, and some practitioners advocate the use of continuous pulmonary artery pressure monitoring during ethanol procedures. Most complications are self-limiting or may be successfully treated with skin grafting; in the case of skin necrosis, however, neurologic complications can be permanent. Ethanol blood levels correlate directly with the amount of ethanol injected, regardless of the type of malformation [102, 108]. General anesthesia should be used in children when using alcohol due to its possible local and systemic effects.

2.2.2.2
Cyanoacrylate

The tissue adhesives or glue are fast and efficient non-resorbable, non-radiopaque embolic material, based on polymerization of the acrylate monomer. Cyanoacrylate is composed of an ethylene molecule with a cyano group and an ester attached to one of the carbons. Isobutyl 2-cyanoacrylate was used previously but its production has been stopped after detection of sarcomas in animals exposed to large doses. N-butyl 2-cyanoacrylate or glue (Histoacryl; B. Braun, Melsungen, Germany) is the most used in Europe. TruFill (Cordis Neurovascular, Miami Lakes, FL) is another N-butyl cyanoacrylate (NBCA) that has been approved by the FDA. Glue starts to polymerize on contact with anionic substances such as plasma, blood cells, endothelium or saline. When in contact of the vessel, glue provokes an inflammatory reaction resulting in fibrosis [109].

Special skill and experience are required to assess the proper dilution of N-butyl cyanoacrylate in iodized oil (Ethiodol or Lipiodol) to opacify the acrylate but also to control vascular penetration. Control of time and place of polymerization depends on many factors such as blood flow, caliber of vessel, dilution of the acrylate, velocity of injection, etc. The speed of polymerization is affected by the concentration of iodized oil. Thus, in a rapid or high flow situation, pure glue or a solution with a lower concentration of Ethiodol should be used. In case of slow flow, a solution with a larger concentration of Ethiodol can be used (80%/20%). Tantalum or tungsten can be added to the solution before injection, to increase the radio-opacity of the agent. Embolization with glue is always performed through microcatheter. The microcatheter is typically changed after the injection. It needs to be positioned as close as possible to the embolization target. The microcatheter may be glued to the vessel. This is a potential complication that might occur in case of reflux, early polymerization or delayed removal of the microcatheter. This issue is less frequent with hydrophilic-coated microcatheters. In case this occurs, the microcatheter is simply cut off and buried in the groin so that it will endothelialized.

The use of glue in peripheral indications was not very popular. However, there is an increasing interest for using glue in peripheral indications. Glue has been used for AVMs, arteriovenous fistulae, GI bleeding from the GDA, portal vein embolization for tissue regeneration, bleeding varicose veins in patients with portal hypertension, varicocele, endoleaks and priapism [110, 111]. It might be used for distal flow directed embolization in GI bleeding or pseudo-aneurysms that are out of range for a sandwich technique occlusion. If the bleeding artery can be catheterized to the point of rupture (and eventually beyond into the bowel lumen), slow deposition of highly concentrated glue might be safe [112]. The catheter tip should be wedged proximally from the bleeding point to achieve excellent control of the glue penetration. This technique can be particularly useful in upper GIH bleeding to achieve occlusion of the bleeding vessel and the connection points with the collaterals.

Deep and diffuse penetration can cause ischemia or even infarction of neighboring tissue. The use of an overly diluted solution can result in delayed polymerization with risk of distal artery or draining vein occlusion. A drip of glue can be attached to the microcatheter which can eventually be embolized to a non-targeted location during retraction of the catheter.

With the introduction of Glubran2 (GEM, Italy) (a mixture of N-butyl 2-cyanoacrylate and methacryloxysulfolane) the acrylate seems more stable in the mixture with Lipiodol and less "sticky", which, has improved the control over the polymerization.

2.2.2.3
Ethibloc

Ethibloc (Ethnor Laboratories/Ethicon Inc., Norderstedt, Germany) is not available in the US. This biodegradable solution is a mixture of zein (a water-insoluble prolamine derived from corn gluten), alcohol, poppy seed, propylene glycol oil and contrast medium. It polymerizes on contact with ionic fluids developing a consistency similar to chewing gum, and subsequently hardens further. Ethibloc provokes thrombosis, necrosis and a fibrotic reaction with a giant cell inflammatory reaction that may produce pain and fever. The product is available in a preloaded syringe. Pump flushing through a three-way stopcock can emulsify the mixture; 10 ml of Ethibloc are mixed with 0.5 ml of Lipiodol. This mixture does not dissolve catheters. The system must be primed with a nonionic fluid, such as 50% glucose to prevent solidification in the delivery device. It can be mixed with Lipiodol (Laboratoire Guerbet, Paris, France) to allow for improved visualization. The embolization endpoint is stasis of the injected substance. It is important to slowly retract the delivery device while injecting the mixture. No significant complication has been reported. Ethibloc seems safer than alcohol because of its fewer complication rate. Also, it is much less painful than alcohol during the injection and does not require general anesthesia [113].

2.2.2.4
Onyx

Onyx, (Micro Therapeutics, Irvine Ca), is a biocompatible liquid embolic agent. It is an ethylene vinyl alcohol copolymer dissolved in various concentrations of dimethyl sulfoxide (DMSO) and opacified with micronized Tantalum powder. When this mixture contacts aqueous media, such as blood, the DMSO rapidly diffuses away, with resulting in situ precipitation and solidification of the polymer. It forms a soft elastic embolus without adhesion to the vascular wall or the catheter [114]. The polymerization process is time dependent and is mainly influenced by the amount of ethylene in the mixture, with less ethylene polymer becomes softer. Onyx is available in several different concentrations; the higher concentration is more viscous. Using a higher concentration makes it easier to prevent the liquid from getting too far from the catheter tip. Since the polymer will solidify on contact with aqueous media the delivery catheter must be pre-flushed with DMSO. A 'DMSO-compatible' catheter is required; DMSO will degrade most currently available catheters. Onyx is non-adhesive, allowing for easy removal of the delivery catheter, and of the polymer itself. Unfortunately it is quite expensive. This agent is mainly used for intracranial aneurysms. In peripheral, Onyx has been successfully used for the treatment of endoleak [115].

2.2.2.5
Detergent-Type Sclerosants

The detergent-type sclerosants includes: aetoxisclerol (polidocanol 1%–3%), sodium tetradecyl sulphate (STS), sodium morrhuate, and ethanolamine. Theses detergents can be used in liquid or foam. They act specifically on endothelium provoking its maceration. Sclerosis therapy requires a contact between the endothelium and a highly concentrated agent to be successful. It is therefore more effective in lesions with little flow. If used in high flow situations, the use of tourniquet or other compression techniques is of primary importance. They have been used in variety of indications in medicine including in GI bleeding, vascular malformations, and varicose veins.

2.2.2.5.1
Polidocanol (Aetoxisclerol) (1%–3%)

This agent is used for the small venous malformations and small venous varicosities [116–120]. Polidocanol is effective by altering the endothelium and promoting thrombosis. In addition, it has strong tissue fibrosis effect after tissue damage. Polidocanol is a urethane anesthetic and unique among sclerosing agents in that it is painless to inject [116]. Basically, general anesthesia is not necessary.

Injection volume and concentration of sclerosant depend on the size of the lesion and the flow rate. Some authors used it as sclerosing foam by mixing sclerosant and CO2 or air [117, 118] (see also Sect. 2.2.2.5.2). The German manufacture of polidocanol recommends a maximum daily dose of 2 mg/kg [117]. Some authors described that the maximum recommended dose in the treatment of varicose veins is 6 ml of 3% polidocanol [118]. This agent is associated with less severe allergic and inflammatory reactions [119]. Skin necrosis is rare. However, Cabrera reported skin necrosis in 6% of cases with venous malformations. One reversible cardiac arrest was reported [121].

2.2.2.5.2
Sodium Tetradecyl Sulfate (Sotradecol)

Sodium tetradecyl sulphate damages the endothelium resulting in thrombosis and fibrosis. This agent can be used in a liquid solution or by creating a foam with air. The main difference between liquid solution and foam is the long life of the foam in the vein and by the clear separation obtained between the blood and the sclerosant. Its injection is not painful. Usually, the Sotradecol is mixed with Lipiodol and air (5 cc of Sotradecol, 2 cc of Lipiodol and 20 cc of air). Using two plastic syringes and a three-way stopcock, and a 1:4 or 1:5 ratio of sclerosant to air, a stable and compact foam is obtained [122–124]. There is no agreement on the maximum dose of Sotradecol. Skin necrosis is a well-known complication related to the use of this substance [125]. Percutaneous injection of STS has been reported to provoke thrombosis of localized vascular lesions, facilitating their surgical identification and removal [125].

2.2.2.5.3
Ethanolamine Oleate

Ethanolamine oleate is a mixture of 5% ethanolamine oleate (synthetic mixture of ethanolamine and acid oleic) and iodized oil (Lipiodol) (ratio 5:1–5:2). It is a salt of an unsaturated fatty acid and has been used as a sclerosing agent because it has excellent thrombosing properties [126]. The oleic acid is responsible for the inflammatory response. The sclerosing action is dose-dependent, due to the diffusion of the solution through the venous wall, provoking mural necrosis, thrombosis, and fibrosis. The conjoint use of coils embolization as well as inflated balloons within the internal jugular vein in cases of cervicofacial venous malformations in order to prevent the systemic passage of the sclerosant has been reported with a 92% success rate [127]. The complications include anaphylactic shock, temporary trismus, pleural effusion, pneumonia, and hemolytic reactions [128]. Approximately 50% of oleic acid combines with serum proteins within 30 min that can cause renal toxicity in association with a marked intravascular hemolysis, hemoglobinuria, and hepatotoxicity [126, 129].

2.2.3
Coils and Metallic Embolization

Chapter 3 of this volume will discuss the use of coils for peripheral embolotherapy in more detail. Accurate catheter or microcatheter placement is essential to the performance of coil embolization. A sizing arteriogram is first performed to insure that the coil is appropriately sized. The coil should be about

15%–20% larger than the imaged vessel in order to prevent the distal migration of the device. Coils have been commonly utilized in trauma or in cases where the occlusion of an artery greater than 2 mm is desired to accomplish the clinical end. When there are large vascular structures such as aneurysms that need to be occluded, the combination of large coils and 30-cm sections of movable core guidewires with the cores removed have been reported to be utilized as fillers to take up the available space so that thrombosis will occur. A relatively new device, the Amplatz spider (Cook, Inc., Bloomington, IN) has been utilized to form the framework that will allow the placement of somewhat smaller coils into large vascular structures to occlude them (Fig. 2.10).

Coils are available in a wide variety of sizes from 2 mm to 15 mm in size and are made from either stainless steel or platinum and may have Dacron fibers placed at right angles to the long axis of the coil to increase the surface area and thereby to increase the speed and permanence of thrombosis. In practice, most coils utilized in microcatheters are platinum and those in 4- to 5-F catheters, stainless steel. It should be noted that all coils are permanent devices and should be utilized when the desired occlusion is permanent. Coils should not be used in combination with particulate embolization for the treatment of tumors, as they will occlude the access for further treatment. Coils may, on the other hand, be utilized with Gelfoam embolization in the treatment of pelvic bleedings allowing the hemorrhage to be halted quickly and permanently.

It should also be noted that when larger vessels are occluded with coils, collateral arteries form relatively rapidly and the distal vascular bed is still perfused but at a lower pressure than before the embolization. This is the theory behind the proximal occlusion of the splenic artery to halt splenic hemorrhage. The use of these coils presupposes the existence of collaterals. For example, embolization of the renal artery will most likely not result in viable renal tissue as the kidney is an end-organ and will not have a collateral arterial system that will support the kidney.

Other types of coils are those that have a controlled release either due to a mechanical release or that of electrochemical dissolution of an attachment joint. These GDC-type coils have the advantage that trial placement is used to accurately size the coil and the ill-sized coil can be removed without danger of distal embolization. The disadvantage is in their high cost which has prevented their widespread use outside of intra-cranial aneurysm embolization.

2.2.3.1
Coil Anchors

These are devices used to allow the stable deployment of coils into a large vessel with high flow or high wall compliance. Its main purpose is to allow a tight formation of coils to be deposited while maintaining a stable position in high flow vessels such as the aorta or iliac arteries or in highly compliant vessels such as large veins. These devices are also particularly useful for occlusion of large arteriovenous fistulas in the lungs, and large portosystemic collaterals [130]. While many devices have been used to accomplish this goal such as modified stents or vena cava filters, a number of devices have been specifically designed for this application.

2.2.3.1.1
Amplatz Spider

This device consists of a stainless-steel self-expanding spider shaped object which can be introduced through a guiding catheter or vascular sheath. The spider blocks the movement of steel coils and allows rapid occlusion of the vessel while minimizing the risk of inadvertent non-target embolization (Fig. 2.10). One modification allows the spider to be screwed onto a threaded guidewire before loading into the catheter allowing it to be retrieved and repositioned to ensure accurate placement. In some difficult applications multiple spiders may be deployed to provide a stable matrix for securing subsequent coils, sometimes in staged procedures [130–132].

2.2.3.1.2
Coil Cage

This is essentially a modified Gianturco Z stent modified to function as a cage to trap the coils within it against the direction of blood flow, while also reducing the risk of proximal or distal coil embolization. It is deployed through a long 8-F introducer sheath [133].

2.2.3.1.3
Retrievable Coil Anchor

This is a new design that offers the advantage of improved safety due to ability to retrieve and redeploy suboptimally placed devices. It is also intended to enhance the occlusive efficacy by allowing retaining a high density of occlusive material without

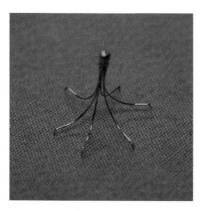

Fig. 2.10. Spider Amplatz device. (Courtesy of Cook inc.)

compromising the self-anchoring capability of the nested coils, which also enhances safety. This is important because of the high-risk locations where such devices are usually required to be deployed. Preliminary in vivo experience with one design in a swine model has shown promise [134].

2.2.4
Balloons

Detachable balloons were on the market in the US several years ago but were recalled due to both manufacturing problems and the difficulties in accurately placing the balloons. The use of these devices has been replaced by the GDC-type coils which allow the trial placement of a coil and its exchange for another size if the first is incorrect.

2.2.5
Stent Grafts

Stent grafts or covered stents are not embolic materials. However, in some clinical indication of embolization, they can be very useful. Stent grafts are composed of a metallic frame covered by either native venous grafts or synthetic materials such as Dacron or PTFE, sewn into the inner or outer portion of the metallic stent frame. These devices can be used in large vessel injuries, aneurysms, or arteriovenous fistulas resulting in an endoluminal bypass. After a series of homemade devices, the Cragg endoprosthesis was the first stent graft that became commercially available. These Nitinol based stent graft was used in different clinical indications. Many other self-expandable and balloon-expandable stent grafts have been since developed

and are currently used in clinical practice. When using a stent graft, proper sizing and precision of deployment are critical for technical and clinical success. Balloon-expandable stent grafts are very useful as they can be placed very precisely with no shortening. An important drawback with most of available stent grafts is their larger profile, making their use much more difficult in tortuous vessels. The balloon expandable stent grafts, however, have a smaller profile than the self-expandable stent graft but they are less flexible. It is anticipated that future advances in material and engineering will result in lower profile and more flexible self-expanding stent-graft systems that will pose comparable technical demands to bare stents.

2.3
Microcatheters

Microcatheters are commonly utilized to facilitate placement as they are more maneuverable and can be placed much more distally than the usual 4- or 5-F diagnostic catheter. One must insure that the guiding catheter can utilize at least a 0.035-in. guidewire so that the catheter can be reliably placed through it. A Touhy-Borst rotating hemostatic valve can be placed on the guiding catheter to allow a continuous flush of saline around the catheter and intermittent contrast injections to visualize the embolization. Microcatheters, like diagnostic catheters, come in a variety of sizes from the larger bore (outer diameter 3 F) to standard size (2.7 F) to very small bore (2 F). The two largest bores are widely utilized when particulate embolization is performed, as the catheters do not become easily obstructed. The smallest bore is most often used in neurointerventional applications with either coil or liquid embolics. The microcatheter has to combine flexibility and tractability to allow distal catheterization of target vessels. There are many microcatheter dedicated to peripheral indication combining these features and kink resistance as well as accepting high flow injection rate (Fig. 2.11).

The wires utilized are similar to those in diagnostic catheters but of 0.018, 0.016, 0.014, and 0.010 in diameter. The ends of these wires are usually straight and need a 45°–90° bend placed in it in order to select the desired vessels. This bend can be placed by pulling the wire against the thumbnail or the introducer in the package. As a practical matter, it is usually easier to place the bend in the wire after it is initially loaded into the microcatheter. The microwires usually have platinum or gold at their tips to aid in visualizing the tip of the wire under fluoroscopy. Excellent fluoroscopy and digital imaging are necessary to fully utilize the microcatheters.

Power injection through the largest bore microcatheters can usually be performed with flow rates of 3–4 ml/s at a pressure limit of 300 psi. This depends on the viscosity of the contrast and the diameter of the microcatheter. With some current microcatheters, high flow rates can be given up to a pressure of 750 psi (Fig. 2.11). Good distal diagnostic angiography can be performed through these catheters. It is still important to continuously visualize the catheter tip during the embolization procedure since movement of the tip can result in non-target embolization.

When using a microcatheter, care must be taken to avoid plugging the lumen with embolic agent, particularly with PVA or resin microspheres, by increasing the dilution of the particles. Embolization is usually performed using 3-ml syringes to achieve adequate pressure. If the catheter becomes completely obstructed, an attempt to pass a wire through the catheter to clear it may be made but such an obstruction usually necessitates removal of the microcatheter and its replacement.

Flow-directed microcatheters are also good tools developed for treating distal brain AVMs. These catheters are more flexible and smaller than the regular microcatheters. They can be carried distally by flowing blood. Also, the use of a 2-cc syringe filled with contrast can help the progression of the flow-directed microcatheter. These catheters can be used in some peripheral clinical indications such as in GI bleeding.

Microcatheters and -wires have revolutionized interventional radiology allowing the placement of embolic agents in more distal locations as well as more accurately so that normal tissues are spared and the therapeutic effect is enhanced.

2.4 Conclusion

The use of embolization to treat a myriad of differing conditions and diseases will only accelerate due to the new devices being developed and the newly found acceptance of loco-regional therapy.

References

1. Grindlay JH, Claggett OT (1949) Plastic sponge prosthesis for use after pneumonectomy: preliminary report. Proc Mayo Clin 24:1538–1539
2. Chardack WM, Brueske DA, Santomauro AP, et al. (1962) Experimental studies on synthetic substitutes for skin and their use in the treatment of burns. Ann Surg 155:127–139
3. Boutsis C, Ellis H (1974) Ivalon-sponge wrap operation for rectal prolapse: experience with 26 patients. Dis Colon Rectum 17:21–37
4. Payne WS. Kirklin JW (1961) Late complication after plastic reconstruction of outflow tract in tetralogy of Fallot. Ann Surg 154:53–57
5. Tadavarthy SM, Moller JH, Amplatz K (1975) Polyvinyl alcohol (Ivalon): a new embolic material. AJR Am J Roentgenol 125:609–616
6. Derdeyn CP, Moran CJ, Cross DT, et al. (1995) Polyvinyl alcohol particle size and suspension characteristics. AJNR Am J Neuroradiol 16:1335–1343
7. Tadavarthy SM, Coleman CC, Hunter D, et al. (1984) Polyvinyl alcohol (Ivalon) as an embolization agent. Semin Intervent Radiol 1:101–109
8. Germano IM, Davis RL, Wilson CB, et al. (1992) Histopathological follow-up study of 66 cerebral arteriovenous malformations after therapeutic embolization with polyvinyl alcohol. J Neurosurg 76:607–614
9. Tadavarthy SM, Knight L, Ovitt TW, et al. (1974) Therapeutic transcatheter arterial embolization. Radiology 111:13–16
10. Latchaw RE, Gold LHA (1979) Polyvinyl foam embolization of vascular and neoplastic lesions of the head, neck, and spine. Radiology 131:669–679
11. Tadavarthy SM, Castaneda-Zuniga WR, Zollikofer C, et al. (1981) Angiodysplasia of the right colon treated by embolization with Ivalon (polyvinyl alcohol). Cardiovasc Intervent Radiol 4:39–42
12. Sun S, Lang EV (1998) Bone metastases from renal cell carcinoma: preoperative embolization. J Vasc Interv Radiol 9:263–269
13. Tomashefski JF, Cohen AM, Doershuk CF (1988) Long-term histopathologic follow-up of bronchial arteries after therapeutic embolization with polyvinyl alcohol (Ivalon) in patients with cystic fibrosis. Hum Pathol 19:555–561

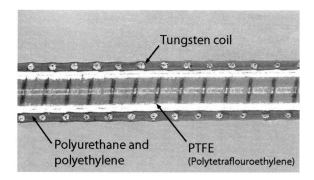

Fig. 2.11. Progreat microcatheter. (Courtesy of Terumo)

14. Goktas S, Tahmaz L, Atac K, et al. (1996) Embolization therapy in two subtypes of priapism. Int Urol Nephrol 28:723–727

15. Pisco JM, Martins JM, Correia MG (1989) Internal iliac artery embolization to control hemorrhage from pelvic neoplasms. Radiology 172:337–339

16. Poppe W, Van Assche FA, Wilms G, et al. (1987) Pregnancy after transcatheter embolization of a uterine arteriovenous malformation. Am J Obstet Gynecol 156:1179–1180

17. Goodwin S, McLucas B, Lee M, et al. (1999) Uterine artery embolization for the treatment of uterine leiomyomata: midterm results. J Vasc Interv Radiol 10:1159–1165

18. Spies JB, Ascher SA, Roth AR, et al. (2001) Uterine artery embolization for leiomyomata. Obstet Gynecol 98:29–34

19. Walker WJ, Pelage JP (2002) Uterine artery embolisation for symptomatic fibroids: clinical results in 400 women with imaging follow-up. BJOG 109:1262–1272

20. Ravina JH, Aymard A, Ciraru-Vigneron N, et al. (2003) Uterine fibroid embolization: results about 454 cases. Gynecol Obstet Fertil 31:597–605

21. Brown KT, Nevins AB, Getrajdman GL, et al. (1998) Particle embolization for hepatocellular carcinoma. J Vasc Interv Radiol 9:822–828

22. Solomon B, Soulen MC, Baum RA, et al. (1999) Chemoembolization of hepatocellular carcinoma with cisplatin, doxorubicin, mitomycin-C, ethiodol, and polyvinyl alcohol: prospective evaluation of response and survival in a U.S. population. J Vasc Interv Radiol 10:793–798

23. Salman HS, Cynamon J, Jagust M, et al. (2002) Randomized phase II trial of embolization therapy versus chemoembolization therapy in previously treated patients with colorectal carcinoma metastatic to the liver. Clin Colorectal Cancer 2:173–179

24. Choe DH, Moon HH, Gyeong HK, et al. (1997) An experimental study of embolic effect according to infusion rate and concentration of suspension in transarterial particulate embolization. Invest Radiol 32:260–267

25. Aziz A, Petrucco OM, Mikinoda S, et al. (1998) Transarterial embolization of the uterine arteries: patient reactions and effects on uterine vasculature. Acta Obstet Gynecol Scand 77:334–340

26. McLucas B, Goodwin SC, Kaminsky D (1998) The embolised fibroid uterus. Min Invas Ther & Allied Technol 7:267–271

27. Quisling RG, Mickle JP, Ballinger WB, et al. (1984) Histopathologic analysis of intraarterial polyvinyl alcohol microemboli in rat cerebral cortex. AJNR Am J Neuroradiol 5:101–104

28. Castaneda-Zuniga WR, Sanchez R, Amplatz K (1978) Experimental observations on short and longterm effects of arterial occlusion with Ivalon. Radiology 126:783–785

29. White R, Stranberg JV, Gross G, et al. (1977) Therapeutic embolization with long-term occluding agents and their effects on embolized tissues. Radiology 125:677–687

30. Link DP, Strandberg JD, Virmani R, et al. (1996) Histopathologic appearance of arterial occlusions with hydrogel and polyvinyl alcohol embolic material in domestic swine. J Vasc Interv Radiol 7:897–905

31. Davidson GS, Terbrugge KG (1995) Histopathologic long-term follow-up after embolization with polyvinyl alcohol particles. AJNR Am J Neuroradiol 16:843–846

32. Siskin GP, Eaton LA, Stainken BF, et al. (1999) Pathologic findings in a uterine leiomyoma after bilateral uterine artery embolization. J Vasc Interv Radiol 10:891–894

33. Kepes JJ, Yarde WL (1995) Visualization of injected embolic material (polyvinyl alcohol) in paraffin sections with Verhoeff-van Gieson elastic stain. Am J Surg Pathol 19:709–711

34. Sorimachi T, Koike T, Takeuchi S, et al. (1999) Embolization of cerebral arteriovenous malformations achieved with polyvinyl alcohol particles: angiographic reappearance and complications. Am J Neuroradiol 20:1323–1328

35. Siskin GP, Dowling K, Virmani R, et al. (2003) Pathologic evaluation of a spherical polyvinyl alcohol embolic agent in a porcine model. J Vasc Interv Radiol 14:89–98

36. Lasjaunias P (1980) Nasopharyngeal angiofibromas: hazards of embolization. Radiology 136:119–123

37. Vujic I, Pyle R, Parker E, et al. (1980) Control of massive hemoptysis by embolization of intercostal arteries. Radiology 137:617–620

38. Hare WSC, Holland CJ (1983) Paresis following internal iliac artery embolization. Radiology 146:47–51

39. Lang EK (1981) Transcatheter embolization of pelvic vessels for control of intractable hemorrhage. Radiology 140:331–339

40. Chrisman HB, Saker MB, Ryu RK, et al. (2000) The impact of uterine fibroid embolization on resumption of menses and ovarian function. J Vasc Interv Radiol 11:699–703

41. Repa I, Moradian GP, Dehner LP, et al. (1989) Mortalities associated with use of a commercial suspension of polyvinyl alcohol. Radiology 170:395–399

42. Laurent A, Beaujeux R, Wassef, M, et al. (1996) Trisacryl gelatin microspheres for therapeutic embolization, I: development and in-vitro evaluation. Am J Neuroradiol 17:533–540

43. Obrenovitch A, Maintier C, Sene C, et al. (1982) Microcarrier culture of fibroblastic cells on modified trisacryl beads. Biol Cell 46:249–256

44. Derdeyn CP, Graves VG, Salamant MS, et al. (1997) Collagen-coated acrylic microspheres for embolotherapy: in vivo and in vitro characteristics. Am J Neuroradiol 18:647–653

45. Andrews RT, Binkert CA (2003) Relatives rates of blood flow reduction during Transcatheter arterial embolization with tris-acryl gelatin microspheres or polyvinyl alcohol: quantitative comparison in a swine model. J Vasc Interv Radiol 14:1311–1316

46. Beaujeux R, Laurent A, Wassef M, et al. (1996) Trisacryl gelatin microspheres for therapeutic embolization, II: preliminary clinical evaluation in tumors and arteriovenous malformations. Am J Neuroradiol 17:541–548

47. Bendszus M, Klein R, Burger R, et al. (2000) Efficacy of trisacryl gelatin microspheres versus polyvinyl alcohol particles in the preoperative embolization of meningiomas. AJNR Am J Neuroradiol 21:255–261

48. Yoon W (2004) Embolic agents used for bronchial artery embolization in massive haemoptysis. Expert Opin Pharmacother 5:361–367

49. Pelage JP, LeDref O, Beregi JP, et al. (2003) Limited uterine artery embolization with tris-acryl gelatin microspheres for uterine fibroids. J Vasc Interv Radiol 14:15–20

50. Spies JB, Benenati JF, Worthington-Kirsch RL, et al. (2001) Initial experience with the use of trisacryl gelatin microspheres for uterine artery embolization for leiomyomata. J Vasc Interv Radiol 12:1059–1063

51. Joffre F, Tubiana JM, Pelage JP, et al. (2002) Interest of calibrated microspheres to perform uterine fibroid embolization: results in 85 patients [abstract]. J Vasc Interv Radiol 13[suppl]:S96

52. Spies JB, Allison S, Flick P, et al. (2004) Poly-vinyl alcohol and tris-acryl gelatin microspheres for uterine artery embolization for leiomyomas: results of a randomized comparative study. J Vasc Interv Radiol 15:793–800

53. Pelage JP, Laurent A, Wassef M, et al. (2002) Uterine artery embolization in sheep: comparison of acute effects with polyvinyl alcohol particles and calibrated microspheres. Radiology 224:436–444

54. Laurent A, Wassef M, Chapot R, et al. (2004) Location of vessel occlusion of calibrated tris-acryl gelatin microspheres for tumor and arteriovenous malformation embolization. J Vasc Interv Radiol 15:491–496

55. de Blok S, de Vries C, Prinssen HM, et al. (2003) Fatal sepsis after uterine artery embolization with microspheres. J Vasc Interv Radiol 14:779–783

56. Brown KT (2004) Fatal complications after arterial embolization with 40–120 micron tris-acryl gelatin microspheres. J Vasc Interv Radiol 15:197–200

57. Richard HM, Siskin GP, Stainken BF (2004) Endometritis after uterine artery embolization with gold-colored gelatin microspheres. J Vasc Interv Radiol 15:406–407

58. Laurent A, Wassef M, Pelage JP, et al. (2005) In vitro and in vivo deformation of TGMS and PVA microsphere in relation with their arterial location [abstract]. J Vasc Interv Radiol 16:S77

59. Berenstein A, Russel E (1981) Gelatin sponge in therapeutic neuroradiology: a subject review. Radiology 141:105–112

60. Correll JT, Wise EC (1945) Certain properties of a new physiologically absorbable sponge. Proc Soc Exp Biol Med 58:233

61. Jenkins HP, Senz EH, Owen HW, et al. (1946) Present status of gelatin sponge for the control of hemorrhage. JAMA 132:614–619

62. Speakman TJ (1964) Internal occlusion of a carotid-cavernous fistula. J Neurosurg 21:303–305

63. Bracken RB, Johnson DF, Goldstein HM, et al. (1975) Percutaneous transfemoral renal artery occlusion in patients with renal carcinoma. Urology 6:6–10

64. Feldman F, Casarella WJ, Dick HM, et al. (1975) Selective intraarterial embolization of bone tumors. AJR Am J Roentgenol 123:130–139

65. Katzen BT, Rossi P, Passairello R, et al. (1976) Transcatheter therapeutic arterial embolization. Radiology 120:523–531

66. Eurvilaichit C (1999) Iatrogenic hemobilia: management with transarterial embolization using Gelfoam particles. J Med Assoc Thai 82:931–937

67. Ben-Menachem Y, Coldwell DM, Young JWR, et al. (1991) Hemorrhage associated with pelvic fractures: causes, diagnosis, and emergent management. AJR Am J Roentgenol 157:1005–1014

68. Heaston DK, Mineau DE, Brown BJ, et al. (1979) Transcatheter arterial embolization for control of persistent massive puerperal hemorrhage after bilateral surgical hypogastric artery ligation. AJR Am J Roentgenol 133:152–154

69. Mitty HA, Sterling KM, Alvarez M, et al. (1993) Obstetric hemorrhage: prophylactic and emergency arterial catheterization and embolotherapy. Radiology 188:183–187

70. Greenwood LH, Glickman MG, Schwartz PE (1987) Obstetric and nonmalignant gynecologic bleeding: treatment with angiographic embolization. Radiology 164:155–159

71. Stancato-Pasik A, Mitty HA, Richard HM, et al. (1997) Obstetric embolotherapy: effect on menses and pregnancy. Radiology 204:791–793

72. Abbas FM, Currie JL, Mitchell S, et al. (1994) Selective vascular embolization in benign gynecologic conditions. J Reprod Med 39:492–496

73. Schneider GT (1984) Pelvic arteriography in obstetrics and gynecology: arteriovenous fistulas and embolization. South Med J 77:1494–1497

74. Frates MC, Benson CB, Doubilet PM, et al. (1994) Cervical ectopic pregnancy: results of conservative treatment. Radiology 191:773–775

75. Higgins CB, Bookstein JJ, Davis GB (1977) Therapeutic embolization for intractable chronic bleeding. Radiology 122:473–478

76. Katz RN, Mitty HA, Stancato-Pasik A, et al. (1998) Comparison of uterine artery embolization for fibroids using gelatin sponge-pledgets and polyvinyl alcohol [abstract]. J Vasc Interv Radiol 9:194

77. Mizukami N, Yamashita Y, Matsukawa T, et al. (1999) Use of an absorbable embolic material for arterial embolization therapy for uterine leiomyomas: midterm results on symptoms and volume of leiomyomas [abstract]. Radiology 213:348

78. Katsumori T, Bamba M, Kobayashi TK, et al. (2002) Uterine leiomyoma after embolization by means of Gelatin sponge particles alone: report of a case with histopathologic features. Ann Diagn Pathol 6:307–311

79. Sterling KM, Siskin GP, Ponturo MM, et al. (2002) A multicenter study evaluating the use of Gelfoam only for uterine artery embolization for symptomatic leiomyomata [abstract]. J Vasc Interv Radiol 13(2, Part 2):S19

80. McIvor J, Cameron EW (1996) Pregnancy after uterine artery embolization to control hemorrhage from gestational trophoblastic tumour. Br J Radiol 69:624–629

81. Yamashita Y, Harada M, Yamamoto H, et al. (1994) Transcatheter arterial embolization of obstetric and gynecological bleeding: efficacy and clinical outcome. Br J Radiol 67:530–534

82. Goldstein HM, Wallace S, Anderson JH, et al. (1976) Transcatheter occlusion of abdominal tumors. Radiology 120:539–545

83. Light RU, Prentice HR (1945) Surgical investigation of new absorbable sponge derived from gelatin for use in hemostasis. J Neurosurg 2:435–455

84. Barth KH, Strandberg JD, White RI (1977) Long-term follow-up of transcatheter embolization with autologous clot, oxycel, and gelfoam in domestic swine. Invest Radiol 12:273–280

85. Gold RE, Grace DM (1975) Gelfoam embolization of the left gastric artery for bleeding ulcer: experimental considerations. Radiology 116:575–580

86. Lindstrom PA (1955) Complications from the use of absorbable hemostatic sponges. Arch Surg 71:133–141

87. Cho KJ, Reuter SR, Schmidt R (1976) Effects of experimental hepatic artery embolization on hepatic function. AJR Am J Roentgenol 127:563–567

88. Jander HP, Russinovich NAE (1980) Transcatheter Gelfoam embolization in abdominal, retroperitoneal, and pelvic hemorrhage. Radiology 136:337–344

89. Sieber P (1994) Bladder necrosis secondary to pelvic artery embolization: case report and literature review. J Urol 151:422

90. Vedantham S, Goodwin SC, McLucas B, et al. (1997) Uterine artery embolization: an underused method of controlling pelvic hemorrhage. Am J Obstet Gynecol 176:938–948

91. Gilbert WM, Moore TR, Resnik R. et al. (1992) Angiographic embolization in the management of hemorrhagic complications of pregnancy. Am J Obstet Gynecol 166:493–497

92. Choo YC, Cho KJ (1980) Pelvic abscess complicating embolic therapy for control of bleeding cervical carcinoma and simultaneous radiation therapy. Obstet Gynecol 55[Suppl]:76S–78S

93. Sakamoto I, Aso N, Nagaoki K, et al. (1998) Complications associated with transcatheter arterial embolization for hepatic tumors. Radiographics 18:605–619

94. Barth KH, Strandberg JD, White RI (1977) Long-term follow-up of transcatheter embolization with autologous clot, oxycel, and gelfoam in domestic swine. Invest Radiol 12:273–280

95. DP MacErlean, DG Shanik and EA Martin (1978) Transcatheter embolisation of bone tumour arteriovenous malformations. Br J Radiol 606:414–419

96. DP Harrington, KH Barth, RR Baker, BT Truax, MD Abeloff and RI White Jr (1978) Therapeutic embolization for hemorrhage from locally recurrent cancer of the breast. Radiology 129:307–310

97. Leung JWT, Gotway MB, Sickles EA (2005) Preoperative embolization of vascular phyllodes tumor of the breast. AJR Am J Roentgenol 184[3 Suppl]: S115–S117

98. CB Higgins, JJ Bookstein, GB Davis, DC Galloway and JW Barr (1977) Therapeutic embolization for intractable chronic bleeding. Radiology 122:473–447

99. Carmignani G, Belgrano E, Martorana G, Puppo P (1978) Clots, oxycel, gelfoam, barium, and cyanoacrylates in transcatheter embolization of rat kidney. Invest Urol 16:9–12

100. Sniderman KW, Sos TA, Alonso DR (1981) Transcatheter embolization with Gelfoam and Avitene: the effect of Sotradecol on the duration of arterial occlusion. Invest Radiol 16:501–507

101. Nakao N, Ohnishi M, Shimada T, Saito F, Matsuoka H, Hayashi T, Miura K, Miura T (1991) Transcatheter hepatic arterial embolization with Avitene in dogs. Cardiovasc Intervent Radiol 14:124–128

102. Burrows PE, Mason KP (2004) Percutaneous treatment of low flow vascular malformations. J Vasc Interv Radiol 15:431–445

103. Soulen MC, Faykus MH, Shlansky-Goldberg, et al. (1994) Elective embolization for prevention of hemorrhage from renal angiomyolipoma. J Vasc Interv Radiol 5:587–591

104. Wright KC, Loh G, Wallace S, et al. (1990) Experimental evaluation of ethanol-Ethiodol for transcatheter renal embolization. Cardiovasc Intervent Radiol 13:309–313

105. Drolet BA, Scott LA, Esterly NB, et al. (2001) Early surgical intervention in a patient with Kasabach Merritt phenomenon. J Pediatr 138:756–758

106. Hanafi M, Orliaguet G, Meyer P, et al. (2001) Embolie pulmonaire au cours de la sclerotherapie percutanee d'un angiome veineux sous anesthesie generale chez un enfant. Ann Fr Anesth Reanim 20:556–558

107. Yakes WF, Engelwood CO, Baker R (1993) Cardiopulmonary collapse: sequelae of ethanol embolotherapy. Radiology 189:145

108. Hammer FD, Boon LM, Matheurin P, Vanwijck RR (2001) Ethanol sclerotherapy of venous malformations: evaluation of systemic ethanol contamination. J Vasc Interv Radiol 12:595–600

109. White RI, Standberg JV, Gross GS, Barth KH (1977) Therapeutic embolization with long-term occluding agents and their effects on embolized tissues. Radiology 125:677–687

110. Lang EK (1992) Transcatheter embolization in management of hemorrhage from duodenal ulcer. Long-term results and complications. Radiology 182:703–707

111. Pollak JS and White RI (2001) The use of Cyanoacrylate adhesives in peripheral embolization. J Vasc Interv Radiol 12:907–913

112. Kish JW, Katz MD, Marx MV, et al. (2004) N-butyl cyanoacrylate embolization for control of acute arterial hemorrhage. J Vasc Interv Radiol 15:689–695

113. Dubois J, Sebag GH, De Prost Y et al. (1991) The treatment of soft tissue venous malformation in children: percutaneous sclerotherapy with Ethibloc. Radiology 180:195–198

114. Numan F, Omeroglu A, Kara B, Cantasdemir M, Adaletli I, Kantarci F. (2004) Embolization of peripheral vascular malformations with ethylene vinyl alcohol copolymer (Onyx). J Vasc Interv Radiol 15:939–46

115. Martin ML, Dolmatch BL, Fry PD, Machan LS (2001) Treatment of type II endoleaks with Onyx. J Vasc Interv Radiol 12:629–32

116. Weiss RA, Goldman MP (1995) Advances in sclerotherapy. Dermatol Clin 13:431–445

117. Rabe E, Pannier-Fischer F, Gerlach H, Breu FX, Guggenbichler S, Zabel (2004) Guidelines for sclerotherapy of varicose veins (ICD 10: I83.0, I83.1, I83.2, and I83.9). Dermatol Surg 30:687–693

118. Cabrera J, Cabrera J Jr, Garcia-Olmedo MA, Redondo P (2003) Treatment of venous malformations with sclerosant in microfoam form. Arch Dermatol 139:1409–1416

119. Yamaki T, Nozaki M, Sasaki K (2000) Color duplex-guided sclerotherapy for the treatment of venous malformations. Dermatol Surg 26:323–328

120. Jain R, Bandhu S, Sawhney S, Mittal R (2002) Sonographically guided percutaneous sclerosis using 1% polidocanol in the treatment of vascular malformations. J Clin Ultrasound 30:416–423

121. Marrocco-Trischitta MM, Guerrini P, Abeni D, Stillo F (2002) Reversible cardiac arrest after polidocanol sclerotherapy of peripheral venous malformation. Dermatol Surg 28: 153–155

122. Tessari L, Cavezzi A, Frullini A (2001) Preliminary experience with a new sclerosing foam in the treatment of varicose veins. Dermatol Surg 27:58–60

123. Tessari L (2000) Nouvelle technique d'obtention de la scléro mousse. Phlébographie 53:129

124. Rabe E, Pannier-Fischer F, Gerlach H, et al. (2004) Guidelines for sclerotherapy of varicose veins (ICD 10: I83.0, I83.1, I83.2, and I83.9). Dermatol Surg 30:687–693, 53:129

125. O'Donovan JC, Donaldson JS, Morello FP, et al. (1997) Symptomatic hemangiomas and venous malformations in infants, children, and young adults: treatment with percutaneous injection of sodium tetradecyl sulfate. AJR Am J Roentgenol 169:723–729

126. Choi YH, Han MH, O-Ki K, et al. (2002) Craniofacial cavernous venous malformations: percutaneous sclerotherapy with use of ethanolamine oleate. J Vasc Interv Radiol 13:475–482

127. Konez O, Burrows PE, Mulliken JB (2002) Cervicofacial venous malformations: MRI features and interventional strategies. Interv Neuroradiol 8:227–234

128. Goldman MP (1991) A comparison of sclerosing agents. Clinical and histologic effects of intravascular sodium Morrhulate, Ethanolamine Oleate, hypertonic saline (11.7%), and Sclerodex in the dorsal rabbit ear vein. J Dermatol Surg Oncol 17:354–362

129. Sukigara M, Omoto R, Miyamae T (1985) Systemic dissemination of ethanolamine oleate after injection sclerotherapy for esophageal varices. Arch Surg 120:833–836

130. Lund G, Cragg AH, Rysavy JA, Castaneda F, Castaneda-Zuniga WR, Amplatz K (1983) Detachable stainless-steel spider. A new device for vessel occlusion. Radiology 148:567–568

131. Robinson DL, Teitelbaum GP, Pentecost MJ, Weaver FA, Finck EJ (1993) Transcatheter embolization of an aortocaval fistula caused by residual renal artery stump from previous nephrectomy: a case report. J Vasc Surg 17:794–797

132. Bates MC, Almehmi A (2004) High-output congestive heart failure successfully treated with transcatheter coil embolization of a large renal arteriovenous fistula. Catheter Cardiovasc Interv 63:373–376

133. Wilson MW, Gordon RL, LaBerge JM, Saavedra J, Kerlan RK (2000) Intravascular occluding device using a modified Gianturco stent as a coil cage. JVIR 11:221–224

134. Kónya A, Wright KC (2005) New retrievable coil anchors: preliminary in vivo experiences in swine. Cardiovasc Intervent Radiol 28:228–241

3 Controlled Delivery of Pushable Fibered Coils for Large Vessel Embolotherapy

Robert I. White Jr. and Jeffrey S. Pollak

CONTENTS

3.1 Introduction

Pushable fibered coils have been the material of choice for large vessel occlusion for the past 30 years, since their introduction by [1]. Their simplicity, reliability, and availability have led to their widespread acceptance by interventional radiologists throughout the world.

A number of significant modifications to the original stainless steel coils with wool fibers were developed. It was realized early on that wool led to occlusion followed by an intense chronic inflammatory reaction [2]. This led manufacturers to substitute polyester (Dacron) for wool fibers. Dacron fibers proved to have excellent platelet aggregation properties without causing the marked inflammatory response associated with wool. Currently, the basic fibered coil consists of a length of guidewire with multiple polyester threads attached transversely along most of its length. Fibered coil emboli are preshaped into a variety of different configurations, such as a helix, and then stretched out in a cartridge for delivery into a catheter (Fig. 3.1a,b).

Since the introduction of pushable fibered coils, detachable balloons, both silicone and latex, were developed for large vessel occlusion and more recently the Grifka large vessel occlusion device and the Amplatzer vascular Plug [3–7]. All of these devices were unique in that they were retrievable before detachment and animal studies proved that long term occlusion was possible as a result of cross sectional occlusion at the time of their placement. Detachable balloons are no longer available and the Gianturco-Grifka occlusion device has limited usage because of its size.

Improvements were made to pushable fibered coils, including the introduction of platinum fibered 0.035–0.038 standard and 0.018 in "microcoils" [8, 9]. These later developments, provided a softer and more MRI compatible coil but without the radial force of the original stainless steel coils. In Europe an Inconel coil, with excellent radial force, replaced the stainless steel coils and so high radial force and soft fibered platinum coils for vessel occlusion, became available in Europe. The Inconel, high radial force coil, is not yet available in the USA.

For neurovascular use, the development of the Gugliemi detachable coil (GDC) without fibers was essential for treatment of intracerebral aneurysm [10]. This coil and subsequent variations remains the standard for occlusion of narrow neck aneurysms. Variations of the GDC coil continue to be developed for management of cerebral aneurysm and other narrow neck aneurysms throughout the body [11]. The downside to the widespread use of GDC type coils for occluding arteries and veins are their expense and lack of thrombogenicity [12].

3.2 Techniques

As a result of treating a large number of patients with high flow fistulas of the lung during the past

R. I. White Jr., MD
Yale University School of Medicine, Department of Diagnostic Radiology, 333 Cedar Street, Room 5039 LMP, New Haven, CT 06520, USA
Jeffrey S. Pollak, MD
Yale University School of Medicine, Department of Diagnostic Radiology, PO Box 20842, New Haven, CT 06504-8042, USA

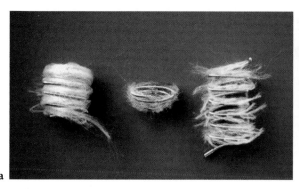
a

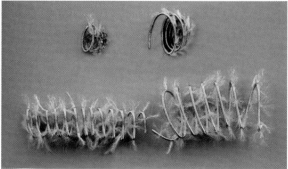
b

Fig. 3.1. a 0.035 High radial force stainless steel, Tornado, and Nester coils. The stainless steel coil (*left*) has a high radial force which is unique among coil manufacturers (Cook Inc., Bloomington, IN). The Tornado coil is a soft platinum shorter coil. Comparable coils include: Trufill (Cordis Corporation Inc., Miami, FL) and Diamond and Vortex (Boston Scientific Corporation, Natick, MA). The Nester coil (*right*) is a long, soft, platinum fibered coil with varying diameters which compresses to 1 cm in length when packed into a blood vessel. **b** *At the top*, 0.018-in. Micro-Tornado coils (Cook Inc.) of 4 and 8 mm are shown. Underneath, 0.018-in. 4 and 8 mm diameter Micronesters are shown. The Micronester is a longer length coil which is packed easily into an occluding mass 1 cm in length. Often both coils are used. After occluding a 1-cm length of a blood vessel with Micronesters, one or two Micro-Tornados may be added if there is a short residual length of blood vessel requiring occlusion

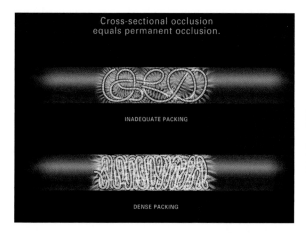

Fig. 3.2. Cross sectional occlusion achieved by packing or nesting soft platinum coils. Image at the *top* demonstrates partially occluded blood vessel with elongated coil. Often the vessel will appear occluded because of associated spasm but on restudy, recanalization will have occurred. Dense packing as shown in the bottom image is necessary to achieve predictable long-term cross sectional occlusion

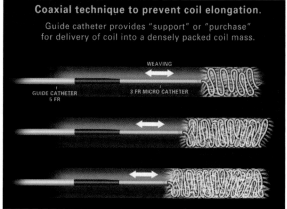

Fig. 3.3. Coaxial technique to prevent coil elongation. In this diagram, a 5-F guide catheter is placed into the vessel to be occluded. A microcatheter is advanced to the site of occlusion and while holding the guide catheter constant, the microcatheter is advanced and the microcoil deployed. The support "purchase" provided by the guide catheter helps the interventionalist to pack the microcoil into a tight coil mass leading to permanent occlusion. The use of guiding catheters is the most important step to preventing coil elongation and uncertain long term occlusion

8 years, we have confirmed the following two principles: Initial cross sectional occlusion provides long term occlusion (Figs. 3.2 and 3.3). Safety and control during deployment of conventional pushable fibered coils is achievable with the use of 6- or 7-F guide catheters. Longer 4- or 5-F catheters are placed coaxially through the guide catheter for deploying 0.035/0.038 in. coils. The shorter guide catheter provides stable position ("purchase") in the artery or

vein to be occluded. The same principle can be utilized when using pushable fibered 0.018-in. micro coils. In this instance a 4- or 5-F catheter is the guide catheter and a longer microcatheter is placed coaxially for deploying the microcoils (Fig. 3.3). In general the first coil selected has a diameter at least 20% larger than the vessel to be occluded.

Experience with follow-up angiograms of patients treated for PAVMs proved that when high flow PAVMs were treated with pushable fibered coils that deployment of one or two coils often produced a temporary occlusion which recanalized over time (Fig. 3.4). It was soon appreciated that initial deployment of the first one or two coils was associated with elongation of the coil and spasm. In simple terms, elongation of the coil during detachment through an endhole catheter was not always associated with long term occlusion.

3.2.1
Nesting/Packing Technique

Cross sectional occlusion of the artery/vein is easily produced when coaxial catheters were used. The elongation of pushable fibered coils is avoided by advancing the coil through the inner 4- or 5-F catheter while holding the outer guide catheter stable in the artery or vein (Fig. 3.3). In this way the soft

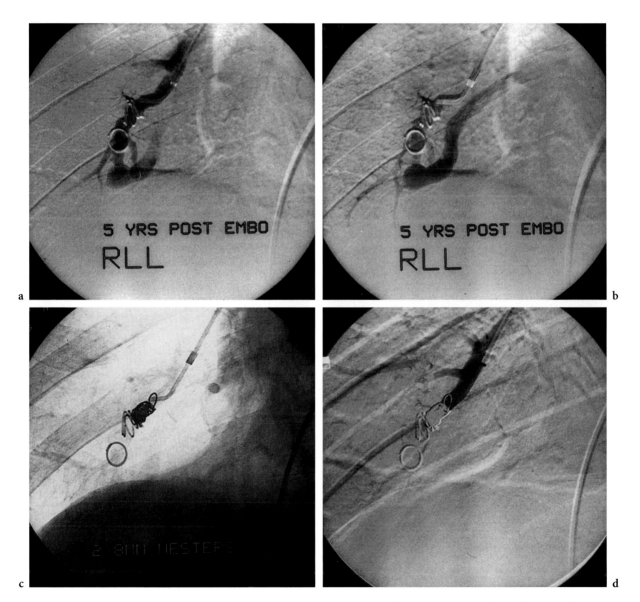

a b c d

Fig. 3.4a–d. A patient with recanalization of a pulmonary arteriovenous malformation (PAVM). **a,b** A selective pulmonary angiogram through the guide and inner catheter demonstrates that the right lower lobe pulmonary malformation is still patent, 5 years later. **c,d** Nesting "packing" of two 8-mm diameter Nester coils are placed just proximal to the recanalized coils, producing cross-sectional occlusion (**d**)

fibered platinum coils are weaved into a tight mass which occludes the vessel. Long term follow-up of our patients proved these two concepts [13].

3.2.2
Anchor Technique

Another benefit of using guide catheters and the improved control they provided when placing pushable fibered coils was the realization that in high flow fistulas in the lung, we could anchor the first 2 cm of a long 14-cm coil in a side branch, close to the aneurysmal sac. Thus, by "anchoring" the coil, we avoided any chance of coil migration and deployment of the remaining coil could be controlled (Fig. 3.5). This technique was very useful in avoiding the potential of paradoxical embolization of the coil through the PAVM. The "anchor" branch was as close to the aneurysmal sac as was possible. This prevented unnecessary occlusion of normal branches since a distal branch is usually sacrificed by whatever occlusion technique is utilized (Fig. 3.6). This technique, while developed for controlled delivery of pushable fibered 0.035 and 0.038 coils for pulmonary arteriovenous malformations (PAVMs), has application throughout the rest of the body when using embolization coils.

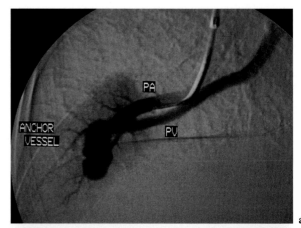

a

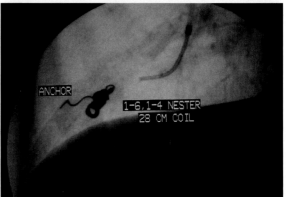

b

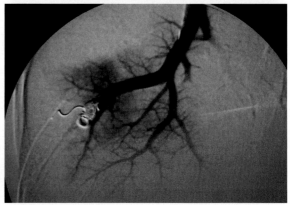

c

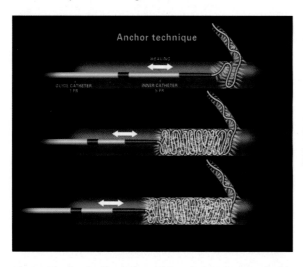

Fig. 3.5. The "anchor" technique. This technique is very valuable for providing safe and distal occlusion when there is a question about instability of pushable fibered coils. Diagrammatically, the guide catheter is placed in the artery to be occluded and a 5-F inner catheter or microcatheter is advanced into a side branch next to the site requiring occlusion. At least 2 cm of a 14-cm standard Nester or Micronester are advanced into the side branch which is normally sacrificed. The rest of the coil is then deployed just proximal to that side branch and additional coils are packed so that cross-sectional occlusion is obtained

Fig. 3.6a–c. In this patient with a high flow pulmonary arteriovenous malformation of the right lower lobe, a number of distal side branches are demonstrated immediately proximal to the aneurysmal sac and fistula. The inner 5-F catheter was advanced into a side branch and 2 cm of the first coil was deployed (b) and then the 5-F catheter was retracted and the remaining 12 cm of the coil was packed into a tight coil mass. One additional 4-mm coil was also packed distally into the 6-mm coil, and the final angiogram in (c) demonstrates a very distal occlusion immediately adjacent to the sac with preservation of most of the normal branches. This technique is used routinely for pulmonary malformations, but is also used for other venous and arterial occlusions when there is concern about migration. Again, the support or "purchase" of the guiding catheter is critical to allow packing of the coil into a tight occlusion mass

3.2.3
Scaffold Technique

In very high flow fistulas with large arteries, this technique is used to achieve a stable matrix, avoiding migration. By first deploying high radial force fibered stainless steel or Inconel coils, a scaffold is formed and the remaining cross sectional occlusion is produced with fibered platinum coils which are "weaved" into the interstices of this "endoskeleton" (Fig. 3.7).

The first, high radial force coils placed to form the scaffold are oversized by 2 mm, i.e. for a 10-mm feeding artery, 12 mm diameter stainless steel or Inconel coils are first placed. These first coils may be anchored as well if there is concern about fixation in the artery. Usually several small diameter high radial force coils are placed as well into the "endoskeleton", followed by several softer platinum coils until cross sectional occlusion is achieved.

In very high flow fistulas with large arteries, 12 mm or larger in diameter, the first coils are often placed through a balloon catheter (Boston Scientific, Natick MA) which has been temporarily inflated in order to stop flow. Once a scaffold is formed the balloon catheter is deflated and exchanged for a standard coaxial guiding catheter and the occlusion is completed with long fibered platinum coils (0.035 or 0.038 Nester. Cook Inc., Bloomington, IN) (Fig. 3.8).

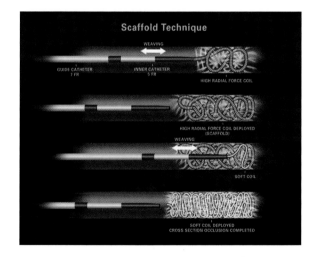

Fig. 3.7. "Scaffold" technique. This technique is used for high flow vessels when there is concern about migration of a softer coil. Initially in this diagram a high radial force coil, with a diameter 2 mm larger than the artery or vein being occluded, is placed. Several high radial force coils may be placed and the occlusion is completed using Nester coils to tightly pack within the "scaffold" or "endoskeleton"

3.3
Guide Catheters

Integral to using pushable fibered coils to produce cross sectional occlusion is the use of coaxial or triaxial guide catheter systems. For venous occlusions (varicocele and/or pelvic congestion) or occlusions of PAVMs, we use standard 7/5 combinations (Pulmonary, Cook) or gonadal (Cordis Inc., Miami FL) with inner 5-F endhole catheters (Fig. 3.9).

For visceral occlusions we use 6-F RDC (Cordis) guide catheters. In Figure 3.10, a splenic false aneurysm is occluded using a 6-F RDC guide catheter placed in the celiac and proximal splenic artery. A 4-F endhole catheter is placed coaxially for standard coils (Fig. 3.10a). A microcatheter for placing microcoils can be placed either through the 4-F catheter, creating a triaxial system, or directly through the 6-F guide catheter (Fig. 3.10b). A coaxial 0.021 lumen microcatheter (Renegade catheter, Boston Scientific) is positioned in the distal splenic artery just beyond false aneurysm and microcoils are placed distal and proximal to the origin of the aneurysm ("trap method" or "closing the back and front door"), thus excluding the point of arterial injury from antegrade or retrograde refilling.

3.4
Microcoil Technique

Controlled delivery of all pushable fibered Micro coils (Cook, Boston Scientific and Cordis) 0.018 in. is possible by using a coaxial guide (4–6 F) and microcatheters [14]. In order to achieve cross sectional occlusion of the artery or vein, the micro coils must be delivered into a tight coil mass. To achieve this, a 0.016 pusher wire (Boston Scientific or Cordis) is used and the same weaving "action" is performed during deployment in order to nest/pack the microcoil into a tight coil mass (Fig. 3.3).

Also, the microcoils are deliverable by the 'Squirt' technique. The Squirt technique is suitable for delivery of all pushable fibered microcoils (0.018 in.) through microcatheters with 0.016- to 0.027-in. endholes. The microcoil is loaded into the microcatheter and preferably a 3-ml luer lock syringe, filled with saline is attached to the hub of the microcatheter. Under fluoroscopic guidance, the microcoil is delivered with small boluses of saline. Final adjustment of the microcoil is accomplished by moving the microcatheter before final deployment of the coil, if

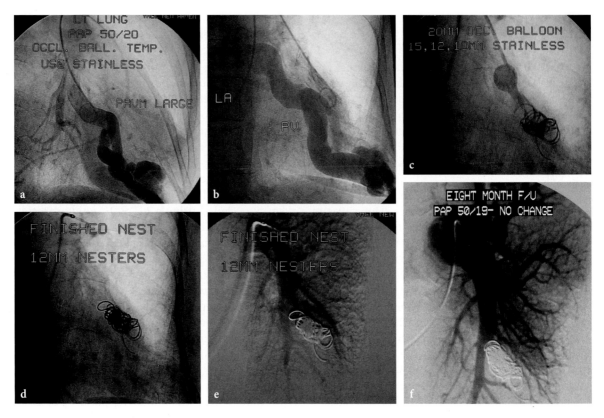

Fig. 3.8a–f. This patient had a very high flow fistula with moderate pulmonary hypertension. The left pulmonary angiogram (**a** and **d**) demonstrated a high flow fistula with a 12-mm diameter artery in the left lower lobe. Using the standard guiding catheter technique, a distal branch for anchoring was not immediately apparent. In order to provide a safe and controlled occlusion, a 20-mm occlusion balloon catheter (Boston Scientific, Natick, MA) was placed and inflated. While fully heparinized, an inner "scaffold" (**c**) was produced, using 15-, 12- and 10-mm diameter stainless steel coils. The balloon catheter was deflated and removed (**d**) and our standard guiding catheter system was placed. The occlusion was completed (**d** and **e**) using 12-mm Nester coils to produce cross-sectional occlusion. A follow-up angiogram 8 months later (**f**) demonstrated permanent occlusion of this large high flow fistula with preservation of normal pulmonary artery branches

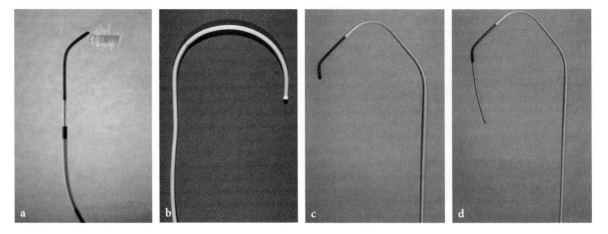

Fig. 3.9a–d. A standard 7-F gonadal guide catheter for occlusion of the left spermatic or ovarian vein (Cordis Inc., Miami, FL) is demonstrated in (**a**) and in (**b**) the 7/5 pulmonary guiding catheter and inner catheter for occlusion of pulmonary arteriovenous malformations is shown. Once the ovarian or internal spermatic vein are catheterized, any standard 100-cm 5-F endhole multipurpose catheter is advanced over a Bentson wire deep into the spermatic or ovarian vein where sclerosants and coils are usually placed. A standard 6-F RDC (Cordis Inc., Miami, FL) guide catheter for visceral embolization is demonstrated with a coaxial 4-F catheter in (**c**) and in (**d**), a triaxial system is demonstrated with an inner 0.021 lumen microcatheter

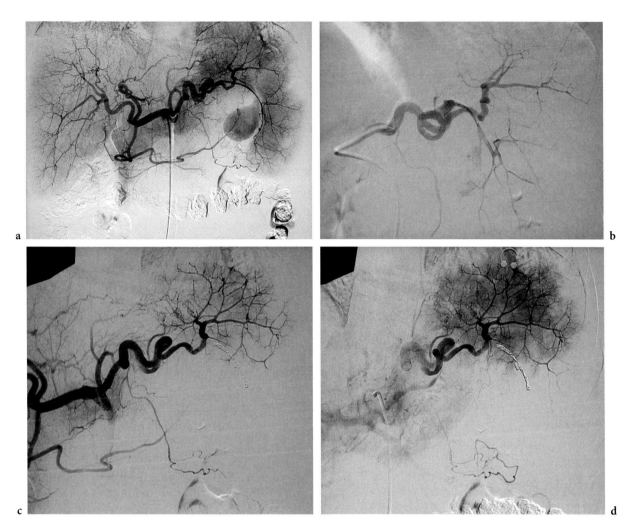

Fig. 3.10a–d. A large splenic artery false aneurysm is demonstrated near the hilum of the spleen (**a**). The 6-F RDC catheter is advanced into the orifice of the splenic artery and a microcatheter is passed to the site of injury in the distal splenic artery (**b**). The microcatheter is advanced distally beyond the site of the communication with the false aneurysm. Micronester coils are placed distal and proximal to the origin of the false aneurysm (**c** and **d**) and the final angiogram demonstrates occlusion of the lower pole of the spleen with preservation of the upper pole

the initial position of the partially delivered coil is distal to the site desired.

Earlier experience with the Squirt technique, using a 1-ml syringe and vigorous force to propel the microcoil can result in the microcatherer moving opposite to the force of injection and the coil deployed proximally or, worse yet, into a non-target vessel. A 3-ml syringe is preferable for delivering microcoils by the squirt technique and of course if there is a fistula or if there is any concern about non-target embolization, a 0.016-in. pusher wire is utilized. The first microcoil placed for closing a fistula should always be placed with a pusher wire for maximizing control.

3.5
Microcoil Usage with New 0.027 Endhole Microcatheters

The development of microcatheters with 0.027 endholes (Renegade Hi-Flo, Boston Scientific, and Mass Transit, Cordis) enabled easier delivery of particulates for embolization of hepatocellular cancer and uterine fibroids. Unfortunately, the 0.016 pusher wires will become trapped between the 0.018 microcoil and the inner diameter of these larger lumen microcatheters. If coil delivery is desirable using a pusher wire, a Teflon coated standard 0.021 wire is utilized. Our preference though is to deliver microcoils through these large lumen microcatheters with the Squirt technique using a 3 ml luer lock saline filled syringe.

Of note though, the Squirt technique should not be used for deployment of the first microcoil for treatment of a PAVM or other fistula. In this instance the coil may pass directly through the fistula.

3.6
Conclusions

Since the development by Gianturco of the first pushable fibered coils over 30 years ago, significant advances in coils and catheters have occurred. It is now possible to deliver pushable fibered standard 0.035 and 0.018 microcoils in a controlled and precise manner. Experience on a day to day basis with high flow fistulas of the lung has enabled us to develop a number of techniques which enable safe deployment and cross sectional occlusion of the vessel.

References

1. Gianturco C, Anderson JH, Wallace S (1975) Mechanical devices for arterial occlusion. Am J Roentgenol 124:428–435
2. Barth KH, Strandberg JD, Kaufman SL et al (1978) Chronic vascular reactions to steel coil occlusion devices. Am J Roentgenol 131:455–458
3. White RI Jr, Ursic TA, Kaufman SL et al (1978) Therapeutic embolization with detachable balloons: physical factors influencing permanent occlusion. Radiology 126:521–523
4. Kaufman SL, Strandberg JD, Barth KH et al (1979) Therapeutic embolization with detachable silicone balloons: long-term effects in swine. Invest Radiol 14:156–161
5. Barth KH, White RI Jr, Kaufman SL et al (1979) Metrizamide, the ideal radiopaque filling material for detachable silicone balloon embolization. Invest Radiol 14:35–40
6. Grifka RG, Mullins CE, Gianturco C et al (1995) New Gianturco-Grifka vascular occlusion device: initial studies in a canine model. Circulation 91:1840–1846
7. Sharafuddin M, Gu X, Umess M et al (1999) The Nitinol vascular occlusion plug: preliminary experimental evaluation in peripheral veins. J Vasc Intervent Radiol 10:23–27
8. Kaufman SL, Martin LG, Zuckerman AM et al (1992) Peripheral transcatheter embolization with platinum microcoils. Radiology 184:369–372
9. Morse SS, Clark RA, Puffenbarger A (1990) Platinum microcoils for therapeutic embolization: nonneuroradiologic applications. Am J Roentgenol 155:401–403
10. Guglielmi G, Vinuela F, Septeka I et al (1991) Electrothrombosis of saccular aneurysms via endovascular approach. I. Electrochemical basis, technique, and experimental results. J Neurosurg 75:1–7
11. Klein GE, Szolar DH, Karaic R et al (1996) Extracranial aneurysm and arteriovenous fistula: embolization with the Guglielmi detachable coil. Radiology 201:489–494
12. White RI Jr, Pollak JS, Picus D (2003) Are Guglielmi detachable coils necessary for treating pulmonary arteriovenous malformations? Letter to the editor. Radiology 226:599–600
13. Pollak JS, Thabet A, Saluja S et al (2005) Clinical and anatomical outcome after embolotherapy of pulmonary arteriovenous malformations. Accepted for presentation SIR 2005, New Orleans, LA, in press J Vasc Intervent Radiol 2006
14. Osuga K, White RI Jr (2003) Micronester: a new pushable fibered microcoil for embolotherapy. Cardiovasc Intervent Radiol 26:554–556

4 Work-up and Follow-up after Embolization

Jim A. Reekers

CONTENTS

4.1 General Work-up

It is important to become familiar with all aspects of the patient's clinical history, as this will ultimately help to determine the appropriateness of the planned intervention and will also help optimize and guide the catheter-based intervention. For example, one should know if the patient is using anti-coagulant medication or other medication, which might alter the clinical presentation of hemorrhaging patient or influence the efficacy of the embolization procedure. It is important to be informed about the patient's medical history and medication. A history of contrast allergy is important, as these patients should be pre-treated with corticosteroids. Since B-blockers might fully mask the hyperdynamic response of hypovolemic shock, appropriate precautions should be taken in patients with elevated creatinine who are using Metformin before contrast medium is given. Patients with renal insufficiency should be pre-treated with hydration, alkalinization and N-acetyl cysteine (600 mg dosing every 6 h, preferably twice before the intervention). Oral anti-coagulants can reduce the prothrombotic effect of coil embolization and, whenever possible, should be stopped or reversed before embolization, or alter-

natively another embolization material should be used, such as occlusion balloon or glue.

Before starting any elective embolization it is important to talk to the patient and obtain informed consent. In talking to the patient, emphasis should not only be on the advantages but also on the risks and complications of embolization therapy. Alternative therapeutic options should be discussed. In both emergency and elective embolization there is no scientific proof that antibiotics should be given prior to embolization. Always work as a team with the referring physician, to have a back-up plan for possible procedure failure or complications.

Needless to say, embolization should only be performed with ample experience and support. Optimal angiographic facilities and all necessary materials should be at hand.

4.2 Work-up for Emergency Embolization

Requests for emergency embolization are usually unexpected and often occur after hours, therefore logistical support must be optimized to provide trained personal who are available on a 24 h basis. In case of an emergency there is usually not much time for full diagnostic work-up. Undoubtedly a CT scan can be very helpful to guide the intervention. In traumatic bleeding essentials like hemodynamic monitoring and live-support should be available. Some basic lab data should also be recorded (Table 4.1). Furthermore, typed and cross match packed red blood cells should be obtained immediately. Fresh frozen plasma and platelets also may be required to correct coagulopathies that develop in severe hemorrhagic shock. Intravenous access and fluid resuscitation are standard. However, this practice has become controversial. For many years, aggressive fluid administration has been advocated to normalize hypotension associated with severe hemorrhagic shock. Recent studies of urban patients

J. A. Reekers, MD, PhD
Academic Medical Centre, University of Amsterdam, Department of Radiology, G1-207, Meibergdreef 9, 1105 AZ, Amsterdam, The Netherlands

with penetrating trauma have shown that mortality increases with these interventions; these findings call these practices into question. Reversal of hypotension prior to the achievement of hemostasis may increase hemorrhage, dislodge partially formed clots, and dilute existing clotting factors. Findings from animal studies of uncontrolled hemorrhage support these postulates. These provocative results raise the possibility that moderate hypotension may be physiologically protective and should be permitted, if present, until hemorrhage is controlled.

For a hemodynamically unstable patient with, for example a pelvic bleeding, timely embolization may be the patient's only chance for survival. Although some of the literature may disagree, it has been our experience that any delay in embolization therapy to allow the application of external or internal pelvic fixators can result in deadly delays. Patients with acute hemodynamic instability do not die in the angio suit, as modern anesthesia can almost always keep them alive during the procedure. They die, however, from the sustained shock and blood transfusions which will lead to multi-organ failure (MOF) days after the initial procedure. There is a direct relation between the amount of blood transfusions and the chance to leave the hospital alive. On the other hand, recently available Velcro-type pelvic binders offer a rapid and effective alternative to time consuming orthopedic fixation procedure in pelvic fractures and may allow stabilization of the patient without delaying indicated angiographic embolization procedures. It is therefore paramount to get the patient to the angiography suite as promptly as possible. It has been the experience in some major trauma centers that an angiography suite next to the trauma bay is a very helpful arrangement. It is important for the interventionist to be present at the emergency department when the patient gets in and to start the preparation for the embolization procedure.

4.3
Semi-Emergency

If there is an acute indication for embolization therapy, but if the patient is hemodynamic stable, a spiral CT can be very beneficial to help planning the intervention. A pseudoaneurysm of a visceral vessel certainly will target the intervention. A retroperitoneal hematoma will suggest potential bleeding sites. Active extravasation can also sometimes be visual-

Table 4.1. Basic data that should be recorded before emergent embolization

- Medication history
- Prothrombin time, activated partial thromboplastin time, and platelets count
- Hemoglobin/hematocrit
- Arterial blood gases, base deficit, and lactate levels (reflect acid-base and perfusion status)

ized on CT, especially newer multi-detector scanners, allowing the angiographer to zoom in on the likely site of major bleeding without a proceeding exhaustive angiographic search. In hemodynamically unstable patients, a focused ultrasound examination of the abdomen while the patient is being prepared for the angiogram can sometimes localize a pelvic or intra-abdominal fluid collection and help guide the intervention. Therefore, we believe that cross-sectional imaging in some form should be performed as a work-up whenever possible.

Other forms of bleeding localization can also be used. In a patient with GI bleeding who was first seen by an endoscopist, as is usually the case, application of a clip to the bleeding site can guide a possible subsequent catheter intervention. Having a good understanding with the endoscopist on this is important. Similarly, in patients presenting with hemoptysis, bronchoscopy can be of great help to determine the bleeding site, along with a cross-sectional imaging study. Again, blood, plasma and at least two large caliber running intravenous lines should always be available. In addition, we have also found that, in these semi-acute patients, professional monitoring by an anesthesiologist is highly advantageous.

4.4
Elective Embolization

Elective embolization can be performed for many indications as will be presented in other chapters in this book. Different indications have different appropriateness criteria and require different work-up and preparations (Table 4.2). For example, preparation for a uterine fibroids embolization procedure varies greatly from preparation for a varicocele embolization. Work-up and preparation includes a focused history with physical examination, evaluation by an appropriate allied clinical specialist (for example, a gynecologist in the case of uterine fibroid embolization), and a proper imaging and laboratory evaluation. Patient education is a crucial part of the preparation procedure, as some of these elective embolization procedures can result in significant complications. The patient needs to be well informed of the indications, alternatives, and the risk of complications.

4.5
Follow-up

The follow-up should be focused on the possible complications and clinical outcome (Table 4.3). In the acute and immediate post-procedural phase, special attention should be directed to the early detection of sequelae of non-target embolization, which can often result in major complications. It is a good practice to routinely conduct a telephone interview with the patient no later than a week after the procedure. Modern interventionists are clinical providers and an interventional clinic follow-up at an appropriate period of time following a major embolization procedure is not an option but a required minimal standard of practice.

After embolization of a uterine fibroid clinical follow-up might be sufficient. However, to prevent an early recurrence, early MR controls might be necessary. Pain control following embolization of a congenital vascular malformation can often be effectively accomplished done with oral analgesics, such as acetaminophen or non-steroidal anti-inflammatory drugs. However, in the case of embolization of a solid organ or tumor, special care should be taken to the management of post-embolization pain that can be severe. In some instances, for example uterine fibroids or kidney tumor embolization, opiates or epidural anesthesia may be required. The interventionist should always check the patient personally as post-embolization pain can sometimes be unpredictable, and may be the source of significant anxiety and negative perception by the patient. Fever, usually below 38.5°C but sometimes as high as 39°C, and nausea are also often seen after embolization due to tissue necrosis. Fever above 39°C is suspect for infection or abscess formation. CT scan guided percutaneous sampling and drainage might be mandatory in some of these cases. Surgical consultation for debridement and drainage may also be needed in extreme cases. Wide spectrum empirical antibiotic therapy should be started whenever infection is suspected. In some embolization applications, like embolization of the splenic artery, there is a higher predilection to abscess formation, which can be treated with antibiotics and percutaneous drainage. It is mandatory to document all of the details surrounding post-operative adverse effect and their management in the medical record.

Table 4.2. Preparation for elective embolization

Application	Work-up	Procedural risks
Vascular malformation	MRI/MRA	Necrosis
Uterine fibroids	MRI/MRA, US	Septicemia/pain and fever
Spermatic vein	US	Recurrence
Endoleaks	Spiral CT, MRI, angiography, duplex US	Recurrence/non-target embolization
Primary liver tumors	CT, angiography	Necrosis/fever/sepsis/recurrence
Metastatic renal cell tumor	CT, angiography	Necrosis/fever/pain
Benign bone tumors	CT	Pain/recurrence
Tumor in general	CT/MR	Necrosis/fever/pain

Table 4.3. Complications of therapeutic embolization

Complication	Referral	Management
Tissue necrosis	Plastic surgeon	Skin grafts/skin transplants
Bowl/parenchyma ischemia/necrosis	Surgeon	CT scan/laparotomy
Sepsis	Interventional radiologist or surgeon	Antibiotics/drainage
Severe pain	Interventional radiologist	NAIDS/morphine

Take Home Points:

- Work-up and follow-up of embolization patients should be specifically tailored to the patient, and the indication for intervention.

- Vital information can be obtained from the patient's medical history.

- The doctor who performs the embolization procedure should be responsible for the follow-up.

- Proper pain management is important after embolization.

- Proper medical documentation is very important.

- A team approach is important.

References

Agnew SG (1994) Hemodynamically unstable pelvic fractures. Orthop Clin North Am 25:715–721

Beers MH, Berkow R (eds) (1999) Hemostasis and coagulation disorders. In: Beers MH, Berkow R (eds) The Merck manual of diagnosis and therapy, 17th edn. Merck, USA

Ben Menachem Y, Coldwell DM, Young JW, Burgess AR (1991) Hemorrhage associated with pelvic fractures: causes, diagnosis, and emergent management. Am J Roentgenol 157:1005–1014

Moore H, List A, Holden A, Osborne T (2000) Therapeutic embolization for acute haemorrhage in the abdomen and pelvis. Australas Radiol 44:161–168

Simons ME (2001) Peripheral vascular malformations: diagnosis and percutaneous management Can Assoc Radiol J 52:242–251

Spies JB, Pelage JP (eds) (2004) Uterine artery embolization and gynecologic embolotherapy. Lippencott, USA

Wilkins RA, Viamonte M (eds) (1982) Interventional radiology. Blackwell, Oxford

GI

5 Upper GI Bleeding

Luc Defreyne

CONTENTS

5.1 Introduction

The first attempts to arrest non-variceal upper gastrointestinal hemorrhage (GIH) by transcatheter embolotherapy were undertaken in the early 1970s. As a low-invasive alternative for the high risk-bearing surgery, embolization had a bright future [1–5]. However, the endoscopic revolution pushed both embolization and laparotomy into the background. From the mid 1980s on, endoscopy had assumed its role of first-line hemostasis, leaving laparotomy for about 10% of refractory bleedings. Unlike in lower GIH, endoscopy rendered diagnostic arteriography in upper GIH redundant. Only at the turn of the cen-

tury, interest in embolotherapy revived. Microcatheter systems and the embolic agents became more efficient and safe. Growing confidence in endovascular techniques contributed to the revival, resulting in an increasing number of promising scientific papers [6–10].

5.2 Epidemiology

With an incidence of 50–100/100 000 and a mortality of 10%–14%, acute upper GIH is recognized world-wide as a clinically significant and expensive health-care issue [11–13].

Acute upper GIH may present as hematemesis (bloody or coffee ground), melena or in rare cases as hematochezia. When a nasogastric tube is placed, aspirate should be blood red. Soon after the initial presentation, a combination of these bleeding manifestations usually occurs.

Over 90% of acute upper GIH are non-variceal [11–13] with peptic ulcer accounting for about 50% of causes. Other major etiologies include erosions and mucosal inflammation such as oesophagitis, gastritis or bulbitis (20%–25%), neoplasms (5%–10%) and vascular malformations such as angiodysplasia, Dieulafoy, aorto-enteral fistula (10%). Despite general availability and vigorous use of endoscopy, 10%–20% of acute upper GIH remain without a documented cause [12, 14].

Although bleeding ceases spontaneously in a high number of cases, there is a consensus that all acute upper GIHs should be investigated by endoscopy [15]. Emergency endoscopic intervention is compulsory in high-risk groups identified by pre-endoscopic stratifications models for rebleeding [16, 17] and mortality [18–21]. In low risk groups, the patients may be held under short observation to undergo endoscopy on a more elective basis. Combined endoscopic injection therapy and thermal coagulation are able to control about 90% of

L. Defreyne, MD, PhD
Department of Vascular and Interventional Radiology, Ghent University Hospital, De Pintelaan 185, 9000 Ghent, Belgium

acute bleedings, thereby significantly reducing the mortality rate [15, 22]. However, 10%–20% of upper GIHs recur or continue to ooze after initial bleeding arrest. In peptic ulcer bleeding, proton pump inhibitors [23, 24] combined with eradication of *Helicobacter pylori* [25, 26] have contributed to a reduction in rebleeding rates. Other endoscopic strategies such as adjunctive prokinetics (erythromycin 250 mg intravenous bolus to induce gastric emptying and improve visibility [27, 28]), hemoclipping and cryotherapy [29–32], aggressive treatment of non-bleeding risk stigmata [33] and scheduled second therapeutic endoscopy [34–37] seem promising or are still under investigation.

Despite these advances in medical treatment and endoscopic intervention, mortality in acute upper gastrointestinal bleeding varies between 10% to 15% and seems not to have declined for more than a decade [12, 38]. Besides age and severe co-morbidity, endoscopic failure to stop upper GIH and post-endoscopic rebleeding are highly associated with mortality [12].

5.3
Indications for Arteriography

When facing an endoscopic refractory upper GIH, two practical questions arise. Firstly, should we recommend rescue arteriography in every case or, if not, which cases should be reserved for surgery or which ones for embolization? Secondly, what is the optimal timing of a diagnostic arteriography? Both issues are controversial and have not yet received a definite answer.

5.3.1
Arteriography Versus Surgery

If the endoscopic and surgical literature are to be believed, arteriography hardly plays a role in salvage of endoscopically unmanageable upper GIH [39–42]. On the contrary, enthusiastic interventional radiologists stated that every uncontrollable upper GIH should be an indication for arteriography and embolization [8, 43]. The involved disciplines seem to indulge in navel-gazing. As is so often the case, the truth lies somewhere in the middle. For lack of scientific evidence (no randomized prospective studies available), decision making should be based on individual parameters and each case discussed with the involved physicians [44, 45]. When a patient is in a frail condition or when surgery has already failed, it is wise to decide for a less invasive arteriographic exploration with the option of embolization. In peptic ulcer bleeding, elderly patients with a high cardiovascular risk and coagulation disorders are likely to profit from embolization [10]. In this study, surgery rescued patients with a lower risk profile and outcome in both therapy groups was similar. However, the study was a retrospective survey which requires cautious interpretation [10]. In an own 10-year retrospective (unpublished) survey, we found that bleeding peptic ulcers visualized at endoscopy were five times more likely to be rescued by surgery. In other cases, the endoscopists did not trust surgical exploration of unclear acute upper GIH. They might be right, since CHENG et al. [46] demonstrated that 50% of the diagnostic failures at endoscopy will remain unclear after surgical rescue. These ultimate diagnostic failures were significantly associated with higher morbidity and mortality [46]. Besides clinical factors, angiographic equipment and expertise in embolization techniques are decisive for interventional radiology to be accepted as a valid option in refractory upper GIH.

5.3.2
Timing of Arteriography

Rapid fall in hemoglobin (Hb) or hematocrit (Hc) blood levels, high transfusion requirements (more than 4 U of packed cells in 24 h) [47–49] and low systolic blood pressure with tachycardia [50] have been postulated as indicators of active bleeding. However, patients will be resuscitated during or after endoscopy and often demonstrate hemodynamic stabilization and/or normalization of Hb and Hc values when they arrive in the angio-suite. In the heat of the fight against shock, the number of transfused blood products may not always reflect the actual severity of bleeding. In an own study, we found a positive arteriography in 36% of GIH episodes with less than 4 U of packed cells transfused. Moreover, 40% of these patients bled actively on arteriography but had no blood transfusion or even shock therapy [51]. In our as well as others' experience, the alertness of the endoscopist facing an intractable bleeding and the rapidity of decision making are crucial to catch the patient while actively bleeding [52].

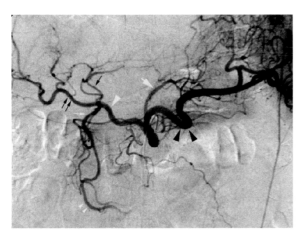

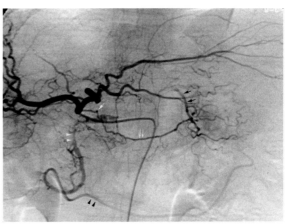

Fig. 5.1. DSA of celiac trunk with a 5-F Cobra catheter. Left gastric artery (*white arrow*), splenic artery (*arrowheads*), common hepatic artery (*white arrowhead*), gastroduodenal artery (*small white arrow*), right gastroepiploic artery (*small white arrowheads*), left (*small arrow*) and right (*double small arrow*) hepatic artery

Fig. 5.2. DSA of the hepatic artery with a 5-F Cobra catheter. Gastroduodenal artery (*white arrowheads*), right gastroepiploic artery (*black arrowheads*), right gastric artery (*white arrow*) branching from the left hepatic artery, arcade (*white arrows*) connecting right and left gastric artery (*black arrows*)

5.4
Gastroduodenal Arteriographic Anatomy

The gastrointestinal tract is supplied by the unpaired visceral arteries branching from the abdominal aorta: the celiac trunk (Fig. 5.1), superior and inferior mesenteric artery.

Each segment or organ of the gastrointestinal tract receives its blood from different so-called organ specific arteries, which are interconnected by arcades.

The stomach is irrigated by the gastric arteries (left and right), the gastroepiploic arteries (left and right) and the short gastric arteries (from the distal splenic artery) (Fig. 5.2).

Between the left and right gastric artery (commonly branching from the left hepatic artery), there is a small anastomotic arcade delineating the small curvature. Connections between the inferior esophageal and cardiac left gastric branches may be observed occasionally during left gastric arteriography or by direct injection of a lower esophageal branch (Fig. 5.3).

The right gastroepiploic artery is the continuation of the gastroduodenal artery running along the major curvature and becoming the left gastroepiploic artery when approaching the splenic hilus. Here one can find constant collaterals to the splenic artery. The fundus of the stomach is supplied by several short gastric arteries branching from the distal splenic artery. Finally, multiple connections

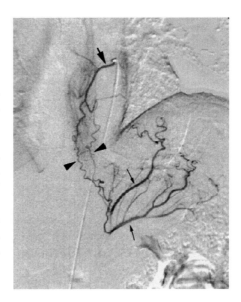

Fig. 5.3. DSA with a 5-F Cobra catheter of an inferior esophageal artery (*arrow*) showing anastomoses with cardiac branches (*arrowheads*) of the left gastric artery (*arrows*)

between the tributaries of the major gastric arteries complete the anastomosing network.

The duodenum is supplied by the pancreaticoduodenal arteries, consisting of two, sometimes three or more trunks bridging the gastroduodenal and superior mesenteric artery. One pancreaticoduodenal arcade is located anteriorly (mostly as a continuation of the gastroduodenal artery) and one posteriorly, with multiple anastomoses between them and other pancreatic arteries, building a rich collateral plexus (Fig. 5.4).

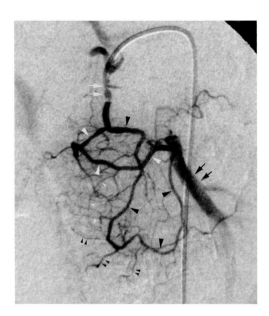

Fig. 5.4. DSA of the gastroduodenal artery with a 5-F Cobra catheter (*white arrows*). Anterior (*black arrowheads*) and posterior (*white arrowheads*) pancreaticoduodenal arcades originating with superior and inferior common trunks. Multiple interconnected mural arteries (*small black arrowheads*) build loops (*small white arrowheads*) between the upper and the lower arcade, completing the dual duodenal supply. Superior mesenteric artery (*black arrows*)

5.5
Diagnostic Arteriography

In stable and cooperative patients, the diagnostic arteriography is performed under local anesthesia via a transfemoral access and in the classical Seldinger technique. Celiac trunk and the superior mesenteric artery (SMA) are catheterized with preshaped single-use 4- or 5-F catheters of the "Cobra" or "side-winder" type. Iodinated nonionic iso-osmolar contrast medium (25–35 ml at a rate of 4–6 ml/s) is injected by a power injector into the celiac trunk and SMA. In patients with renal insufficiency, contrast allergy or hyperthyroidism gadolinium chelates (MRI contrast medium) have been suggested as a substitute for iodinated contrast medium [53], but reports on its use in the visceral arteries are still awaited.

The arteriograms of the celiac trunk and superior mesenteric artery should completely map the gastroduodenal blood supply. Anatomical variants should be searched for (esophageal, phrenic, hepatic arteries branching from the aorta, direct origin of the left gastric from the aorta, etc.). If all territories are visualized and no bleeding source

is found, hemobilia and wirsungorrhagia are excluded, the investigation should be completed with an abdominal aortography to trace an aortoduodenal fistula. Furthermore, we generally finish the arteriography with a repeat study of the most suspected region.

Using X-ray equipment, the passage of the contrast medium in the arteries, the parenchymal staining and the portal-venous return are recorded in one series by successive shots. In the digital subtraction technique, the contrast-filled vessels are automatically subtracted from the background. At this point, it becomes of utmost importance that the empty "background" mask remains spatially matched with the "filled" images. Therefore, the patients are asked to stop breathing and not to move during the recording. Moreover, bowel gas and peristalsis should be anticipated by the administration of 20–40 mg of butylhyoscine. When the patient's condition does not allow co-operation, general anesthesia should be readily available.

After each series, the images are examined on the display to look for extravasation of contrast medium or a pseudoaneurysm. When bowel movement is disturbing, images should also be examined in the non-subtraction mode. Since NUSBAUM and BAUM investigated gastrointestinal bleeding in a canine model, it has been generally accepted that extravasation of contrast medium becomes visible when the blood loss exceeds 0.5 ml/min [54–56].

Only the demonstration of contrast medium extravasation provides proof of the site of vessel rupture. The detection of an aneurysm provides strong evidence, contrary to other structural abnormalities, which are potential bleeding sources. In Table 5.1, we have summarized the angiographic findings in upper GIH and correlated them with the most commonly involved diseases.

GIH is often intermittent and of varying rates, accounting for a considerable number of negative angiographic studies [57]. In recent large retrospective studies the diagnostic yield hardly exceeded 50% [7, 8, 49, 51, 58]. If no contrast extravasation is detected, provocation of bleeding with intra-arterial or intravenous injection of vasodilators, heparin or even fibrinolytics has been proposed, albeit with inconsistent success [59–61]. Occasionally, more selective catheterization may provoke bleeding and visualization of contrast extravasation (Fig. 5.5).

Carbon dioxide has been proposed as an alternative (negative) contrast medium for arteriography of GIH. Carbon dioxide has a very low viscos-

Table 5.1. Angiographic findings and clinicopathologic correlations in upper GIH

Angiographic finding	Clinical correlation
Contrast extravasation	Active bleeding (> 0.5 ml/min)
Aneurysm	Iatrogenic trauma (post-operative, post-bile duct intervention, post-liver biopsy) Accidental trauma Pancreatitis (proteolysis, pseudocyst) Mycotic Arteriitis (polyarteriitis nodosa etc.) Collagen tissue disorder (Ehler Danlos etc.)
Arteriovenous shunt	Dieulafoy lesion Arteriovenous malformation and fistula Rendu-Weber-Osler (HTT) telangiectasia
Focal/spot-like mucosal hyperaemia	Ulcer Small arteriovenous malformation Rendu-Weber-Osler (HTT) telangiectasia
Segmental mucosal hyperaemia	Post-operative (anastomotic, stomal) Gastroduodenitis Hypertensive gastropathy Tuberculosis/granuloma (sarcoidosis)
Neovascularisation/extramucosal hyperaemia	Benign tumor (leiomyoma etc.) Malignant tumor (carcinoma, lymphoma etc.) Metastatic tumor (renal cell cancer etc.)
Pooling of contrast medium	Malignant, metastatic tumor Cavernous/capillary hemangioma Tuberculosis
Arterial wall alterations	Tumor infiltration and erosion Proteolytic erosion (pancreatitis) Atheromatosis

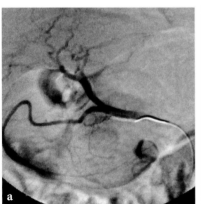 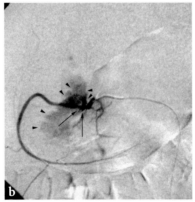 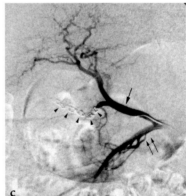

Fig. 5.5a–c. A 55-year-old male with known liver cirrhosis and portal hypertension, presenting with melena. Endoscopy revealed gastroesophageal varices Grade II, but without bleeding stigmata. Blood inundated duodenum did not allow adequate view. **a** DSA of the common hepatic artery with a 5-F Cobra catheter without evidence of contrast medium extravasation or pseudoaneurysm. Note the reduced liver size with arterialization. **b** Selective DSA of the gastroduodenal artery suddenly demonstrates extravasation (*arrowheads*), most probably caused by erosion of the main trunk (*arrows*). **c** Control DSA of the hepatic artery after sandwich embolization of the gastroduodenal artery with 0.038-in. (5 mm diameter, 5 cm length) stainless steel coils (*arrowheads*), delivered through the 5-F catheter. The gastroduodenal artery is occluded distal to the origin of the superior pancreaticoduodenal artery. The hepatic artery (*arrow*) aberrantly originated from the superior mesenteric artery (*double arrow*). Control endoscopy confirmed duodenal ulcer with adherent clot. No rebleeding, but patient died of multi-organ failure

ity allowing detection of much smaller amounts of extravasation [62]. However, the few clinical reports on carbon dioxide in GIH are casuistic and not convincing [63, 64]. Furthermore, the initial enthusiasm was damped by the difficulties and side effects encountered with the administration of CO2 into visceral arteries [64–66].

5.6
Alternatives to Diagnostic Catheter Arteriography

Nuclear medicine became involved in detection of gastrointestinal bleeding in the late 1970s. Two competing imaging tracers were developed: Technetium (Tc-99m) sulfur colloid [67] and Tc-99m labeled red blood cells (RBC) [68]. Although Tc-99m sulfur colloid scintigraphy should detect bleeding rates as low as 0.05–0.1 ml/min, it is rapidly cleared from the blood pool in the reticuloendothelial system (half time of 2.5–3.5 min) limiting its applicability to the active bleeding period. To prolong the level of radioactivity, in vivo labeling of RBC with Tc-99m was developed, with slightly lower bleeding detection rates of 0.2 ml/min [68, 69]. Timing of scanning sequences is optimized to detect extremely rapid bleedings (immediate "radionuclide angiogram"), intermittent bleedings (every 30 s for 60–90 min digitally compiled in a "movie mode"), as well as low-grade bleedings (delayed scanning up to 24 h) [70]. In delayed bleedings occurring during a reduced level of radioactivity, injection of a second dose of radio-labeled RBCs can be helpful [71].

Most of the work with Tc-99m labeled RBC scintigraphy has been carried out for detection of lower GIH with the rationale to avert blind bowel or colonic resection. However, investigators still disagree on the usefulness of radionuclide methods to detect and localize bowel bleeding, guide surgery or screen patients for arteriography [72–77].

Contrast-enhanced computer tomography angiography (CTA) is a challenging modality to localize contrast extravasation in acute bleeding without catheterization. In GIH, multislice CTA seems promising for detection of acute small and large bowel bleeding. A preliminary report calculated a CTA sensitivity of 62.5% (15 of 24 patients) for locating the bleeding site [78]. Moreover, in 41.7% of the cases, CTA disclosed the nature of the bleeding lesion [78]. In upper GIH, detection of the bleeding by enhanced CT scan might be less relevant, but is nevertheless possible (Fig. 5.6a,b).

Fig. 5.6a–n. A 40-year-old man suffering a syncope and melena. He had taken a NSAID for a flue-like malaise 1 day previously. Endoscopy showed a spurting artery adjacent to the papilla. Two attempts at injection and sclerotherapy were unsuccessful. **a** Enhanced CT scan showed extravasation (*black arrow*) at D2, without identifiable cause. Anterior (*white arrow*) and posterior pancreaticoduodenal arcade (*white arrowhead*) are indicated. **b** Emergency DSA of the superior mesenteric artery (5-F Cobra catheter) confirms extravasation at D2 (*arrowheads*). Although anterior (*double arrow*) and posterior (*arrow*) pancreaticoduodenal arcades are fully visualized, the bleeding artery can not be differentiated. Note flow reversal in the gastroduodenal artery because of celiac trunk stenosis. **c** Selective DSA of the common origin of the inferior pancreaticoduodenal arteries: contrast extravasates (*arrowhead*) from a mural artery (*arrow*) branching from the anterior pancreaticoduodenal arcade (*double arrow*) at the transition from the lower to the upper course. **d** Superselective DSA of the mural branch at its origin with a 2.7-F microcatheter, confirming rupture of its distal segment (*arrowheads*). However, the bleeding vessel can not be followed due to reflexive bowel contractions. **e** After a 5-min wait, bowel movements ceased and the course of the mural artery becomes visible again. Tip of the microcatheter (*arrow*) and extravasation (*arrowheads*). **f** Control DSA after injection of 0.2 ml of PVA 150–250 μ shows occlusion of the distal segment. Glue was not a good option as the supplied area is too large. Platinum microcoils would occlude too proximally allowing distal collateralization. Finally, a more distal catheterization of this small and tortuous branch was not attempted to avoid vasospasm and loss of free flow. **g** Control DSA of the common inferior pancreaticoduodenal trunk reveals persisting contrast extravasation (*arrowheads*), probably from a mural branch of the posterior pancreaticoduodenal arcade (*arrow*). Anterior arcade (*double arrow*). **h** DSA of the celiac trunk with a 5-F Simmons-1 catheter shows contrast dilution in the common hepatic artery (*arrows*) due to flow reversal in the gastroduodenal artery. The 2.7-F microcatheter was introduced into the gastroduodenal artery and all side-branches were "blindly" investigated until the one with a distal rupture was found. If we had kept the catheter in the mesenteric artery and had performed a contralateral puncture and catheterization of the celiac trunk, microcatheterization guidance would have been easier. **i** Tip of the microcatheter (*small arrow*) positioned in front of the rupture site (*arrow*): contrast medium escapes immediately into the duodenal lumen (*arrowheads*). An ultimate site-branch of the ruptured mural artery is indicated (*small arrowhead*). Embolization was performed with 0.6 ml of 1/3 diluted glue (Gluebran2/lipiodol). **j** Control DSA of the superior mesenteric artery no longer demonstrates contrast extravasation. Most of the polymerized glue is located in the bowel lumen, adherent to the duodenal wall (*arrowheads*). During embolization visibility was blurred due to piling up of the extravasated glue in the duodenal lumen, accounting for the unusually large amount required to stop the bleeding. **k** Duodenoscopy immediately after embolization reveals clean and blood free duodenum with adherent glue pellet (*arrowheads*). **l** Endoscopic view of D2 after intensive flushing and washing shows a crateriform mucosal lesion (*arrows*) with a shape similar to that of the extravasated contrast depot in (**a**). The glue plug was hosed and washed away (*white arrowheads*). **m** Digital image post endoscopy confirms that the glue (*arrowheads*) was dislodged from the bleeding wall defect (landmarked by the arterial glue cast, *small arrows*) and moved downwards into the duodenum. **n** Retrospectively, one single DSA sequence already revealed that the bleeding (*large arrow*) was located on a mural loop connecting both embol- ▷

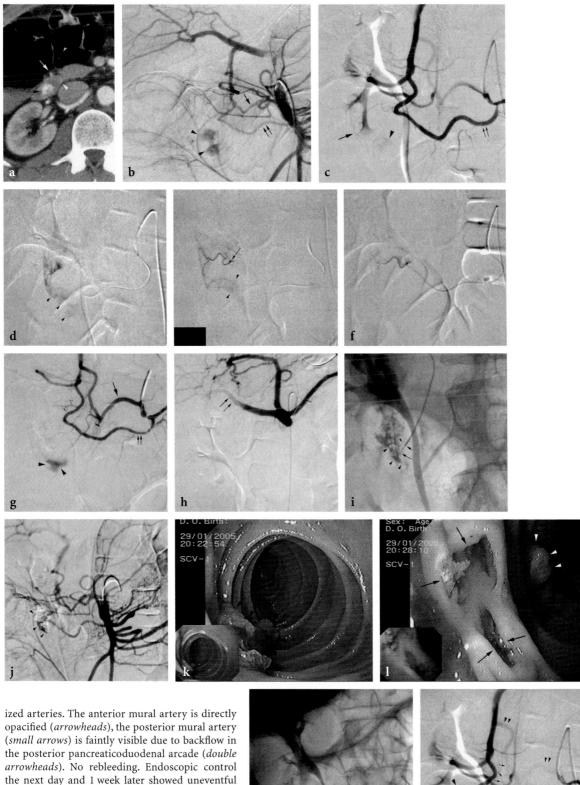

ized arteries. The anterior mural artery is directly opacified (*arrowheads*), the posterior mural artery (*small arrows*) is faintly visible due to backflow in the posterior pancreaticoduodenal arcade (*double arrowheads*). No rebleeding. Endoscopic control the next day and 1 week later showed uneventful healing of the mucosal erosion. Comment: In view of the patient's young age, non-compromised clinical status and the technical difficulties encountered during embolization, surgical salvage would have been a reasonable alternative. (Endoscopic images courtesy by Prof. Dr. Isabelle Colle, gastroenterologist at the Ghent University Hospital)

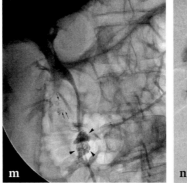

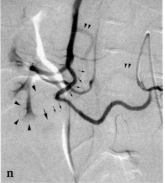

5.7
Therapeutic Arteriography

There are several ways to stop gastrointestinal bleeding by catheter intervention: infusion of vasoconstrictive drugs (vasopressin), embolization and intentional induction of vasospasm.

Vasoconstriction and local vasospasm are physiological defenses against exsanguinations. When the bleeding has ceased and no extravasation is visible, focal vasospasm at arteriography sometimes indicates the bleeding site.

Therapeutic vasopressin infusion into the main arterial trunks induces visceral vasospasm, enhancing the physiological vasoconstrictive reaction against bleeding. Initial enthusiasm about vasopressin infusion ebbed away because of less favorable results compared to embolization [79–81], and the systemic side effects [82]. Vasopressin infusion has been shown more effective in lower than in upper GIH.

Proximal vasospasm induced by manipulations of the diagnostic catheter in the main branches or arcades was a major problem in the early days of visceral catheterization [83]. Modern diagnostic catheters have smaller diameters (4–5 F compared to the older 6–7 F) and softer tips. Proximal catheter induced vasospasm is less frequently encountered. In contrast, distal vasospasm often occurs during superselective catheterization due to micro-guidewire manipulations. Iatrogenic vasospasm is irritating as it may once and for all preclude entering of the spurting artery [6, 84, 85]. Because iatrogenic vasospasm frequently results in instant bleeding arrest, some have induced it intentionally to stop extravasation in lower GIH [86]. Although preliminary results are promising (93% of bleeding stopped), the durability of this haemostatic act should be confirmed in other studies, also dealing with upper GIH. Nevertheless, we should be less alarmed when iatrogenic vasospasm of the previously bleeding artery limits further catheterization.

Embolization goes beyond vasospasm and aims at definitive occlusion of the bleeding artery.

5.8
Embolization

Superselective embolization is the endovascular analogue to surgical vessel clipping. The technical success of embolization is determined by the ability of superselective vessel catheterization and the use of appropriate embolic agents.

5.8.1
General Technical Aspects

All efforts should be made to obtain assessable arteriographic images of the upper GI tract. In hemodynamically unstable patients or in patients who are unable to cooperate, tracheal intubation and general anesthesia arc mandatory. At our institution, the angiography protocol for acute bleeding includes a request for anesthesiological assistance.

The primary goal of arteriography is to locate the bleeding site. Revealing the nature of the bleeding lesion will be more difficult and, in planning embolization, is of subordinate importance. Arteriographic results might be subdivided into three categories: (1) normal findings, (2) contrast medium extravasation proving active bleeding and (3) structural arterial abnormalities. In each of these situations, the technique of embolization will differ.

If no abnormalities are detected, one should consider blind [48] or so-called "prophylactic" [87] or "empiric"[49] embolization of the left gastric or gastroduodenal artery (Table 5.2). Blind embolization was first applied with poor success by REUTER et al. in 1975 [2], reinvigorated by LANG et al. in 1992 [87], criticized by DEMPSEY et al. in 1999 [48] and recently highly advocated in larger retrospective studies by ANIA et al. [7] and SCHENKER et al. [8]. Blind embolization is tempting because of its technical simplicity and safety (see 5.8.2.3 Gelfoam embolization). However, one should keep in mind that effectiveness of blind embolization has not been proved against a control group. In view of the considerable number of spontaneous bleeding arrests that may occur after non-therapeutic arteriography [51], the outcome of such a comparative study might be quite unpredictable. In daily practice however, we agree with LANG et al. to recommend deliberate use of blind embolization only when there is definite prior identification of a lesion in the vascular territory [87].

If contrast medium extravasation is demonstrated, the location on the arterial tree determines the technique of embolization (Table 5.2). If blood spurts from a main artery such as the gastroduodenal, then embolic hemostasis should be performed at the site of rupture to be effective and safe. If the bleeding point cannot be reached, embolization by injection of Gelfoam "from a distance" might be safe yet uncertain as the bleeding might stop only temporarily.

Table 5.2. Contrast extravasation/aneurysm in upper GIH: technique of embolization according to vascular anatomy

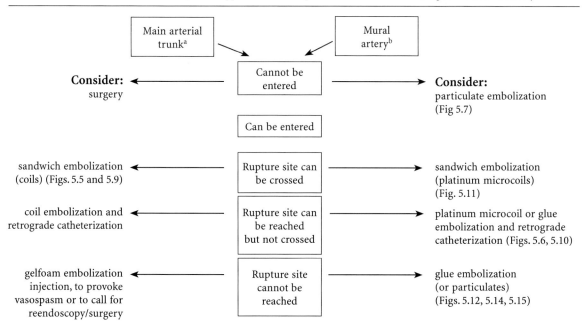

aGastroduodenal, pancreaticoduodenal arcade.
bAlso called muscular branches.

if bleeding point is close to
main artery consider sandwich
technique coiling (Fig. 5.11)

Glue embolization of major arteries is very effective but contains a high risk of ischemic complications. Thus if, in major artery rupture, the bleeding point is beyond the range of catheterization, alert the gastroenterologist to get a control endoscopy or, even wiser, get a surgeon for a definitive salvage.

If the bleeding is located on a mural artery or its tributaries, then we have more options (Table 5.2). The mucosal area supplied by a mural artery is delimited. Branches from adjacent mural arteries contribute to a more or less extended dual supply. Therefore, ischemic complications after embolization in the mural tree are assessable. Flow directed remote injection of particulates or even glue is a valid technique if the rupture site cannot be reached.

Any aneurysm detected on the arterial tributaries located in the bleeding area should be considered as a pseudoaneurysm and therefore treated as a contrast medium extravasation.

If structural abnormalities such as vascular malformations, hypervascular tumors, vessel wall irregularities suggesting erosion etc., are visualized, then we may try for a palliative embolization with Gelfoam or particulates. Rarely, curative embolization of an arteriovenous malformation or fistula is achievable with non-resorbable agents, such as glue or detachable balloons.

5.8.2
Specific Technical Aspects

Embolic agents can cause permanent or temporary occlusion. According to their behavior in the bloodstream, embolic agents may be categorized as mechanically either proximally or distally occlusive and distally flow-dependent occlusive. In case of a (pseudo-)aneurysm, endosaccular embolization might be an option, similar to coiling of intracranial aneurysms (Table 5.3).

Properties of the microcatheters and microguidewires we use are listed in Table 5.4. Most companies offer adequate coaxial systems. We do not adhere to specific brands and have used all kinds of microcatheters and microguidewires over the years.

If vasospasm due to microcatheter manipulation occurs, patience is required; eventually withdraw the catheter a little. Superselective manipulations often irritate the bowel wall, which then contracts, obscuring the vessel course. Intravenous butylhyoscine may reduce wall reactivity, but even better is taking a rest and the opportunity to study the arteriogram, while flushing the microcatheter (Fig. 5.6d,e).

Table 5.3. Embolic agents, mechanism of occlusive action and applicability in upper GIH

Embolic agents/ embolisation technique	Mechanical proximal occlusion[a]	Mechanical distal occlusion[a]	Flow dependent distal occlusion[b]	Endo-saccular occlusion	Applicability in upper GIH
Particles					
Non-calibrated PVA	–	+	++	–	Yes
Calibrated PVA or gelatin spheres	–	–	+++	–	?
Gelatin sponge					
Plugs (> 2mm)	++	+	+	–	Yes
Powder	–	+	+++	–	(Yes)
Coils					
Macrocoils (0.035-0.038 inch)	+++	+	–	++	yes
Microcoils (0.018 inch)	–	+++	+	++	Yes
Detachable microcoils	++	+++	–	+++	?
Liquids					
N-butyl 2- cyanoacrylate	–	+	++	+	Yes
Ethylene polyvinyl alcohol	–	+	++	++	?
Ethanol/polidocanol	–	–	+++	–	No

[a] "Mechanical" is defined as occlusive at or close to the point of delivery.
[b] "Flow dependent" means that the embolic agent will be carried by the bloodstream to occlude remote from the catheter tip.
–, Not applicable;   + to +++, not typical to very characteristic action;   ?, no experience reported.

5.8.2.1
Particulate Embolization

Particulate embolization is an option when contrast extravasates and the bleeding branch is beyond the reach of superselective catheterization (Fig. 5.7). Non-calibrated polyvinyl alcohol particles (PVA) in sizes of 150–250 μ to 250–350 μ or even larger should be used. The amount of particles should be kept as low as possible to avoid diffuse distal embolization. After each injection of 0.1–0.2 ml (up to a maximum of 1 ml) of a dilution of PVA, control arteriography should verify that the bleeding point has been occluded. If extravasation is no longer visible, injection should be stopped and occlusion confirmed after 10–15 min (Fig. 5.6f).

Bleeding from hypervascular tumors, such as duodenal metastasis of renal cell carcinoma, can be stopped by palliative particulate embolization (Fig. 5.8), although other authors preferred Gelfoam [88, 89].

- Mechanism of action: flow-directed distal embolization, shunting of particles to the point of least resistance (rupture site), cluttering and plug formation of particles (no deep penetration).

Table 5.4. Cookbook: Properties of catheters and guidewires used in upper GIH embolization

	Configuration	Caliber (French/inch)	Length (cm)	Hydrophilic coating	Radiopacity
Sheath	Straight	4–5	10	-	-
Catheter	Cobra I/sidewinder I or II[a]	4–5	60–100[b]	Optional	Distal part
Guidewire	J-tip	0.035	150–170	Yes	Yes
Microcatheter	Straight (steam shapeable)	2.4–3.0[c]	130–150	Yes	Tip marker
Microguidewire	J-tip (45°–90°) or straight if shapeable	0.014–0.021[d]	150–180	Yes	Yes

[a] For a transbrachial approach, also consider a vertebral or headhunter catheter; we rarely use guiding catheters.
[b] For transbrachial approach.
[c] Only in rare occasions we resorted to smaller French-size microcatheters.
[d] Some companies offer microcatheter-microguidewire sets.

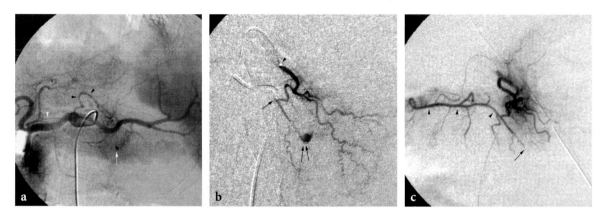

Fig. 5.7a–c. A 52-year-old man with hematemesis after a suicide attempt with corrosive fluid. On gastroscopy no visualization of a lesion due to massive bleeding. **a** Celiac trunk DSA demonstrating contrast medium extravasation (*white arrow*) from a distal branch of the left gastric artery (*arrowheads*). Note the course of the right gastric artery branching off the left hepatic artery (*white arrowhead*). **b** Selective DSA of the left gastric artery with a 2.7-F microcatheter (*arrowhead*): route to the ruptured artery (*double arrow*) too tortuous for superselective catheterization. Proximal coil embolization would obviously allow inflow via the collateral arcade to the right gastric artery (*small arrow*). Therefore, flow directed embolization with small amounts (0.5 ml) of PVA particles (150–250 μ) was performed. **c** Post-embolization DSA showing distal occlusion of the bleeding artery (*arrow*) and adjacent mural arteries. Reverse flow into the right gastric artery (*arrowheads*). No rebleeding until 3 weeks later oozing from a small ulcer at the same location was easily treated by sclerotherapy. The patient died 8 months later of a gastric carcinoma

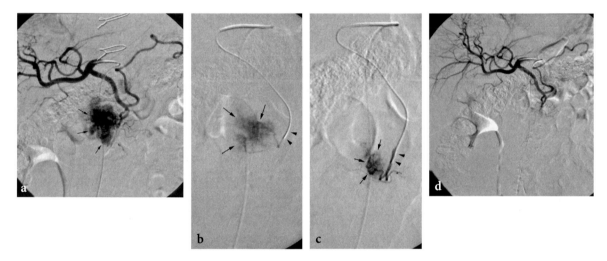

Fig. 5.8a–d. A 79-year-old male, who underwent a left nephrectomy for renal cell cancer 1 year previously, now presents with melena from bleeding duodenal metastases. **a** DSA of the common hepatic artery showing hypervascular tumor blush (*arrows*) in the duodenum, supplied by hypertrophied duodenal branches of the gastroduodenal artery. **b,c** Superselective visualization of two different tumor compartments (*arrows*) with a 2.7-F microcatheter (*arrowheads*). **d** Control DSA after injection of several millilitres of PVA 150–250 μ and 250–355 μ in four tumor feeders (two of them shown here), confirming tumor devascularization. After each injection of 0.5–1 ml of PVA, superselective DSA was performed to control flow arrest and prevent reflux of particulates. Patient stopped bleeding for about 7 months and was then retreated

- Major disadvantages: proximal occlusion due to cluttering of particles may leave major collaterals and distal circulation patent. Late recanalization after PVA embolization is described but is not a matter of concern in acute GIH.
- Adverse effects: low risk of ischemic complications when the guidelines for size and injected volume of particles are respected.
- Future perspectives: calibrated particles of polyvinyl alcohol or gelatin penetrate deeper into the vascular system due to lower viscosity. Risk of ischemia is probably higher, but no clinical experience reported. Palliative tumor embolization might be more efficient with calibrated particles, in analogy with uterine fibroid embolization.

5.8.2.2
Coil Embolization

Large-caliber stainless steel or so-called Gianturco coils are coated with strands of Dacron. They are compatible with most 4- to 5-F diagnostic catheters (0.035 or 0.038 inner diameter). They are used to embolize in large size arteries (left gastric, gastroduodenal or hepatic arteries) (Fig. 5.5) [90]. Under favorable anatomical conditions, a small bleeding branch of the pancreaticoduodenal arcade can be entered with a diagnostic 5-F catheter and eventually occluded by a small (1–2 mm) stainless steel coil.

Platinum microcoils have a core of 0.018 in. and are compatible with 2.7- to 3.0-F microcatheters. Different manufacturers provide coils in different shapes (straight, helical, complex, crescent, omega etc.) and lengths (1 to several cm). Ideally, the ruptured vessel segment should be endovascularly "ligated" by placing microcoils on each side of the rupture point, averting retrograde collateralization (Fig. 5.9).

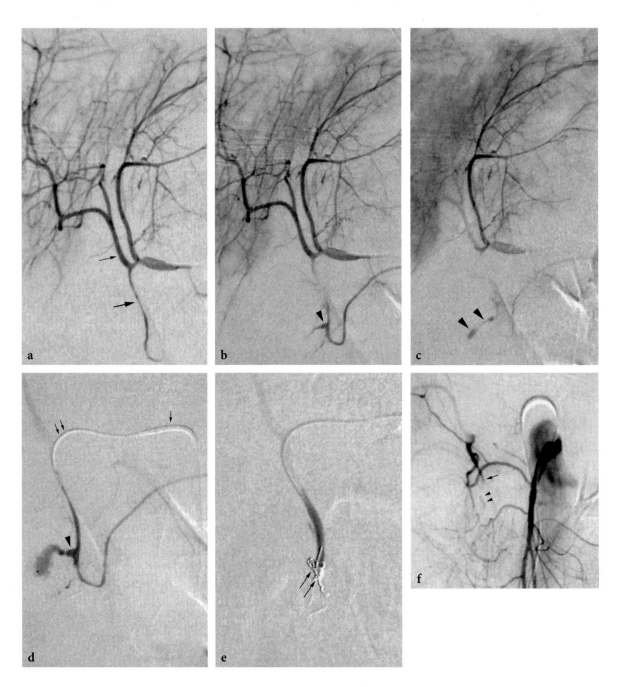

To perform this so-called sandwich technique, the bleeding point must be crossed, which in small mural arteries might be difficult if not impossible. In such cases, direct proximal occlusion might also work (Fig. 5.10). Microcoils are pushed into and out of the microcatheter by a flexible guidewire with a stiff and flattened tip ("coil pusher"). Alternatively, short, straight microcoils can be pushed and ejected by contrast medium injection. With this latter technique, one can try to "shoot" the coils more distally in the bleeding artery (Fig. 5.10). Moreover, always check that all pancreaticoduodenal arcades are visualized to exclude dual supply of the ruptured segment. Eventually, sandwich embolization can be accomplished by approaching from both sides (Fig. 5.6g).

If, due to small caliber or tortuosity, the mural artery cannot be catheterized, sandwich technique occlusion of the main artery might be a solution (Fig. 5.11), provided the bleeding point is very near to the branching point and no collaterals are visible. However, even if angiographically not apparent, the distal tract of the ruptured artery will be patent in many cases, allowing collateral retrograde re-perfusion. If embolization has not occluded potential anastomoses, early post-embolization endoscopy to ensure sustained hemostasis is mandatory (Fig. 5.11).

For treatment of upper GIH, stainless steel coils and platinum microcoils were found to be more effective if combined with Gelfoam or PVA [7, 87].

In lower GIH, platinum microcoils placed in or near to the bleeding artery have served as a landmark for surgical exploration. In upper GIH, there is little indication of such guidance, as gastroduodenal anatomy does not present particular difficulties during laparotomy.

Microcoils can be used to protect the distal circulation by blocking and reversing the bloodstream when flow-directed particulate or glue embolization is considered (Fig. 5.12).

- Mechanism of action: local mechanical obstruction of blood flow and promotion of thrombus formation (Dacron strands).
- Major disadvantage: Flow may be restored if coil embolus is loose (thrombus organization) or patient has a coagulation disorder (failing thrombus formation). Therefore, coil embolus should be as compact as possible by filling up the dead space between the large diameter coils with smaller ones. Angiographic flow arrest is no guarantee that occlusion will be permanent.
- Adverse effects/complications: Coils delivered at the rupture site may perforate the vessel wall (or pseudo-wall in case of an aneurysm) and aggravate the bleeding. Coil placement may also provoke or increase vasospasm.
- Future perspectives: Detachable coils can be repositioned until a focal and compact mechanical obstruction is achieved. Detachable coils may be covered with small Dacron strands to promote thrombus formation or with an expanding hydrogel to minimize dead space between the coil loops. Although dedicated detachable coils are available for intracranial aneurysm embolization, the high cost of these coils precludes its routine use in non-neurointerventional indications.

5.8.2.3
Gelfoam Embolization

Introduced as early as 1975, surgical gelatin or Gelfoam is still widely used for embolization of upper GIH because of its availability and easy handling combined with quick and so-called safe occlusion [2, 91]. Gelfoam is an absorbable non-radiopaque non-permanent embolic agent consisting of dry gelatin. Control angiogram performed several days to weeks after embolization will demonstrate recanalization of the occluded trunk [92]. Practically,

---

Fig. 5.9a–f. A 64-year-old patient with hematemesis. Gastroscopic hemostasis of bleeding bulboduodenal ulcer failed as well as emergency surgery. Rebleeding after 4 days with shock. a-c Common hepatic DSA shows vasospastic gastroduodenal artery (*large arrow*) branching from the right hepatic artery (*small arrow*). Contrast medium extravasation from the distal third of the gastroduodenal artery becomes slowly visible (*arrowheads*). d Because of the vasospasm the option was to catheterize the gastroduodenal artery with a 2.7-F microcatheter (*double arrows*) instead of with the 5-F diagnostic Cobra catheter (*arrow*). Rupture of the main vessel is demonstrated (*arrowhead*). e After plugging the gastroduodenal artery with several platinum microcoils (*arrows*) in sandwich technique, the extravasation stops. f Control DSA of the superior mesenteric artery excludes retrograde collateralization of the gastroduodenal artery, which is occluded (*arrows*). Shadow of coils is visible (*arrowheads*). Persistent shock with rebleeding from gastric lesion 5 days later, treated again with left gastric artery embolization. Patient died in septic shock 7 days later

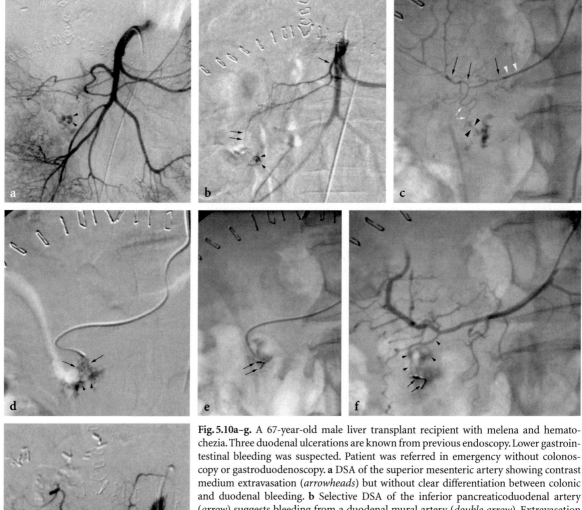

Fig. 5.10a–g. A 67-year-old male liver transplant recipient with melena and hemato-chezia. Three duodenal ulcerations are known from previous endoscopy. Lower gastroin-testinal bleeding was suspected. Patient was referred in emergency without colonos-copy or gastroduodenoscopy. **a** DSA of the superior mesenteric artery showing contrast medium extravasation (*arrowheads*) but without clear differentiation between colonic and duodenal bleeding. **b** Selective DSA of the inferior pancreaticoduodenal artery (*arrow*) suggests bleeding from a duodenal mural artery (*double arrow*). Extravasation (*arrowheads*). **c** Superselective non-subtracted DSA of the anterior pancreaticoduodenal arcade (*arrows*) with a 2.7-F microcatheter (*white arrowheads*): bleeding (*arrowheads*) from a mural branch (*white arrows*) of the horizontal duodenal segment: Note the dis-crepancy between the superselective picture and the overviews: the course of the artery might have been altered by peristalsis or the initially suspect mural artery is not involved. **d** DSA of the bleeding mural artery demonstrating extravasation (*arrowhead*) and intra-mural (*arrows*) contrast medium due to the wedged catheter position. **e** Three straight platinum microcoils (2 mm by 10 mm) (*long arrows*) were placed by injection. **f** Control DSA in non-subtracted reconstruction: patent bleeding mural artery (*arrowheads*) with distal stop caused by the platinum microcoils (*arrows*). **g** Control DSA of the pancrea-ticoduodenal trunk: contrast extravasation is no longer observed. Coils (*arrowheads*). Control duodenoscopy the next day: no bleeding in D3, no lesion observed

Gelfoam fragments, cubes, plugs or pledgets are manually cut to stripes of variable sizes from flat blocks of branded surgical sponge. These "torpe-does" are back-loaded into a 1- or 2-ml syringe after removing the plunger. A small amount of contrast medium is sucked in just to soak the torpedo for radio-opacity [3]. The pledget is then injected into the 4- to 5-F diagnostic catheter. Other investigators prefer the dry method of loading and lancing the Gelfoam torpedo [93]. Under fluoroscopic control, the Gelfoam pledget is expelled by force into the target vessel. The first pledget will be drawn into the main trunk and stuck at the point of vessel tapering or at the first bifurcation. The next torpedoes will pile up proximally to the first one. The pledgets should be sized according to the diameter of the

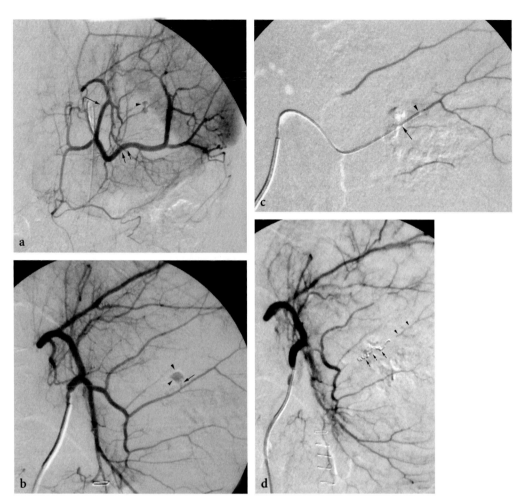

Fig. 5.11a–d. A 32-year-old female underwent terminal ileostomy for bowel complications after laser therapy for endometriosis. Postoperative bleeding from gastric tube and fall in hematocrit. Gastroscopy revealed large organized clot at the major curvature. **a** Contrast medium extravasation (*arrowhead*) on celiac trunk DSA. Left gastric artery (*arrow*); splenic artery (*double arrow*). **b** DSA of the left gastric artery: extravasation (*arrowheads*) from a tiny side-branch near its origin (*arrow*). We opted for a sandwich embolization of the main vessel. **c** Superselective catheterization with a 2.7-F microcatheter of the main artery, positioning the tip (*arrowhead*) distally to the origin of the rupture branch (*arrow*). **d** Post-embolization DSA shows platinum microcoils (*arrows*) proximally and distally from the bleeding point, preventing backflow (*arrowheads*) and potential reperfusion. No retrograde opacification of the tiny ruptured artery was observed. Control gastroscopy at day 1 postembolization: adherent clot; at day 2 arterial oozing treated with adrenaline injection and bipolar coagulation with permanent hemostasis. Progressive retrograde collateralization of the ulcer artery was the likely cause. Nowadays, we would have injected a droplet of glue (or PVA) after placing the distal coils, occluding the tiny side branch as well

vessel to occlude. Usually, to occlude the main trunk of the left gastric artery three or four torpedoes of 2–3 mm by 1–2 cm are sufficient. After each injection, a control angiogram should verify that flow has stopped (Fig. 5.13). Applied in this way, Gelfoam remains very appropriate for proximal occlusion of the left gastric artery and gastroduodenal artery if no contrast extravasation is visible [87, 92]. Until the plug is resorbed, blood pressure distally will be lowered, enabling clots to be formed and organized. Moreover, if bleeding recurs, a possible con-trast medium extravasation in the same territory might still be suitable for embolization, since the main trunk might be opened again [92].

- Mechanism of action: mechanical proximal occlusion with thrombus formation.
- Major disadvantage: Flow will be restored within days or weeks after resorption of the gelatin and organization of the clot.
- Adverse effects/complications: Overly small gelatin pledgets may cause diffuse distal embolization and subsequently ischemia. For the same

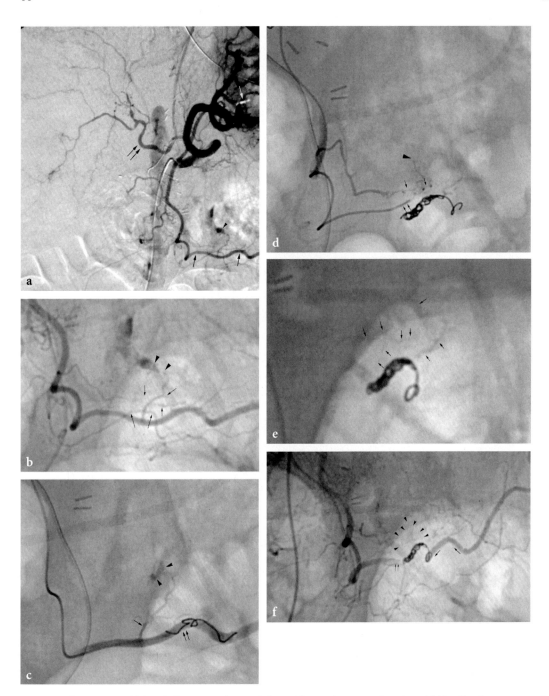

Fig. 5.12a–f. A 58-year-old female liver transplant recipient with massive upper GIH. Arterial bleeding from preantral ulcer with attempt of endoscopic clipping. **a** DSA of celiac trunk confirming contrast medium extravasation (*arrowhead*) from a side-branch of the right gastroepiploic artery (*arrows*). Donor hepatic artery (*double arrow*) shows intrahepatic wall irregularities. Dislocated hemoclip from previous endoscopic intervention (*white arrow*). **b** Non-subtracted DSA demonstrates extravasation (*arrowheads*) and potential collaterals to the ruptured branch (*arrows*). **c** Non-subtracted DSA showing extravasation (*arrowhead*). As the antral branch (*arrow*) might be too small for superselective catheterization, we first performed a coil block of the gastroepiploic artery (*double arrow*) distal to the branch (*arrow*). Either a particulate embolization from the main artery or glue injection was then considered. **d** Non-subtracted DSA: the bleeding branch is entered over a few millimeters with the 2.7-F microcatheter (*double arrow*) and vasospasm (*arrowhead*) has developed. No further catheterization possible. Wedge angiography demonstrates collaterals (*arrows*). **e** Non-subtracted image of glue cast (*arrows*) after injection of a 1:3 diluted Gluebran2/Lipiodol UF mixture. **f** Non-subtracted DSA shows devascularized antral area (*arrowheads*). Also visible is a small thrombus (*double arrows*) due to reflux of glue into the epiploic artery after withdrawing the microcatheter. Flow in the epiploic artery distally to the safety coils is reversed (*black arrows*)

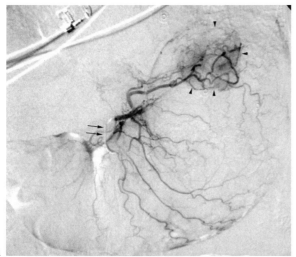
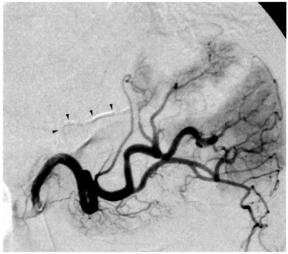

a b

Fig. 5.13a,b. A 91-year-old male with hematemesis and hemorrhagic shock. Stomach filled with fresh blood blurring the endoscopic view. **a** 5-F Cobra catheter in the left gastric artery (*arrows*): DSA reveals a hypervascular tumoral lesion (*arrowheads*) in the fundus. **b** Control DSA and non-subtracted image after injection of four somewhat undersized Gelfoam torpedoes (soaked with contrast medium, *arrowheads*) confirming occlusion of the main trunk of the left gastric and the major tumor artery. Tumor blush is no longer visible. An alternative but more elaborate option was superselective particulate embolization of the tumor. We choose a proximal Gelfoam embolization to avoid any risk of ischemia and because surgery was planned after patient's stabilization. Patient did not rebleed but unfortunately died from multi-organ failure

reason, we do not advise the use of scraped Gelfoam particles or Gelfoam powder for blind embolization.

- Future perspectives: We are not aware of any product innovation in this field.

5.8.2.4
Glue Embolization

The tissue adhesive N-butyl 2-cyanoacrylate or glue (Histoacryl) is a fast and efficient non-resorbable, non-radiopaque embolic material, based on polymerization of the acrylate monomer. Special skill and experience are required to assess the proper dilution of N-butyl cyanoacrylate in lipiodol (Lipiodol-UF, Guerbet, oily contrast medium) to control vascular penetration and avoid ischemia. Therefore, it is not surprising that reporting on the use of glue in the gastrointestinal tract is scarce [4, 94]. Glueing of the microcatheter, once a classical problem, is no longer an issue due to its hydrophilic coating. Glue might be used for flow-directed permanent distal embolization in extravasation or pseudo-aneurysms that are out of range for a sandwich technique occlusion (Fig. 5.14).

Massive bleeding from duodenal ulcers might be treated with glue embolization of the gastrodu-odenal artery or muscular/mural branches, as suggested by LANG [94]. However, this technique entailed an increased risk for acute bowel infarction and chronic stenotic complications [94]. If the bleeding artery can be catheterized to the point of rupture (and eventually beyond into the bowel lumen), slow deposition of highly concentrated glue might be safe [95]. However, in such cases, glue might escape immediately into the bowel lumen blurring the view on the arterial site (Fig. 5.6i,j). If possible, the catheter tip should be wedged proximally from the bleeding point to achieve excellent control of the glue penetration. This technique can be particularly useful in upper GIH bleeding to achieve occlusion of the bleeding vessel and the connection points with the collaterals (Figs. 5.12 and 5.15).

Arterial devascularization of a small area (usually less than 1 cm2) is well tolerated in the stomach and duodenum due to the rich dual collateral supply and healing capacities of the mucosa. Ischemic effects of penetration or reflux of glue might be anticipated by placement of protective microcoils (Fig. 5.12) [95, 96].

- Mechanism of action: Rapid polymerization after contact with ions in blood to create an elastic and adherent plug.
- Major disadvantages: Control of time and place of polymerization depends on many factors such as

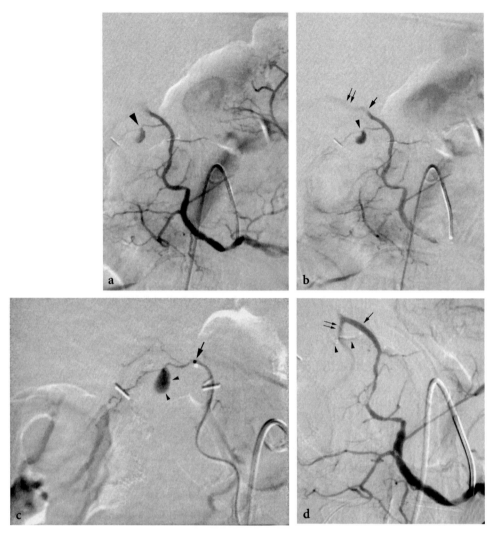

Fig. 5.14a–d. A 68-year-old male with massive bleeding from duodenal Petzer drain after a complicated gastrectomy for dysplastic ulcer. **a** DSA of the inferior anterior pancreaticoduodenal artery reveals extravasation (*arrowhead*) from a mural artery branching from the upper segment of the arcade. **b** Late arterial phase shows accumulation of contrast in a pseudoaneurysm (*arrowhead*). The gastroduodenal artery is very short (*arrow*) and there is reflux into the hepatic artery (*double arrow*). **c** Superselective DSA of the mural artery with a 2.7-F microcatheter (*arrow*) shows extravasation or staining of a pseudoaneurysm (*arrowheads*) **d** Control DSA of the arcade after injection of 0.1 cc of 1 to 3 diluted glue demonstrates occlusion of the mural artery with glue cast (*arrowheads*). Superior anterior (*arrow*) and posterior arcade (*double arrow*) are opacified. No rebleeding.

blood flow, caliber of vessel, dilution of the acrylate, velocity of injection etc.. The microcatheter may be glued in the embolus.

- Adverse effects/complications: Deep and diffuse (>1 cm2) penetration can cause ischemia or even infarction.
- Future perspectives: With the introduction of Glubran2 (GEM, Italy) (mixture of N-butyl 2-cyanoacrylate and methacryloxysulfolane) the acrylate seems more stable in the mixture with lipiodol and less "sticky", which, in our opinion, has improved the control over the polymerization.

5.8.2.5
Other Embolic Agents

Sclerotic agents such as ethanol and polidocanol are pure liquids which penetrate into the capillary bed, causing coagulation necrosis [97] and therefore are not suitable for transarterial embolization. Detachable balloons are very helpful in the rare case of an arteriovenous fistula [98].

- Future perspectives: Superselective intra-arterial infusion of platelets has been successful in patients with GIH suffering refractory thrombo-

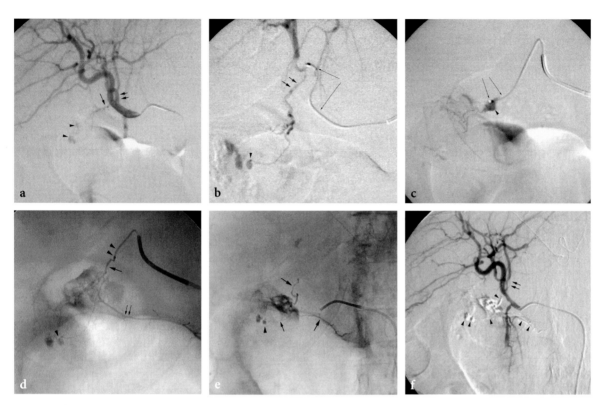

Fig. 5.15a–f. A 74-year-old female with hematemesis after aortic valve replacement. Massive bleeding on endoscopy without visible lesion. **a** DSA of the common hepatic artery revealing contrast medium extravasation (*arrowheads*) from the right gastric artery (*arrow*), branching from the left hepatic artery (*double arrows*). **b** Selective DSA of the left hepatic artery with a 2.7-F microcatheter (*arrows*): distal extravasation from a pyloric branch (*arrowhead*) of the right gastric artery (*double arrows*). **c** Superselective catheterization of the small tortuous right gastric artery results in wedging the catheter tip (*arrows*) in a proximal pyloric branch. Contrast medium partially penetrates into the pyloric wall (*arrowhead*). **d** Non-subtracted DSA after withdrawing the microcatheter (*arrowheads*) into the main right gastric artery (*arrow*): ruptured site (*arrowhead*) as well as the right-to-left gastric arcade (*double arrow*) are clearly visualized. Because of the tortuosity and small dimensions, we decided to perform a flow directed distal occlusion to prevent backward filling via the gastric arcade or the proximal pyloric artery. **e** Digital image of the glue cast (*arrows*). The 1:3 diluted glue penetrated into the ruptured artery to the point of extravasation (*arrowhead*), and into the gastric arcade. **f** Post-embolization DSA of the hepatic artery confirming occlusion of the right gastric artery. Shadows of the glue cast (*arrowheads*). Left hepatic artery remains patent (*arrows*). No rebleeding and no ischemic complication at endoscopy

cytopenia [99, 100]. Ethylene/vinyl alcohol co-polymer or Onyx (MTI, USA) is used as an alternative for glue in embolization of intracranial AVMs. Because penetration of the copolymer into the AVM nidus can be accurately monitored, this liquid embolic plastic has the potential of improving target arterial devascularization in the GI tract.

5.9
Complications

Since the introduction of the microcatheter systems, ischemic complications or infarction are rarely encountered in upper GIH embolization. Prudence is called for when arterial supply has been altered by previous surgery or by arteriosclerotic narrowing or occlusions. Back flow or reflux of Gelfoam into the hepatic or splenic artery may cause organ infarctions, which fortunately are seldom clinically relevant [7, 8]. Overdosing the amount of particulates or glue can occlude too many collateral vessels and hence provoke irreversible ischemia. Also, overdosing may result in reflux of embolic agents into adjacent non-involved territories. Chronic duodenal stenosis has been described as a late complication of glue embolization of the gastroduodenal artery or its muscular side-branches [94].

The contribution of contrast medium overload to renal complications is not well documented, but appears low. Renal insufficiency is multifactorially related to hypovolemic shock or concomitant diseases and mostly transient [7, 8].

Intimal damage during (micro-)catheterization with subsequent dissection and flow arrest can occur after forced entry in tortuous trunks or side-branches. Although rarely reported, every interventionist should be prepared for it, since it may preclude any hemostatic action [8, 10].

5.10
Outcome

Devascularization of the target area, confirmed by angiographic cessation of extravasation or flow arrest in the vessel believed to supply the bleeding source, is achieved in 90%–95 % of cases [6–9, 58]. In 15%–25% of primary vessel occlusions, major collateral flow to the bleeding site will persist, requiring a second or third vessel embolization [6–8, 49]. Proximal anatomical obstacles, such as celiac trunk stenosis or occlusion, may be the cause of technical failures.

Primary clinical success, defined as cessation of bleeding within 30 days of embolization, ranges from 58%–78% [7–10, 51, 58, 97, 102]. After secondary rescue by repeat endoscopy, surgery, re-embolization or a combination of interventions, bleeding can be controlled in about 90% of patients [7, 51, 58].

The mortality rate after embolization for refractory upper GIH varies between 25%–35% [7, 8, 10, 51]. Mortality is associated with underlying disease, multi-organ failure and rebleeding after embolization. Schenker et al. [8] calculated that patients with a clinically successful embolization were 13.3 times more likely to survive, independently of their clinical condition.

5.11
Perspectives

In several studies, attempts have been made to explain the high primary failure rate. The use of coils as the only embolic agents was found to be associated with rebleeding [7]. Other investigators did not confirm an association with procedural parameters. Coagulopathy [7, 8, 102], multi-organ failure or shock [6, 8] and corticosteroid use [6] are clinical risk factors for recurrence of bleeding after embolization.

All associated parameters counteract intrinsic hemostasis and induce rebleeding when embolization does not permanently plug the vessel at the site of rupture. During devascularization of the target area, the embolic agent often does not enter the ruptured segment. Although contrast extravasation may disappear, the abundant collateral circulation will get an opportunity to re-supply the unplugged hole in the ruptured artery. In blind or proximal embolization, which essentially relies on the effect of pressure drop and clot formation, this mechanism of failure is even more relevant. Because associated clinical factors may be difficult to correct, refinement of the technique is a key to improving clinical success of embolization. In our experience, if a "spot weld" embolization cannot be achieved, the embolic agent should be pushed into the target area to penetrate the rupture site. For this purpose, minimal and adequately diluted glue has proved to be efficacious. It may be that other liquid or particulate embolic agents (ethylene/vinyl alcohol, calibrated PVA or gelatin particles, thrombin etc.) may achieve the same goal, but experience has not yet been reported. If this technique is anatomically impossible or unsafe and another occlusive method has to be chosen, early endoscopic control is another key to preventing failure.

5.12
Conclusion

Transcatheter embolization has the potential to further reduce mortality in acute non-variceal upper GIH, provided we continue our efforts to optimize the occlusive technique and enhance the haemostatic effect. Furthermore, increasing angiographic sensitivity, which in our opinion depends much on the alertness of the involved endoscopist, will reduce the need for non-targeted blind embolization. Whether transcatheter techniques can replace surgical salvage in upper GIH remains to be established by prospective randomized studies.

References

1. Katzen BT, McSweeney J (1975) Therapeutic transluminal arterial embolization for bleeding in the upper part of the gastrointestinal tract. Surg Gynecol Obstet 141:523–527
2. Reuter SR, Chuang VP, Bree RL (1975) Selective arterial embolization for control of massive upper gastrointestinal bleeding. Am J Roentgenol Radium Ther Nucl Med 125:119–126
3. Goldman ML, Land WC, Bradley EL, et al. (1976) Transcatheter therapeutic embolization in the management of massive upper gastrointestinal bleeding. Radiology 120:513–521
4. Goldman ML, Freeny PC, Tallman JM, et al. (1978) Transcatheter vascular occlusion therapy with isobutyl 2-cyanoacrylate (bucrylate) for control of massive upper-gastrointestinal bleeding. Radiology 129:41–49
5. Castaneda-Zuniga WR, Jauregui H, Rysavy J, et al. (1978) Selective transcatheter embolization of the upper gastrointestinal tract: an experimental study. Radiology 127:81–83
6. Defreyne L, Vanlangenhove P, De Vos M, et al. (2001) Embolization as a first approach with endoscopically unmanageable acute nonvariceal gastrointestinal hemorrhage. Radiology 218:739–748
7. Aina R, Oliva VL, Therasse E, et al. (2001) Arterial embolotherapy for upper gastrointestinal hemorrhage: outcome assessment. J Vasc Interv Radiol 12:195–200
8. Schenker MP, Duszak RJ, Soulen MC, et al. (2001) Upper gastrointestinal hemorrhage and transcatheter embolotherapy: clinical and technical factors impacting success and survival. J Vasc Interv Radiol 12:1263–1271
9. Patel TH, Cordts PR, Abcarian P, et al. (2001) Will transcatheter embolotherapy replace surgery in the treatment of gastrointestinal bleeding?(2)(2). Curr Surg 58:323–327
10. Ripoll C, Banares R, Beceiro I, et al. (2004) Comparison of transcatheter arterial embolization and surgery for treatment of bleeding peptic ulcer after endoscopic treatment failure. J Vasc Interv Radiol 15:447–450
11. Rockall TA, Logan RF, Devlin HB, et al. (1995) Incidence of and mortality from acute upper gastrointestinal haemorrhage in the United Kingdom. Steering Committee and members of the National Audit of Acute Upper Gastrointestinal Haemorrhage. BMJ 311:222–226
12. van Leerdam ME, Vreeburg EM, Rauws EA, et al. (2003) Acute upper GI bleeding: did anything change? Time trend analysis of incidence and outcome of acute upper GI bleeding between 1993/1994 and 2000. Am J Gastroenterol 98:1494–1499
13. Longstreth GF (1995) Epidemiology of hospitalization for acute upper gastrointestinal hemorrhage: a population-based study. Am J Gastroenterol 90:206–210
14. Vreeburg EM, Snel P, de Bruijne JW, et al. (1997) Acute upper gastrointestinal bleeding in the Amsterdam area: incidence, diagnosis, and clinical outcome. Am J Gastroenterol 92:236–243
15. Barkun A, Bardou M, Marshall JK (2003) Consensus recommendations for managing patients with nonvariceal upper gastrointestinal bleeding. Ann Intern Med 139:843–857
16. Blatchford O, Murray WR, Blatchford M (2000) A risk score to predict need for treatment for upper-gastrointestinal haemorrhage [In Process Citation]. Lancet 356:1318–1321
17. Cameron EA, Pratap JN, Sims TJ, et al. (2002) Three-year prospective validation of a pre-endoscopic risk stratification in patients with acute upper-gastrointestinal haemorrhage. Eur J Gastroenterol Hepatol 14:497–501
18. Rockall TA, Logan RF, Devlin HB, et al. (1996) Selection of patients for early discharge or outpatient care after acute upper gastrointestinal haemorrhage. National Audit of Acute Upper Gastrointestinal Haemorrhage [see comments]. Lancet 347:1138–1140
19. Vreeburg EM, Terwee CB, Snel P, et al. (1999) Validation of the Rockall risk scoring system in upper gastrointestinal bleeding. Gut 44:331–335
20. Phang TS, Vornik V, Stubbs R (2000) Risk assessment in upper gastrointestinal haemorrhage: implications for resource utilisation. N Z Med J 113:331–333
21. Oei TT, Dulai GS, Gralnek IM, et al. (2002) Hospital care for low-risk patients with acute, nonvariceal upper GI hemorrhage: a comparison of neighboring community and tertiary care centers. Am J Gastroenterol 97:2271–2278
22. Cook DJ, Guyatt GH, Salena BJ, et al. (1992) Endoscopic therapy for acute nonvariceal upper gastrointestinal hemorrhage: a meta-analysis. Gastroenterology 102:139–148
23. Sung JJ, Chan FK, Lau JY, et al. (2003) The effect of endoscopic therapy in patients receiving omeprazole for bleeding ulcers with nonbleeding visible vessels or adherent clots: a randomized comparison. Ann Intern Med 139:237–243
24. Enns RA, Gagnon YM, Rioux KP, et al. (2003) Cost-effectiveness in Canada of intravenous proton pump inhibitors for all patients presenting with acute upper gastrointestinal bleeding. Aliment Pharmacol Ther 17:225–233
25. Rauws EA, Tytgat GN (1990) Cure of duodenal ulcer associated with eradication of Helicobacter pylori. Lancet 335:1233–1235
26. Gisbert JP, Khorrami S, Carballo F, et al. (2004) H. pylori eradication therapy vs. antisecretory non-eradication therapy (with or without long-term maintenance antisecretory therapy) for the prevention of recurrent bleeding from peptic ulcer. Cochrane Database Syst Rev 2: CD004062
27. Frossard JL, Spahr L, Queneau PE, et al. (2002) Erythromycin intravenous bolus infusion in acute upper gastrointestinal bleeding: a randomized, controlled, double-blind trial. Gastroenterology 123:17–23
28. Coffin B, Pocard M, Panis Y, et al. (2002) Erythromycin improves the quality of EGD in patients with acute upper GI bleeding: a randomized controlled study. Gastrointest Endosc 56:174–179
29. Lee YC, Wang HP, Yang CS, et al. (2002) Endoscopic hemostasis of a bleeding marginal ulcer: hemoclipping or dual therapy with epinephrine injection and heater probe thermocoagulation. J Gastroenterol Hepatol 17:1220–1225
30. Park CH, Sohn YH, Lee WS, et al. (2003) The usefulness of endoscopic hemoclipping for bleeding Dieulafoy lesions. Endoscopy 35:388–392
31. Yamaguchi Y, Yamato T, Katsumi N, et al. (2001) Endoscopic hemoclipping for upper GI bleeding due to Mallory-Weiss syndrome. Gastrointest Endosc 53:427–430
32. Kantsevoy SV, Cruz-Correa MR, Vaughn CA, et al. (2003) Endoscopic cryotherapy for the treatment of bleeding mucosal vascular lesions of the GI tract: a pilot study. Gastrointest Endosc 57:403–406
33. Jensen DM, Kovacs TO, Jutabha R, et al. (2002) Rand-

omized trial of medical or endoscopic therapy to prevent recurrent ulcer hemorrhage in patients with adherent clots. Gastroenterology 123:407–413

34. Lau JY, Sung JJ, Lam YH, et al. (1999) Endoscopic retreatment compared with surgery in patients with recurrent bleeding after initial endoscopic control of bleeding ulcers. N Engl J Med 340:751–756

35. Marmo R, Rotondano G, Bianco MA, et al. (2003) Outcome of endoscopic treatment for peptic ulcer bleeding: is a second look necessary? A meta-analysis. Gastrointest Endosc 57:62–67

36. Chiu PW, Lam CY, Lee SW, et al. (2003) Effect of scheduled second therapeutic endoscopy on peptic ulcer rebleeding: a prospective randomised trial. Gut 52:1403–1407

37. Romagnuolo J (2004) Routine second look endoscopy: ineffective, costly and potentially misleading. Can J Gastroenterol 18:401–404

38. Rollhauser C, Fleischer DE (2004) Nonvariceal upper gastrointestinal bleeding. Endoscopy 36:52–58

39. Laine LA, Peterson WL (1994) Bleeding peptic ulcer. N Engl J Med 331:717–727

40. Elta GH (2002) Acute nonvariceal upper gastrointestinal hemorrhage. Curr Treat Options Gastroenterol 5:147–152

41. Monig SP, Lubke T, Baldus SE, et al. (2002) Early elective surgery for bleeding ulcer in the posterior duodenal bulb. Own results and review of the literature. Hepatogastroenterology 49:416–418

42. Conrad SA (2002) Acute upper gastrointestinal bleeding in critically ill patients: causes and treatment modalities. Crit Care Med 30:S365–368

43. Funaki B (2002) Endovascular intervention for the treatment of acute arterial gastrointestinal hemorrhage. Gastroenterol Clin North Am 31:701–713

44. Aabakken L (2001) Nonvariceal upper gastrointestinal bleeding. Endoscopy 33:16–23

45. Huang CS, Lichtenstein DR (2003) Nonvariceal upper gastrointestinal bleeding. Gastroenterol Clin North Am 32:1053–1078

46. Cheng CL, Lee CS, Liu NJ, et al. (2002) Overlooked lesions at emergency endoscopy for acute nonvariceal upper gastrointestinal bleeding. Endoscopy 34:527–530

47. Koval G, Benner KG, Rosch J, et al. (1987) Aggressive angiographic diagnosis in acute lower gastrointestinal hemorrhage. Dig Dis Sci 32:248–253

48. Dempsey DT, Burke DR, Reilly RS, et al. (1990) Angiography in poor-risk patients with massive nonvariceal upper gastrointestinal bleeding. Am J Surg 159:282–286

49. Walsh RM, Anain P, Geisinger M, et al. (1999) Role of angiography and embolization for massive gastroduodenal hemorrhage. J Gastrointest Surg 3:61–65; discussion 66

50. Nicholson AA, Ettles DF, Hartley JE, et al. (1998) Transcatheter coil embolotherapy: a safe and effective option for major colonic haemorrhage. Gut 43:79–84

51. Defreyne L, Vanlangenhove P, Decruyenaere J, et al. (2003) Outcome of acute nonvariceal gastrointestinal haemorrhage after nontherapeutic arteriography compared with embolization. Eur Radiol 13:2604–2614

52. Whitaker SC, Gregson RH (1993) The role of angiography in the investigation of acute or chronic gastrointestinal haemorrhage. Clin Radiol 47:382–388

53. Wagner HJ, Kalinowski M, Klose KJ, et al. (2001) The use of gadolinium chelates for X-ray digital subtraction angiography. Invest Radiol 36:257–265

54. Nusbaum M, Baum S (1963) Radiographic demonstration of unknown sites of gastrointestinal bleeding. Surg Forum 14:374–375

55. Grace DM, Gold RE (1978) Angiography in determining the cause and treatment of gastrointestinal bleeding. Can J Surg 21:171–174

56. Thorne DA, Datz FL, Remley K, et al. (1987) Bleeding rates necessary for detecting acute gastrointestinal bleeding with technetium-99m-labeled rcd blood cells in an experimental model. J Nucl Med 28:514–520

57. Sos TA, Lee JG, Wixson D, et al. (1978) Intermittent bleeding from minute to minute in acute massive gastrointestinal hemorrhage: arteriographic demonstration. AJR Am J Roentgenol 131:1015–1017

58. De Wispelaere JF, De Ronde T, Trigaux JP, et al. (2002) Duodenal ulcer hemorrhage treated by embolization: results in 28 patients. Acta Gastroenterol Belg 65:6–11

59. Rosch J, Keller FS, Wawrukiewicz AS, et al. (1982) Pharmacoangiography in the diagnosis of recurrent massive lower gastrointestinal bleeding. Radiology 145:615–619

60. Glickerman DJ, Kowdley KV, Rosch J (1988) Urokinase in gastrointestinal tract bleeding. Radiology 168:375–376

61. Ryan JM, Key SM, Dumbleton SA, et al. (2001) Nonlocalized lower gastrointestinal bleeding: provocative bleeding studies with intraarterial tPA, heparin, and tolazoline. J Vasc Interv Radiol 12:1273–1277

62. Hawkins IF, Caridi JG (1998) Carbon dioxide (CO2) digital subtraction angiography: 26-year experience at the University of Florida. Eur Radiol 8:391–402

63. Textor HJ, Wilhelm K, Strunk H, et al. (1997) [The diagnosis of intra-abdominal hemorrhages with CO2 as the contrast medium.] Rofo Fortschr Geb Rontgenstr Neuen Bildgeb Verfahr 166:51–53

64. Sandhu C, Buckenham TM, Belli AM (1999) Using CO2-enhanced arteriography to investigate acute gastrointestinal hemorrhage. AJR Am J Roentgenol 173:1399–1401

65. Rundback JH, Shah PM, Wong J, et al. (1997) Livedo reticularis, rhabdomyolysis, massive intestinal infarction, and death after carbon dioxide arteriography. J Vasc Surg 26:337–340

66. Spinosa DJ, Matsumoto AH, Angle JF, et al. (1998) Transient mesenteric ischemia: a complication of carbon dioxide angiography [see comments]. J Vasc Interv Radiol 9:561–564

67. Alavi A, Dann RW, Baum S, et al. (1977) Scintigraphic detection of acute gastrointestinal bleeding. Radiology 124:753–756

68. Pavel DG, Zimmer M, Patterson VN (1977) In vivo labeling of red blood cells with 99mTc: a new approach to blood pool visualization. J Nucl Med 18:305–308

69. Markisz JA, Front D, Royal HD, et al. (1982) An evaluation of 99mTc-labeled red blood cell scintigraphy for the detection and localization of gastrointestinal bleeding sites. Gastroenterology 83:394–398

70. Zettinig G, Staudenherz A, Leitha T (2002) The importance of delayed images in gastrointestinal bleeding scintigraphy. Nucl Med Commun 23:803–808

71. Jacobson AF (1991) Delayed positive gastrointestinal bleeding studies with technetium-99m-red blood cells: utility of a second injection. J Nucl Med 32:330–332

72. McKusick KA, Froelich J, Callahan RJ, et al. (1981) 99mTc

red blood cells for detection of gastrointestinal bleeding: experience with 80 patients. AJR Am J Roentgenol 137:1113–1118

73. Gupta S, Luna E, Kingsley S, et al. (1984) Detection of gastrointestinal bleeding by radionuclide scintigraphy. Am J Gastroenterol 79:26–31

74. Nicholson ML, Neoptolemos JP, Sharp JF, et al. (1989) Localization of lower gastrointestinal bleeding using in vivo technetium-99m-labelled red blood cell scintigraphy. Br J Surg 76:358–361

75. Hunter JM, Pezim ME (1990) Limited value of technetium 99m-labeled red cell scintigraphy in localization of lower gastrointestinal bleeding. Am J Surg 159:504–506

76. Bentley DE, Richardson JD (1991) The role of tagged red blood cell imaging in the localization of gastrointestinal bleeding. Arch Surg 126:821–824

77. Voeller GR, Bunch G, Britt LG (1991) Use of technetium-labeled red blood cell scintigraphy in the detection and management of gastrointestinal hemorrhage. Surgery 110:799–804

78. Ernst O, Bulois P, Saint-Drenant S, et al. (2003) Helical CT in acute lower gastrointestinal bleeding. Eur Radiol 13:114–117

79. Rose SC, Dunnick NR (1987) Angiographic treatment of gastrointestinal hemorrhage: comparison of vasopressin infusion and embolization. Invest Radiol 22:354–356

80. Gomes AS, Lois JF, McCoy RD (1986) Angiographic treatment of gastrointestinal hemorrhage: comparison of vasopressin infusion and embolization. AJR Am J Roentgenol 146:1031–1037

81. Pennoyer WP, Vignati PV, Cohen JL (1996) Management of angiogram positive lower gastrointestinal hemorrhage: long term follow-up of non-operative treatments. Int J Colorectal Dis 11:279–282

82. Darcy M (2003) Treatment of lower gastrointestinal bleeding: vasopressin infusion versus embolization. J Vasc Interv Radiol 14:535–543

83. Ring EJ, Oleaga JA, Frieman D, et al. (1977) Pitfalls in the angiographic management of hemorrhage: hemodynamic considerations. AJR Am J Roentgenol 129:1007–1013

84. Peck DJ, McLoughlin RF, Hughson MN, et al. (1998) Percutaneous embolotherapy of lower gastrointestinal hemorrhage. JVIR 9:747–757

85. Bandi R, Shetty PC, Sharma RP, et al. (2001) Superselective arterial embolization for the treatment of lower gastrointestinal hemorrhage. J Vasc Interv Radiol 12:1399–1405

86. Cynamon J, Atar E, Steiner A, et al. (2003) Catheter-induced vasospasm in the treatment of acute lower gastrointestinal bleeding. J Vasc Interv Radiol 14:211–216

87. Lang EV, Picus D, Marx MV, et al. (1992) Massive upper gastrointestinal hemorrhage with normal findings on arteriography: value of prophylactic embolization of the left gastric artery. AJR Am J Roentgenol 158:547–549

88. Gordon B, Lossef SV, Jelinger E, et al. (1991) Embolotherapy for small bowel hemorrhage from metastatic renal cell carcinoma: case report. Cardiovasc Intervent Radiol 14:311–313

89. Blake MA, Owens A, O'Donoghue DP, et al. (1995) Embolotherapy for massive upper gastrointestinal haemorrhage secondary to metastatic renal cell carcinoma: report of three cases. Gut 37:835–837

90. Granmayeh M, Wallace S, Schwarten D (1979) Transcatheter occlusion of the gastroduodenal artery. Radiology 131:59–64

91. Palmaz JC, Walter JF, Cho KJ (1984) Therapeutic embolization of the small-bowel arteries. Radiology 152:377–382

92. Morris DC, Nichols DM, Connell DG, et al. (1986) Embolization of the left gastric artery in the absence of angiographic extravasation. Cardiovasc Intervent Radiol 9:195–198

93. Walker WJ, Goldiin AR, Shaff MI, et al. (1980) Per catheter control of haemorrhage from the superior and inferior mesenteric arteries. Clin Radiol 31:71–80

94. Lang EK (1992) Transcatheter embolization in management of hemorrhage from duodenal ulcer. Long-term results and complications. Radiology 182:703–707

95. Kish JW, Katz MD, Marx MV, et al. (2004) N-butyl cyanoacrylate embolization for control of acute arterial hemorrhage. J Vasc Interv Radiol 15:689–695

96. Yamakado K, Nakatsuka A, Tanaka N, et al. (2000) Transcatheter arterial embolization of ruptured pseudoaneurysms with coils and n-butyl cyanoacrylate. J Vasc Interv Radiol 11:66–72

97. Latshaw RF, Pearlman RL, Schaitkin BM, et al. (1985) Intraarterial ethanol as a long-term occlusive agent in renal, hepatic, and gastrosplenic arteries of pigs. Cardiovasc Intervent Radiol 8:24–30

98. Defreyne L, De Schrijver I, Vanlangenhove P, et al. (2002) Detachable balloon embolization of an aneurysmal gastroduodenal arterioportal fistula. Eur Radiol 12:231–236

99. Hvizda JL, Wood BJ (2001) Selective transcatheter platelet infusion for gastrointestinal bleeding after failed embolization with resistant thrombocytopenia. J Vasc Interv Radiol 12:549–550

100. Madoff DC, Wallace MJ, Lichtiger B, et al. (2004) Intraarterial platelet infusion for patients with intractable gastrointestinal hemorrhage and severe refractory thrombocytopenia. J Vasc Interv Radiol 15:393–397

101. Carreira JM, Reyes R, Pulido-Duque JM, et al. (1999) Diagnosis and percutaneous treatment of gastrointestinal hemorrhage. Long-term experience. Rev Esp Enferm Dig 91:684–692

102. Encarnacion CE, Kadir S, Beam CA, et al. (1992) Gastrointestinal bleeding: treatment with gastrointestinal arterial embolization. Radiology 183:505–508

6 Embolization for Lower GI Bleeding

Michael Darcy

6.1
Introduction

Whereas endoscopic therapy can often be used to manage upper gastrointestinal bleeding, these techniques are difficult to apply to lower gastrointestinal (LGI) bleeding. Thus angiographic techniques assume greater importance in managing LGI hemorrhage. For many years the primary interventional technique utilized was vasopressin infusion. With the development of microcatheters and embolic agents that can be used with them, embolization has assumed a more prominent role and in our practice and has become the procedure of choice.

Although embolotherapy in lower gastrointestinal (LGI) tract has been a topic of great interest

M. Darcy, MD
Professor of Radiology and Surgery, Mallinckrodt Institute of Radiology, Washington University School of Medicine, 510 S. Kingshighway Blvd., St. Louis, MO 63110–1076, USA

in the recent literature, this is actually not a new concept. Embolization to treat LGI bleeding was first described in 1974 [1]. These authors reported three cases of small bowel embolization followed in 1978 by a report of two cases of colonic diverticular bleeding embolized with autologous clot [2]. There were several initial reports of high rates of clinical success, terminating bleeding in 80%–96% of cases [3–5].

Unfortunately, the early attempts at LGI embolization were hindered by an unacceptable rate of colonic infarction which was as high as 10%–20% in some series. Thus for LGI bleeding, embolization was largely abandoned in favor of vasopressin infusion which is usually reversible if the therapy results in bowel ischemia. Since the early 1990s, technological advances both in microcatheters as well as embolic agents have considerably altered the technique so that embolization is now a safe and viable option for managing LGI hemorrhage.

6.2
Physiopathology

6.2.1
Underlying Principles

Vasopressin infusions and embolization differ fundamentally in the mechanism by which they work. With vasopressin infusion the goal is to decrease the head of pressure to the bleeding site and allow stable clot to form. Vasopressin infusions diffusely constrict all the arteries leading to the bleeding site and the specific vessel that was bleeding is not really targeted by this therapy. This mechanism allows the treatment to be carried out by simple selective catheterization of the main trunk of the visceral artery. Thus the difficulty of the catheter manipulation is usually minimal. Even with the older forms of embolization using autologous clot and gelfoam, the treatments targeted more central vessels and relied on decreasing the arterial pressure to the general region of the hemorrhage rather than specifically targeting the actual site of bleeding.

A major disadvantage of vasopressin therapy is that vascular constriction occurs only during the infusion. Once the infusion is stopped the vasoconstriction quickly dissipates Thus in order to provide time for stable clot to form at the bleeding site, the infusion catheter must be maintained in the artery for a day or 2. Catheter-related complications such as peri-catheter bleeding, thrombosis, or dissections can result from this prolonged catheterization. Also since the vasoconstriction ends when the infusion is stopped, the incompletely healed lesion is soon subjected to normal arterial flow. This is likely what accounts for the high rate of recurrent bleeding (up to 50%) that occurs after vasopressin therapy. Vasopressin also causes vasoconstriction in other vascular beds and can cause coronary vasoconstriction leading to angina and even myocardial infarction.

With modern embolotherapy, however, the goal has shifted towards direct mechanical blockage of the specific branch vessel from which the bleeding arises. This is accomplished by super-selective catheterization. While this technique does require a higher level of skill to achieve the more selective catheter position, the modern super-selective techniques sometimes allow the catheter to be advanced right up to the actual point of extravasation in the bowel wall (Fig. 6.1). This eliminates many of the problems associated with vasopressin infusion and should lead to both fewer systemic effects and less effect on the surrounding normal bowel. An added benefit to a very peripheral embolization is that this should decrease the potential for collateral flow to the defect in the artery where the extravasation originates. Theoretically one would expect that this would lead to improved efficacy.

6.2.2
Type of Lesion

While technology changes have altered the pathophysiologic approach underlying the therapy, the type of lesion from which the bleeding originates also has important pathophysiologic implications. In some conditions like a bleeding colonic diver-

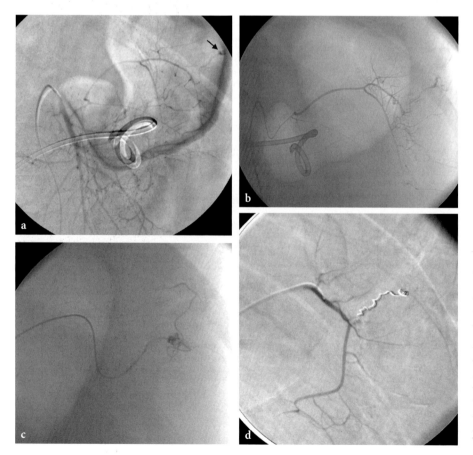

Fig. 6.1. a SMA arteriogram with contrast extravasation (*arrow*) in the splenic flexure. **b** More selective contrast injection done through a microcatheter in the middle colic artery. **c** The microcatheter has been maneuvered to within a few millimeters of the point of extravasation. **d** Arteriogram post embolization showing the microcoil out beyond the marginal artery and occlusion of only the specific branch that was bleeding

ticulum or a focal ulcer, the lesion is small and consequently the vascular anatomy tends to be simple. The bleeding will often arise from a single small branch.

Other conditions like inflammatory bowel disease or tumors often affect larger areas and multiple arterial branches may supply the bleeding site. The bleeding may be a diffuse ooze rather than a focal source of extravasation. In this setting, it is less likely that one could occlude all the branches feeding the bleeding site without compromising a significant number of branches and risking bowel ischemia.

Although angiodysplasias are usually small, they also have an increased number of small arterial branches that intercommunicate and make it difficult both to embolize very focally but also to effectively terminate the bleeding. Several authors have implicated angiodysplasias as the cause of clinical failure despite technical success at depositing embolic agents in the target vessels. BANDI et al. [6] noted that rebleeding occurred in 50% (three of six) of angiodysplasias treated with embolization. While it can be argued that angiodysplasias are a pathologic condition not suitable for embolization, there are some reports of embolization providing successful control of angiodysplasia bleeding [7–9]. Also, even if definitive bowel resection is still warranted, embolization may control bleeding long enough to allow a patient to be medically stabilized and undergo a bowel prep prior to resection.

6.3
Clinical Considerations

Prior to all interventional procedures, a careful assessment of the patient is crucial. As with all angiographic procedures, a history of contrast allergy or renal dysfunction should be sought. If present, the arteriogram may need to be delayed in order to allow adequate pre-treatment. However, the decision to delay needs to be tempered by the magnitude of the bleeding. For patients with massive hemorrhage, the need to stop the bleeding may out-weigh the need for a prolonged course of steroids or hydration.

When contemplating LGI embolization there are some unique aspects of the history that need to be investigated. Knowing the past surgical history is important since prior intestinal surgery may have disrupted potential arterial collateral pathways and will increase the risk of an ischemic complication. If the patient has had radiation therapy to the abdomen, the risk of ischemic complications may be increased since radiation therapy may obliterate small arterioles that can potentially provide collateral flow to maintain the viability of an embolized segment. Although one may be planning to utilize embolization, sometimes the initial arteriogram will reveal that the lesion is not amenable to embolization. It then becomes important to know if vasopressin infusion is a reasonable alternate therapy. Thus a history of coronary disease should also be sought since this is a relative contraindication to vasopressin infusion.

The pre-procedure evaluation should also include assessment of the patient's coagulation parameters and bleeding history. Any coagulopathy or thrombocytopenia should be corrected if possible since the clinical efficacy of LGI embolization is significantly diminished in patients with clotting abnormalities [10, 11]. In one small series [10], LGI hemorrhage was controlled by embolization in all patients with a normal coagulation profile. However, all three patients with coagulation abnormalities suffered recurrent bleeding.

Finally, it may be useful to have a surgical evaluation simultaneously during the interventional radiologic pre-procedure evaluation. Fortunately, complications requiring surgical correction are quite rare; however, if bowel infarction does occur and surgical correction is not an option, then this complication could very well lead to death. Having a surgeon consult at the front end allows better coordination of care should surgical intervention be required. Also, if the patient is deemed to not be a surgical candidate, then the irreversible nature of an ischemic complication assumes greater significance during the consent process.

6.4
Anatomy

The superior mesenteric artery (SMA) supplies the entire small bowel, cecum and colon usually up to the splenic flexure. As such this is the vessel that is commonly studied first if there are no clues that the bleeding is coming from the inferior mesenteric artery (IMA) distribution. The primary branches of the SMA have numerous interconnections both in the mesentery and via the arcade along the mesenteric margin of the bowel. This communication between mesenteric branches may provide more than one pathway to reach a site of extravasation (Fig. 6.2).

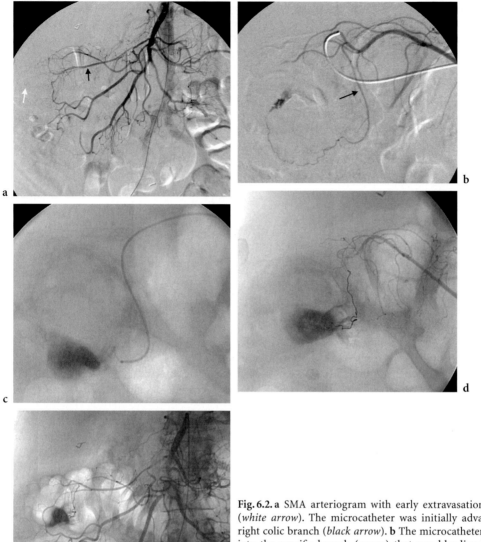

Fig. 6.2. a SMA arteriogram with early extravasation in the hepatic flexure (*white arrow*). The microcatheter was initially advanced through the high right colic branch (*black arrow*). **b** The microcatheter could not be advanced into the specific branch (*arrow*) that was bleeding because of unfavorable angles. **c** The bleeding branch was easily catheterized after re-approaching the area through the middle colic artery. **d** A microcoil has been deposited right at the point of bleeding. **e** Final arteriogram shows cessation of bleeding but good preservation of the arterial arcade along the mesenteric border of the bowel

The IMA supplies colon distal to the splenic flexure including the descending colon, sigmoid colon, and rectum. When embolizing rectal branches off of the superior hemorrhoidal branch of the IMA, one must remember the rich collateral network around the rectum with middle hemorrhoidal branches arising from the internal iliac arteries. The internal iliac arteries should be studied after embolizing a rectal branch to exclude the possibility of collateral flow to the bleeding site.

Although the celiac artery is rarely considered when dealing with LGI bleeding, there is an uncom-mon anatomic variant in which portions of the transverse colon can be supplied by a branch arising from the splenic artery or its pancreatic branches. This can be suspected when comparison of the SMA and IMA arteriograms reveals a relative lack of perfusion in the left half of the transverse colon. A celiac arteriogram will demonstrate a branch to the left transverse colon that supplies the bowel in the gap between the SMA and IMA distributions.

The LGI tract is quite long and there is significant diversity in the peripheral aspects of the different mesenteric arteries. In the small bowel, particularly the jejunum, there are a great number of interconnections between arterial branches in the mesentery. In the colon, there is communication along the marginal artery but fewer branches in the mesentery leading up to the marginal artery. Thus there are fewer potential collateral pathways (Fig. 6.3). However, in the rectum the potential for collateral flow increases again since the rectum also receives arterial supply from the middle and inferior hemorrhoidal arteries.

Lesions in the LGI segments that have increased collateral potential are probably more prone to

recurrent bleeding due to greater collateral perfusion around the embolic agents. This has been implicated as a possible explanation for the higher rate of clinical failure in some anatomic segments. PECK et al. [12] reported that rebleeding was more common after embolizing jejunal and cecal lesions. The higher incidence in the jejunum was felt to relate to better collateral perfusion in that area. The higher incidence of rebleeding in the cecum was not felt to relate to the vascular supply but rather was felt to reflect the higher incidence of angiodysplasias in the cecum.

Differences in segmental arterial supply probably also impact on the risk of infarction. The rectum is likely to tolerate embolization better than other regions since it has a dual blood supply with the superior hemorrhoidal artery off of the inferior mesenteric artery and middle hemorrhoidal arteries arising from the internal iliac circulation. This translates into increased potential for collateral blood flow and thus decreased risk of ischemia. The cecum may be more prone to ischemia since there is not a well developed arcade along the mesenteric border of the cecum and instead there are separate anterior and posterior cecal branches. The tissue supplied by these individual branches may be more susceptible to ischemia and in fact infarction of the cecum (even after microcatheter embolization) has been reported [13].

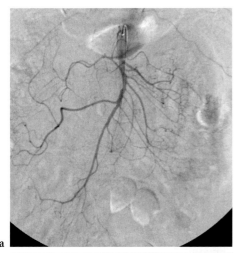

a

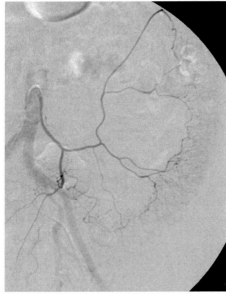

b

Fig. 6.3. a SMA arteriogram showing numerous inter-connections in the mesentery between the small bowel branches. **b** IMA arteriogram showing that aside from the marginal artery, there are relatively few potential collateral connections between the major IMA branches

6.5
Technique

An access sheath is a useful adjunct and usually automatically placed when starting a LGI hemorrhage case. The sheath will decrease the friction between the angiographic catheter and the arterial wall at the entry site and will allow better control over the manipulation of the catheter. When performing embolization a sheath also helps prevent loss of arterial access if the catheter should become plugged by the embolic agent and need to be removed. This is less of an issue with modern LGI embolization since a microcatheter is typically used coaxially through the outer 5-F angiographic catheter. If the microcatheter becomes occluded by the embolic agent, it can be removed through the outer 5-F catheter with out losing arterial access. Usually a 6-F sheath is used even though the initial catheter used to engage the visceral arteries is most often 5 F. This allows slightly easier manipulation of the catheter plus the sheath can be more easily flushed to prevent thrombus formation around the catheter. A 5-F catheter occupies so much of the lumen of a 5-F sheath that IV fluids attached to the sheath side port often will not flow well.

6.5.1
Initial Mesenteric Catheter

Typically the procedure starts with a 5-F angiographic catheter which is used to select the main trunk of the visceral artery. This is used both for performance of the diagnostic arteriogram as well as to provide a conduit to direct the microcatheter into the visceral artery. The choice of the initial 5-F catheter depends greatly on personal preference but also depends on the particular shape of the target artery the target artery.

For an SMA, the primary catheter chosen is most often a cobra or a Sos Omni (Angiodynamics, Queensbury, NY) re-curved catheter. Which one will perform best depends on the orientation of the proximal segment of the SMA. If the proximal SMA has a downward course, then a recurved catheter like a Sos or Simmons 1 will most easily seat down into the SMA trunk. When the SMA is oriented so that the proximal trunk comes straight off the aorta at a right angle, the Sos or the cobra will likely work equally well. Occasionally the proximal SMA actually heads cephalad before turning in a caudal direction. For this type of SMA a cobra works better.

The cobra shape has one advantage for work in the SMA in that it can be advanced well beyond the SMA origin. It can even be used to engage individual small bowel or colic branches. This can be advantageous in two situations. First, if the SMA trunk is capacious and the branch you need to go out arises from the SMA at an acute angle, micro catheters (which are exceedingly floppy) will sometimes just buckle in the main SMA rather than go around the corner into the desired branch. In this setting, it may be necessary to engage the first order branch with the cobra itself before trying to advance the microcatheter. Secondly, if the more peripheral branches are very tortuous and the microcatheter needs to be pushed a little harder, it will sometimes start to buckle in the main SMA. Advancing the cobra closer to the first order branch will provide additional support for the microcatheter and decrease buckling (Table 6.1).

Compared to the SMA, the IMA origin tends to be more constant and almost always is directed acutely downward immediately after it originates from the

Table 6.1. Materials cookbook for embolization of SMA bleeding

First line tools:

Standard 6-F access sheath

0.035-in. Bentson guidewire

5-F Sos Omni catheter (Angiodynamics) to engage SMA

MassTransit microcatheter with integrated wire to advance out to bleed

In case of failure to engage SMA trunk:

5-F Cobra or Simmons type II to seat into SMA

4-F Glide Cobra for particularly small or acutely angled SMAs

0.035-in. glidewire (Terumo) to help engage or seat into SMA

In case of difficult advancement out into peripheral branches:

Alternate wire: Transend wire (Boston Scientific)

Alternate microcatheter: Renegade (Boston Scientific)

aorta. However, the aorta is also smaller in diameter here compared to the level of the SMA. For this reason a Sos catheter often is not the best choice despite the caudal orientation of the proximal IMA. The smaller aortic caliber will sometimes compress the curve of the Sos and keep the catheter tip from engaging the IMA origin. A catheter that works more consistently to engage the IMA is the RIM (Roesch Inferior Mesenteric, Cook Inc., Bloomington, IN). Once the RIM engages the IMA origin, the catheter is pushed minimally into the body to seat the catheter tip slightly into the IMA trunk (Table 6.2).

These general catheter trends may be altered by the presence of large atherosclerotic plaques in the aorta. Sometimes this will distort the vessel origin such

Table 6.2. Materials cookbook for embolization of IMA bleeding

First line tools:

Standard 6-F access sheath

0.035-in. Bentson guidewire

5-F RIM catheter (Cook Inc.)

MassTransit microcatheter with integrated wire to advance out to bleed

In case of failure to engage IMA trunk:

5-F Sos Simmons type II to seat into IMA

0.035-in. glidewire (Terumo) to help engage or seat into SMA

In case of difficult advancement out into peripheral branches:

Alternate wire: Transend wire (Boston Scientific)

Alternate microcatheter: Renegade (Boston Scientific)

that the usual catheters will not work. Large plaques around the IMA origin can distort the ostium sufficiently that a cobra or even a straighter catheter like an MPA (Cook Inc., Bloomington, IN) have occasionally been needed to engage the IMA ostium. When the usual catheters fail to engage the IMA ostium, a brief flush aortogram may be needed. This not only confirms that the IMA is actually patent but will also delineate the location and orientation of the IMA origin. This is best performed with the flush catheter positioned down near the lower half of the 3rd lumbar vertebral body to avoid filling SMA branches that might overlap and obscure the IMA origin. A 15–20 degree right anterior oblique projection is useful to profile the IMA origin since the vessel usually courses in a left anterolateral direction.

6.5.2
Microcatheters

Once the 5-F catheter has been seated in the origin of the target vessel, a microcatheter is then advanced further out towards the site of extravasation. Modern microcatheters are typically complex constructions that have a stiffer larger section (usually about 3 F) closer to the hub and this stiffer section provides good pushability. Towards the tip of the catheter, it generally becomes smaller (2.7 F) and more flexible to aid maneuvering the catheter through small tortuous arterial branches.

The catheters themselves have no torque control and thus high torque guidewires are used to steer the catheter through the tortuous turns in the mesenteric arteries. These wires are typically 0.018–0.014 in. in diameter in order to readily pass through the microcatheter and tiny peripheral vessels. An example of such a wire is the Transend wire (Boston Scientific, Natick, MA).

While these specialized devices are critical, it is also vital to have a high quality imaging system. Because the goal is a super-selective embolization, it is necessary to precisely localize the bleeding site. Multiple small contrast injections done as the catheter is advanced more selectively and viewing in multiple obliquities both make it easier to identify the specific branch that is bleeding. High quality fluoroscopy is essential to be able to visualize these small injections as well as the manipulation of these micro-devices. Digital road-mapping also helps facilitate directing the catheter into the appropriate branch.

The optimal level of embolization has not been conclusively determined. One study proposed that

embolization at the level of the marginal artery is less effective than embolizing out in the vasa recta [14]. They were able to stop bleeding in all patients when the microcoils were placed beyond the marginal artery, but when the microcoils were placed in the marginal artery itself half of the patients rebled. A critical comparison of two studies provides additional insight [15]. This letter noted that while in both studies [12, 16] initial bleeding was controlled in 71%–86% of patients, the long-term clinical success varied. When emboli were deposited at or proximal to the marginal artery [12] 52% of the patients developed recurrent bleeding. However, when emboli were deposited beyond the marginal artery [16] their recurrent hemorrhage rate was 0%. Another recent study though reported moderate recurrent hemorrhage despite embolizing at the level of the vasa recta [6]. Plus at times it may not be technically possible to embolize distal to the marginal artery (Fig. 6.4). Thus the optimal level of embolization has not clearly been defined and larger clinical trials are needed to clarify this point.

6.5.3
Embolic Agents

Polyvinyl alcohol (PVA) particles have been used in a number of series [6, 10, 17–20]. The particles need to be suspended in iodinated contrast since PVA is not intrinsically radio-opaque otherwise it is not possible to fluoroscopically monitor the embolization. Because the PVA is flow directed, delivery of this embolic agent is less precise than with coils and more subject to local hemodynamics. If the catheter is obturating the feeding artery, the particles will not flow away as readily. Also as the vessel starts to become occluded by the PVA, the resistance to flow increases and hence the potential for reflux to non-target segments of bowel will increase.

PVA size is an important consideration. The particles should be at least 300–500 µm. KUSANO et al. [21] demonstrated that using smaller particles led to a high rate of infarction. Smaller particles occlude the arterioles too peripherally which decreases the potential for collateral flow which in turn is important to maintain enough perfusion to keep the bowel viable.

Probably the more common embolic agent used for LGI embolization is the microcoil. Both microcoils and PVA have been used successfully in reports of LGI embolization and while there have not been any trials to determine if one embolic agent is superior; microcoils do have several advantages over

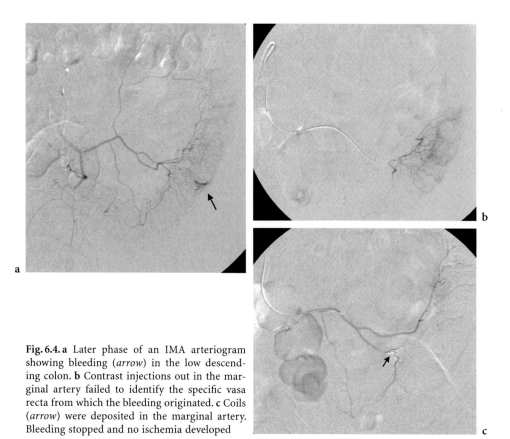

Fig. 6.4. a Later phase of an IMA arteriogram showing bleeding (*arrow*) in the low descending colon. b Contrast injections out in the marginal artery failed to identify the specific vasa recta from which the bleeding originated. c Coils (*arrow*) were deposited in the marginal artery. Bleeding stopped and no ischemia developed

PVA. They are highly visible at fluoroscopy and this allows for precise control over their deployment.

Another advantage is the mechanism of deployment. Unlike PVA which relies on flow direction, microcoils are precisely placed by pushing them out of the microcatheter. Simultaneously this is also a disadvantage of microcoils. In order to achieve this precise placement, the microcatheter needs to be maneuvered right to the desired point of coil deposition. If the vessels are small or tortuous this can be challenging. If the catheter can not be manipulated out into the specific vessel that is bleeding, PVA may be a better choice in that situation (Fig. 6.5).

Precise coil deployment also requires careful selection of coil size. If the coils are sized appropriately they will form into a loose coil spring at the tip of the catheter. Using a coil that is too large for the target artery will cause the coil to not form properly and this can cause the catheter to back out into the feeding vessel. This can lead to occlusion of a larger branch than was intended and increase the potential for ischemia. This is particularly a problem with super-selective LGI embolization. Since the microcoil is often being deposited in a tiny vasa recta, there is often not sufficient space to allow the microcoil to curl

up properly. Thus even the smallest 2-mm microcoils will often assume an elongated stretched out shape.

Some manufacturers of microcatheters also produce coil pushers designed to push coils through the microcatheter. However, some of the microcatheters have lumens with a diameter around 0.025 in. or larger. When using microcoils which are often 0.018 through a microcatheter with a larger internal diameter, it is possible for the usual coil pusher to wedge along side of the coil. This not only may prevent advancing the microcoil out of the catheter, but as the pusher is pulled back it may also pull the trapped microcoil with it.

A 0.025 in hydrophilic wire (Boston Scientific, Natick, MA) is a nice alternative to use instead of the coil pusher. The larger lumen prevents wedging along side of the microcoil. The hydrophilic coating of the glidewire allows the wire to more readily pass around the tortuous curves that the microcatheter may be forced to take.

Sometimes the microcoil will get stuck in the microcatheter so it can not be pushed out into the artery even with a glidewire. In that setting the coil can usually be flushed out of the microcatheter with a firm but short controlled saline injection. This can be achieved by using a 1-cc Luer lock syringe. This

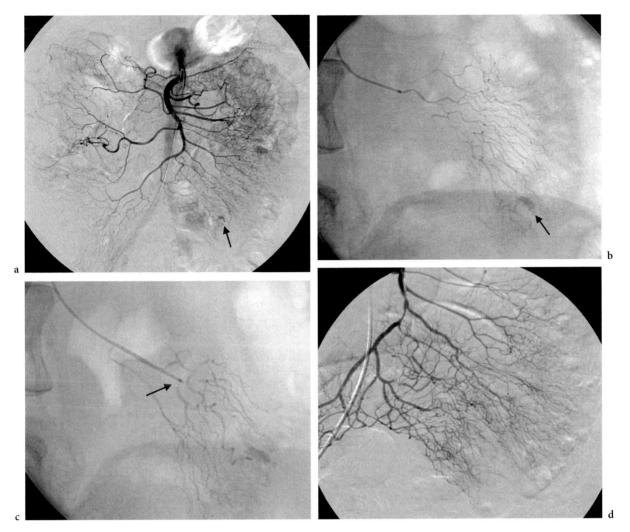

Fig. 6.5. a SMA arteriogram with bleeding (*arrow*) in the ileum. **b** More selective study shows numerous arterial communications before the level of the vasa recta. In addition, the arteries leading to the extravasation (*arrow*) are smaller than the microcatheter. **c** Despite liberal use of nitroglycerin boluses, the catheter tip (*arrow*) was able to be advanced only a little closer to the bleeding. A small volume of 500–700 μm PVA particles were injected at that point. **d** Final arteriogram shows cessation of bleeding and minimal devascularization of the bowel. The patient had no symptoms of ischemic bowel

generates sufficient force to push the coil out of the catheter but the volume is small enough to prevent significant catheter recoil or vessel damage.

6.6
Alternative Therapies

If it is not possible to pass the catheter selectively enough to permit safe embolization, alternate approaches need to be considered. The initial approach may be to fall back to the well established methods of vasopressin infusion. Some of the main benefits of a vasopressin infusion are that it does not require super-selective catheterization, it is fairly effective at stopping bleeding, and the infusion can be stopped if symptoms of ischemic bowel develop. However, the rebleeding rate is very high after stopping the vasopressin infusion and this treatment can not be readily applied to patients with significant coronary vascular disease. The relative benefits and risks of vasopressin therapy versus embolization have been recently reviewed [22].

An alternative to diffusely constricting the whole mesenteric vessel is to purposefully induce local vasospasm by means of catheter manipulation. This technique was discovered fortuitously in some patients in whom spasm was induced accidentally during attempted catheterization for embolization [23]. Although this prevented doing the embolization, some of these patients stopped bleeding as a result of the spasm alone. With this technique the initial maneuver is to wedge the catheter as close to the bleeding as possible and let it sit there for several minutes occluding the vessel. If that alone fails to induce spasm, then the catheter and wire are moved rapidly back and forth to induce spasm. With this technique they were able to initially stop bleeding in all 15 patients in who they attempted this procedure. One patient (6.7%) had recurrent bleeding within 24 h. Complications were minimal. They did have two patients who had dissection of their proximal IMA artery, but no patients had clinically evident bowel ischemia or infarction.

Instead of inducing spasm, another recently described technique that may not require superselective catheterization is intra-arterial platelet infusion. This has been described in a few cases where bleeding was too diffuse to allow safe embolization [24]. In one LGI case, diffuse colonic bleeding was terminated by infusing 4 units of platelets into the proximal SMA. Presumably infusing platelets, which are normally present in the blood, should carry little risk of causing ischemia but both the safety and efficacy of this technique needs to be validated in larger series.

If the patient is a surgical candidate and embolization is not technically feasible, another option is to mark the bowel to localize the lesion and aid resection. The main benefit of this technique is that it will aid identification of lesions, such as angiodysplasias, that can not usually be palpated by the surgeon. Marking the bowel allows precise localization of the bleeding lesion which in turn insures that the proper segment of bowel is resected and that the amount of bowel removed can be more limited.

There are two ways to mark the bowel. One is to deposit a coil in the mesenteric branch leading to the bleeding lesion [25]. During the operation, the surgeon should be able to palpate the coil. If it can not be palpated, an abdominal radiograph will reveal the location of the coil. The surgeon then resects the segment of bowel supplied by the artery containing the coil. Localization can also be done with methylene blue dye. In this technique, the microcatheter is placed close to the bleeding site and the patient is transported to the operating room with the microcatheter in place. Once the bowel has been surgically exposed, methylene blue is injected through the catheter. This brightly stains the bowel allowing the bowel segment containing the lesion to be easily identified. Again this insures resection of the correct bowel segment.

6.7
Results

When discussing the results of LGI embolization one must understand the difference between technical and clinical success. The successful deposition of embolic material in the intended target artery, with occlusion of flow and termination of contrast extravasation is the general definition of technical success. Clinical success on the other hand is successful termination of bleeding as evidenced by no further bloody output, stable vital signs without pressors, and a stable hematocrit.

6.7.1
Technical Success

Technical success for LGI embolization is quite high, generally around 80%–100%, in most series [5, 10, 12, 16, 26–28]. Vessel tortuosity or spasm preventing catheterization of the target vessel are the most commonly cited causes of technical failure. This statistic has not changed much over the past 30 years despite improvements in technology. However this likely reflects the changing goals of LGI embolization. In early studies, flow directed emboli were injected from a less selective position than is currently required for placement of microcoils. However, modern interventional radiologists advance catheters far more peripherally into the artery before embolizing. For example, embolization was considered to be technically successful in only 73% of cases reported in one study [6]; however, they did not embolize if they could not advance the catheter into the vasa recta beyond the marginal artery. Thus in recent series the definition of technical success may just be more stringent and more difficult to achieve. This may explain why the technical success rates have remained unchanged despite improved technology.

6.7.2
Clinical Success

Clinical success (the successful termination of bleeding) depends on more than just the deposition of embolic agents. Some pathology such as inflammatory conditions or tumors, do not have a focal blood supply and may be fed by multiple branches. In that setting, bleeding may continue even after successfully occluding a feeding vessel. Collateral supply around a microcoil may also result in continued bleeding if the coil is placed too proximally. As mentioned earlier, coagulopathy also makes clinical failure more likely. This is because microcoils may not completely occupy a vessel lumen and successful occlusion actually depends partially on formation of thrombus around the coils. Clinical success therefore occurs at a slightly lower rate than technical success. In modern series clinical success is achieved in 71%–100% [10, 12, 16–19, 26, 29].

6.7.3
Recurrent Bleeding

After LGI embolotherapy, the literature reports that anywhere from 0% to 52% of patients will have recurrent hemorrhage [6, 12, 16, 17, 19, 29, 30]. This wide range is partially due to different lengths of follow-up since shorter follow-up may lead to underestimation of the rebleeding rate.

In a recent study [6], twelve of 35 (34%) patients rebled a mean of 74 days (range 2–603 days) after the initial embolization. Perhaps bleeding occurring 603 days after embolization should be considered a separate discreet event instead of recurrent hemorrhage and in fact three of the 12 patients were documented by angiography to be bleeding from sources different from the original site. However, half of the patients were bleeding from the same site that was originally embolized. In the remaining patients the site of bleeding was not determined. In other series, recurrent bleeding was reported to originate from a site different from the one originally treated in as many as 50%–66% of the cases [10, 19].

6.8
Complications

Like other vascular interventions, LGI embolization procedures have potential for puncture site and catheter related complications. Clinically significant puncture site bleeding, hematoma, or occlusions occur in around 1%–2% of cases. Dissection of the target vessel is possible but rare.

The most feared complication is bowel ischemia, but this is the area where we have seen the greatest change between modern embolization techniques and those used in the 1970s and 1980s. In the early series, infarction occurred in 10%–20% of cases and this was the primary reason why embolization for LGI bleeding was largely abandoned. Since the development of microcatheters and suitable embolic agents, the reported rates of major ischemic complications in most series have dropped to close to 0% (range 0%–5.9%) [6, 10, 17, 19, 20, 31].

While overt infarction is very rare, overall complications in the modern series have been reported at an average rate of 21% with the range being as low as 5% up to 70% [10, 12, 16, 18, 19, 26, 29]. While this seems unacceptably high, one must realize that the vast majority of the complications are not clinically significant. Examples of these insignificant complications include self-limited abdominal pain that resolved without therapy or minor patches of ischemic mucosa that were asymptomatic and discovered only on endoscopy done for other reasons. These types of "ischemic complications" have rarely required any kind of therapy.

One unanswered question is if these minor ischemic insults could lead to delayed complications such as stricture formation. BANDI et al. [6] reported no clinically significant complications in their group of 48 patients with follow-up out to 10 years. They had ten patients with clinical follow-up and 25 with objective post-procedure evaluation (endoscopy or surgical pathology). No patient had any symptoms of an ischemic complication including six patients who had minor signs of ischemia identified at endoscopy.

In another study of 14 patients [30], one patient had circular muscular fibrosis identified on histological exam and the authors postulated that this might become an occlusive bowel stenosis. However, this patient also had an extensive embolization procedure with numerous gelfoam pledgets being injected from the proximal arcade of the SMA. Thus the technique used in this case was really not a modern super-selective embolization and was probably more analogous to the older methods of embolization used 20–30 years ago. Thus when using modern super-selective techniques, the risk of significant ischemic complications is now so low that embolization should be considered a reasonable first-line therapy for LGI hemorrhage and should not be avoided because of fear of infarction.

6.9
Future Development and Research

One of the ongoing needs is to continue to improve the ability of microcatheters to track out into very small peripheral branches. Since vessel tortuosity and spasm are the main causes of technical failure, improving catheter characteristics should improve technical success. Alternatively, future research could seek to develop better embolic agents. An agent that could be positioned as precisely as a microcoil without having to get the delivery catheter all the way out to the bowel wall could be another way to overcome the tortuosity and spasm problem.

Another area that needs investigation is to further define the results of embolization stratified by anatomic location within the bowel and type of lesion. Most studies have pooled different types of pathologic conditions. Only a few case reports have focused only on specific pathologic lesions such as angiodysplasias [7, 9]. While these studies mostly report success, the follow-up is generally short and their results are contradicted by other small series that suggest that angiodysplasias are prone to rebleeding after embolization [6, 12].

The vast majority of studies to date have also lumped together bleeding from both small bowel and colonic sources. The differences in vascular anatomy with greater potential for collateral flow in the jejunum and rectum make it unlikely that bleeding in these regions can be terminated as effectively as in regions like the descending colon that have more limited collateral potential. The preliminary work by Peck et al. [12] has suggested that regional differences in efficacy will occur but given that this study had only a few patients in some anatomic regions, larger studies are clearly needed.

Regional anatomic differences may also alter the risk of complications. Gerlock et al. [13] pointed out the lack of a good arterial arcade in the cecal region and that there tend to be independent anterior and posterior cecal branches. They reported a case of cecal infarction and suggested that the unique anatomy in this region may lead to a higher risk of infarction. They cautioned against embolization of the terminal portions of these terminal branches ileocolic artery. Again larger series are needed to be able to stratify risk by anatomic region.

Evaluation of the long term effects of embolization is another area where additional research is needed. The length of follow-up in modern series is quite short. Although this proves short term safety and efficacy, there is little data on longer term rebleeding rates. This will be a difficult task since it may be hard to determine if delayed hemorrhage is coming from the original lesion that was embolized or a different lesion. Although short term safety has been well documented, longer term studies are also needed to determine if these patients will develop more chronic complications such bowel stricture. Finally, it will be important to better define what

role embolization has in patients that are surgical candidates. In these patients it will be important to better document that LGI embolization (for either pre-operative stabilization or as definitive therapy) provides a survival benefit compared to just surgically removing the offending bowel segment.

6.10
Conclusion

Although for many years embolization was felt to be contraindicated in the LGI tract because of the risk of infarction, modern technologic advances in microcatheters have significantly decreased the risks of LGI embolization. Given the advantages of this technique, LGI embolization is rapidly gaining acceptance. While the results to date have been very good, considerable work is needed to better define in what regions, for which lesions, and under what circumstances is LGI embolization best suited.

References

1. Bookstein JJ, Chlosta EM, Foley D, Walter JF (1974) Transcatheter hemostasis of gastrointestinal bleeding using modified autogenous clot. Radiology 113:277–285
2. Bookstein JJ, Naderi MJ, Walter JF (1978) Transcatheter embolization for lower gastrointestinal bleeding. Radiology 127:345–349
3. Chuang VP, Wallace S, Zornoza J, Davis LJ (1979) Transcatheter arterial occlusion in the management of rectosigmoidal bleeding. Radiology 133:605–609
4. Rosenkrantz H, Bookstein JJ, Rosen RJ, Goff WB, Healy JF (1982) Postembolic colonic infarction. Radiology 142:47–51
5. Sebrechts C, Bookstein JJ (1988) Embolization in the management of lower-gastrointestinal hemorrhage. Semin Interv Radiol 5:39–47
6. Bandi R, Shetty PC, Sharma RP, Burke TH, Burke MW, Kastan D (2001) Superselective arterial embolization for the treatment of lower gastrointestinal hemorrhage. J Vasc Interv Radiol 12:1399–1405
7. Bilbao JI, Barettino MD, Longo JM, Aquerreta JD, Larrea JA, Caballero AD (1996) Permanent therapeutic embolization of cecal angiodysplasia (letter). Am J Gastroenterol 91:1287–1288
8. Tisnado J, Cho SR, Beachley MC, Margolius DA (1985) Transcatheter embolization of angiodysplasia of the rectum. Report of a case. Acta Radiol 26:677–680
9. Tadavarthy SM, Castaneda-Zuniga W, Zollikofer C, Nemer F, Barron J, Amplatz K (1981) Angiodysplasia of the right colon treated by embolization with ivalon (polyvinyl alcohol). Cardiovasc Intervent Radiol 4:39–42
10. Bulakbasi N, Kurtaran K, Ustunsoz B, Somuncu I (1999)

Massive lower gastrointestinal hemorrhage from the surgical anastomosis in patients with multiorgan trauma: treatment by subselective embolization with polyvinyl alcohol particles. Cardiovasc Intervent Radiol 22:461–467

11. Encarnacion CE, Kadir S, Beam CA, Payne CS (1992) Gastrointestinal bleeding: treatment with gastrointestinal arterial embolization. Radiology 183:505–508

12. Peck DJ, McLoughlin RF, Hughson MN, Rankin RN (1998) Percutaneous embolotherapy of lower gastrointestinal hemorrhage. J Vasc Interv Radiol 9:747–751

13. Gerlock AJ Jr., Muhletaler CA, Berger JL, Halter SA, O'Leary JP, Avant GR (1981) Infarction after embolization of the ileocolic artery. Cardiovasc Intervent Radiol 4:202–205

14. Curzon IL, Nicholson AA, Dyet JF, Hartley J (1996) Transcatheter coil embolotherapy for major colonic hemorrhage. Cardiovasc Intervent Radiol 19 [Suppl 2]:s83

15. Nicholson T, Ettles DF (1999) Embolization for life-threatening colonic hemorrhage (letter; comment). J Vasc Interv Radiol 10:519

16. Nicholson AA, Ettles DF, Hartley JE, Curzon I, Lee PW, Duthie GS et al (1998) Transcatheter coil embolotherapy: a safe and effective option for major colonic haemorrhage. Gut 43:79–84

17. Kuo WT, Lee DE, Saad WE, Patel N, Sahler LG, Waldman DL (2003) Superselective microcoil embolization for the treatment of lower gastrointestinal hemorrhage. J Vasc Interv Radiol 14:1503–1509

18. Guy GE, Shetty PC, Sharma RP, Burke MW, Burke TH (1992) Acute lower gastrointestinal hemorrhage: treatment by superselective embolization with polyvinyl alcohol particles. AJR Am J Roentgenol 159:521–526

19. Evangelista PT, Hallisey MJ (2000) Transcatheter embolization for acute lower gastrointestinal hemorrhage. J Vasc Interv Radiol 11:601–606

20. Defreyne L, Vanlangenhove P, de Vos M, Pattyn P, van Maele G, Decruyenaere J et al (2001) Embolization as a first approach with endoscopically unmanageable acute nonvariceal gastrointestinal hemorrhage. Radiology 218:739–748

21. Kusano S, Murata K, Ohuchi H, Motohashi O, Atari H (1987) Low-dose particulate polyvinylalcohol embolization in massive small artery intestinal hemorrhage. Experimental and clinical results. Invest Radiol 22:388–392

22. Darcy M (2003) Treatment of lower gastrointestinal bleeding: vasopressin infusion versus embolization. J Vasc Interv Radiol 14:535–543

23. Cynamon J, Atar E, Steiner A, Hoppenfeld BM, Jagust MB, Rosado M et al (2003) Catheter-induced vasospasm in the treatment of acute lower gastrointestinal bleeding. J Vasc Interv Radiol 14:211–216

24. Madoff DC, Wallace MJ, Lichtiger B, Komanduri KV, Ross WA, Narvios AB et al (2004) Intraarterial platelet infusion for patients with intractable gastrointestinal hemorrhage and severe refractory thrombocytopenia. J Vasc Interv Radiol 15:393–397

25. Zuckerman DA, Gaz RD (1991) Catheter-guided intraoperative localization of a jejunal angiodysplasia using the Tracker-18 coaxial catheter system: case report. Cardiovasc Intervent Radiol 14:358–359

26. Luchtefeld MA, Senagore AJ, Szomstein M, Fedeson B, van Erp J, Rupp S (2000) Evaluation of transarterial embolization for lower gastrointestinal bleeding. Dis Colon Rectum 43:532–534

27. Uflacker R (1987) Transcatheter embolization for treatment of acute lower gastrointestinal bleeding. Acta Radiol 28:425–430

28. Waugh J, Madan A, Sacharias N, Thomson K (2004) Embolization for major lower gastrointestinal haemorrhage: five-year experience. Australas Radiol 48:311–317

29. Gordon RL, Ahl KL, Kerlan RK, Wilson MW, LaBerge JM, Sandhu JS et al (1997) Selective arterial embolization for the control of lower gastrointestinal bleeding. Am J Surg 174:24–28

30. Horiguchi J, Naito A, Fukuda H, Nakashige A, Ito K, Kiso T et al (2003) Morphologic and histopathologic changes in the bowel after super-selective transcatheter embolization for focal lower gastrointestinal hemorrhage. Acta Radiol 44:334–339

31. Funaki B, Kostelic JK, Lorenz J, Ha TV, Yip DL, Rosenblum JD et al (2001) Superselective microcoil embolization of colonic hemorrhage. AJR Am J Roentgenol 177:829–836

7 Haemobilia and Bleeding Complications in Pancreatitis

Tony A. Nicholson

7.1
Introduction

Haemorrhage into the biliary tract is called haemobilia. It was first described in 1654 [1], but the condition was not termed 'haemobilia' until 1948 [1, 2]. The majority of cases are due to trauma (50%), operative trauma accounting for 15% [2], though this incidence may have increased with the introduction of laparoscopic biliary surgery [3]. Pancreatitis is a rare cause of haemobilia.

The majority of patients who develop significant bleeding as a complication of pancreatitis do so because of associated upper gastrointestinal ulceration and inflammation. Occasionally portal vein thrombosis can lead to variceal bleeding [4]. Neither of these pathologies is within the remit of this chapter. The estimated incidence of visceral aneurysm development in patients with pancreati-

tis is 5%–10% [5, 6]. Such aneurysms are caused by the actions of pancreatic enzymes such as elastase on adjacent blood vessels released in the course of pancreatitis.

Though spontaneous thrombosis of such aneurysms has been reported [7] mortality from conservative management is said to be more than 90% [8, 9]. The reported mortality when such aneurysms are treated surgically ranges from 12.5% to 40% [10]. Importantly re-bleeding can occur in 6%–10% of patients who survive initial surgery [11]. The first report of successful embolization in this condition was in 1982 [12]. Since then there has been a plethora of articles describing the diagnosis and endovascular treatment of pancreatitis associated visceral aneurysms [8, 13–15].

7.2
Haemobilia

7.2.1
Clinical, Pathophysiological and Anatomical Considerations

The classical triad of gastrointestinal bleeding, right hypochondrial pain and jaundice suggest haemobilia [2]. However it can be difficult to diagnose and if bleeding is of low volume may present as anaemia of unknown cause. Bleeding can also be massive and life threatening. The commonest cause as already stated is blunt and penetrating trauma in 35%. Iatrogenic haemobilia is a complication of all forms of biliary surgery, percutaneous biliary procedures (4%–14%) including stent insertion [16] and biopsy (3%–7%) [17]. In addition an aberrant papillary artery, found in approximately 20% in cadaveric studies, can bleed following endoscopic sphincterotomy [18]. Other causes include gallstone induced cholecystitis, halothane induced liver necrosis, varices secondary to severe portal hypertension, primary and metastatic malignancies of the liver

T. A. NICHOLSON, BScM,Sc, MB, ChB, FRCR
Consultant Vascular Radiologist and Senior Lecturer, Leeds Teaching Hospitals NHS Trust, Great George Street, Leeds LS1 3EX, UK

and biliary tract, arteriovenous malformations in the liver or pancreas and infections and infestations including ascariasis, hydatid and amoebic abscess, and mycotic aneurysms due to any organism [17].

Haemobilia is almost always due to damage to the hepatic artery. As this supplies only about one third of the liver's blood supply it can usually be tied off or embolized with impunity. However if the portal vein is occluded interruption to the hepatic arterial supply may lead to liver infarction. This is not invariable as the hepatic arteries can backfill around the portal triads. This latter feature also means that a proximal tie or embolization may not be effective. Therefore embolization is best done proximal and distal to the pseudoaneurysm or bleeding point.

7.2.2
Imaging and Technical Considerations

Although ultrasound and ERCP can confirm the diagnosis of haemobilia in a few cases, CT is more sensitive, contrast enhanced CT (CECT) diagnosing active blood loss or haematoma and its site of origin in almost 100% of cases . In occult cases increased attenuation of bile in the gall bladder and ducts confirms the diagnosis [17]. Good quality selective and super-selective angiography remains the diagnostic procedure of choice, as it not only confirms the diagnosis, but also localises the site accurately and allows immediate treatment by embolization (Fig. 7.1). It is essential prior to definitive treatment to make sure that the portal vein is patent and this must be imaged on CECT or indirect portography.

Catheterisation of the hepatic artery is usually performed from the femoral artery. The radial or brachial approach may be preferred especially where the patient is thin and the angle with the aorta very acute. A 4- or 5-F Cobra Glidecatheter (Terumo) and hydrophilic wire will usually suffice to diagnose and cross the bleeding point in the hepatic artery. If it is very peripheral, proves difficult or is stenosed or in spasm, a co-axial system will almost always do so. Occasionally patients have a series of intermittent large haematemeses. Though the diagnosis of haemobilia is obvious from their history, ERCP and perhaps CT findings, no pseudoaneurysm or bleeding site can be seen at angiography. Invariably there will be spasm somewhere associated with the temporarily sealed bleeding site or occult pseudoaneurysm. Usually local contrast injection will reveal this but in any case the area should be embolized. This usually requires a coaxial system to negotiate the narrowed segment (Fig. 7.2).

For a list of technical requirements see Table 7.1.

Table 7.1. Cookbook

	Primary	Alternatives	Comments
Preprocedure	1. Prevoius imaging available especially CT 2. Monitoring: pulse BP, pulse oximetry 3. Minimum 18G IVI	1. If acute rupture may be no previous imaging 2. GA with full anaesthetic support	Should not be attempted without full nursing and technical support
Drugs	1. Buscopam 20–40 mg 2. Maxalon and Atropine should be available in case of vomiting or bradycardia	Glucagon 1 ugrm	
Sheath	5-F 11-cm sheath	5-F 45-cm flexisheath if pelvic arteries are tortuous	
Catheters	1. 5-F appropriate femorovisceral glidecatheter e.g. Cobra 2 or Sidewinder 1 or 2 2. Coaxial catheters are often very useful if superselective or distal embolization is necessary	1. 5-F Sos type catheter or Waltman loop often useful in large diameter aortas 2. Multipurpose or Berenstein catheters useful if arm approach	4-F femorovisceral catheters are less torquable than 5-F
Wires	Glidewire (Terumo)	Other hydrophilic wire	
Embolic material	Steel coils Platinum microcoils if co-axial system used	1. Glue 2. Thrombin 3. Long detachable coils or detachable balloons if the aneurysm must be packed	Unless the haemorrhage is immediately life threatening (see Fig. 7.3) do not use: Particles Gelfoam Autologous blood

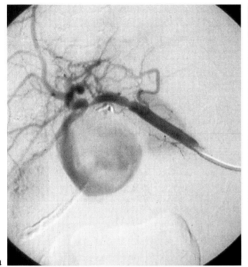

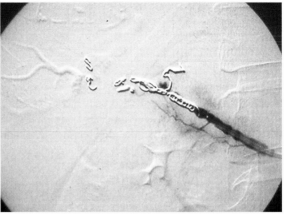

Fig. 7.1a,b. Coeliac angiography in a patient with life threatening haemobilia 24 h post cholecystectomy revealed a large hepatic pseudoaneurysm (**a**) treated successfully by proximal and distal coil embolization (**b**)

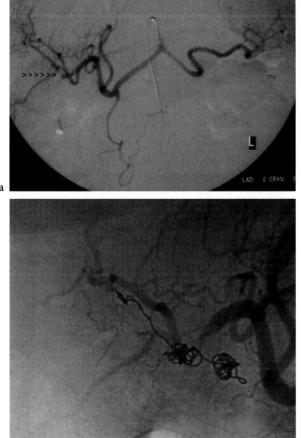

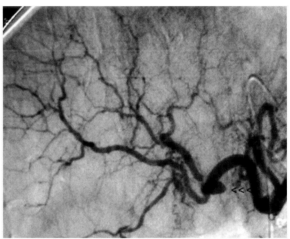

Fig. 7.2a–c. Coeliac angiography on a 53-year-old patient post laparoscopic cholecystectomy who suffered three large haematemeses in the perioperative period. The initial angiogram (**a**) was thought to be normal and no further procedure was carried out. However, note the spasm in the segment 6 artery (*arrowheads*). 24 h later after two more major episodes of bleeding during which the patient became unstable, repeat angiography (**b**) revealed the area of spasm to be due to a pseudoaneurysm (*arrowheads*). This was successfully embolized with steel coils (**c**)

7.2.3
Endovascular Management and Results

Haemobilia requires treatment as spontaneous resolution is exceedingly rare and the mortality from
ruptured pseudoaneurysms is in excess of 90%.
Technically endovascular management is relatively
simple and involves the proximal and distal embolization, with tightly packed steel coils, of the hepatic

artery from where the pseudoaneurysm arises. In
post surgical cases this nearly always involves the
hepatic artery proper (Fig. 7.1a) but in post biopsy or
PTC cases the pseudoaneurysm usually arises from a
right hepatic branch and the main hepatic artery can
be preserved (Fig. 7.3). In acute cases of penetrating injury the bleed may be quite distal and where
bleeding is immediately life threatening particles of
500–1000 μm diameter can be used (Fig. 7.4).

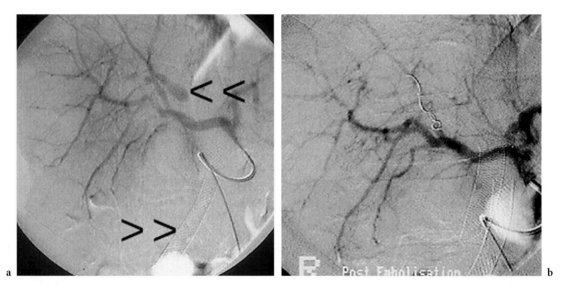

Fig. 7.3a,b. Hepatic arteriogram in a 26-year-old man with a small inoperable neuroendocrine tumour in the head of his
pancreas. The papilla of Vater could not be accessed at ERCP and he underwent a percutaneous stenting procedure at which
two self-expanding stents were inserted (*lower arrowheads*) apparently side by side (**a**). 12 hours later repeat ERCP revealed a
significant haemorrhage from the papilla. The angiogram revealed a segment 4 arterial pseudoaneurysm (*upper arrowheads*)
which was embolized successfully with coils (**b**)

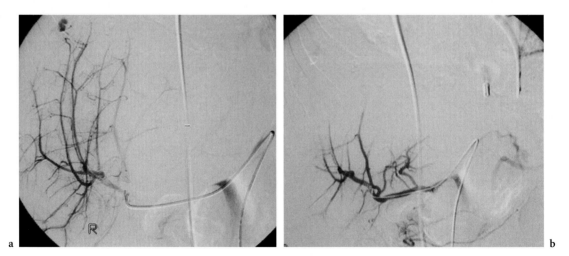

Fig. 7.4a,b. This patient was admitted in haemodynamic shock after a knife wound to the right hypochondrium. Emergency
hepatic angiography revealed a segment 8 haemorrhage (**a**). As the patient had an unrecordable blood pressure at the time
700–900 μm PVA particles were injected selectively (**b**) with immediate improvement in haemodynamic status, the patient was
discharged within 5 days of the procedure

If the portal vein is occluded and the bleeding site is in the hepatic artery proper or at the gastroduodenal artery origin, as is sometimes the case after surgery for pancreatitis or pancreatic carcinoma, treatment decisions become very difficult. Surgery may be possible but has a very high mortality. Packing the aneurysm itself with long detachable coils or detachable balloons has been described [19]. However in the author's experience, whilst this is effective in the short term, the aneurysm may recanalize due to clot retraction and rebleeding may take place. This is may be fatal especially if the patient has been discharged after initially successful embolization. If further elective surgery is definitely contraindicated, proximal and distal hepatic artery embolization is the safest option relying on collateralization of the distal hepatic artery branches in the liver. The use of thrombin, which is described in the next section, has not, to the author's knowledge been used to treat a hepatic pseudoaneurysm causing haemobilia. However it may well be that this will be an effective treatment option.

The results of embolization for haemobilia are reported as being 95%–100% effective [3] even on an intention to treat basis and it should be the treatment of first choice.

7.2.4
Complications

These are very rare. Clearly all the complications relating to arterial catheterization at any site and for whatever reason can occur. Non-target embolization should not happen in the experienced hands of a well trained operator. It is said that fungal abscesses are commoner after hepatic arterial embolization [3] but there is no real evidence for this and most patients have had surgery or a penetrating injury prior to the embolization. Liver infarction as described above is uncommon but a rise in liver enzymes is often observed [3].

7.3
Bleeding Complications in Pancreatitis

7.3.1
Clinical, Pathophysiological and Anatomical Considerations

Pancreatitis associated visceral aneurysms are caused by the action of proteolytic enzymes, released from the necrotic pancreas, on vessel walls and are often associated with pseudocysts. Patients are usually extremely ill with Ranson scores above 3. Prior to rupture most aneurysms are either asymptomatic or cause pain by pressure on local structures that may mimic the pain of pancreatitis. Imaging is therefore vital to their early diagnosis and treatment. The splenic artery is most commonly involved followed by the gastroduodenal and pancreaticoduodenal arteries, although all peripancreatic arteries can develop aneurysms and pseudoaneurysms [20]. Their natural history is to increase in size and ultimately rupture into the upper GI tract, abdominal cavity or the pancreas itself [21]. Occasionally they can erode into the aorta or adjacent venous structures though the latter does not preclude embolization (Fig. 7.5).

7.3.2
Imaging and Technical Considerations

Ultrasound is useful for many aspects of pancreatitis but has a sensitivity of less than 73% for visceral pseudoaneurysm in the condition, whereas contrast enhanced computer tomography (CECT) has a sensitivity of almost 100% [22]. CECT is also very useful in terms of endovascular treatment as it can indicate what type of aneurysm has formed, which artery it has formed from and whether there is more than one.

Angiography was formerly the procedure of choice for identifying the site of visceral aneurysm. It is certainly true that where ultrasound, CECT and endoscopy have failed to diagnose a source of active bleeding, angiography can occasionally do so. In one study angiography identified 90 out of 93 arterial pathologies [8]. However, it is the author's experience that some aneurysms within pseudocysts are not associated with a specific named artery and even when obvious on CECT, cannot be diagnosed accurately by angiography (Fig. 7.6). It is probable that such aneurysms are either the result of erosion within the arteriolar or capillary bed or have a significant venous contribution.

Catheterisation of coeliac and superior mesenteric arteries is usually performed from the femoral artery. The radial or brachial approach may be preferred especially where the patient is thin and the angle with the aorta very acute. A 4- or 5-F visceral curved Glidecatheter (Terumo) and hydrophilic wire will allow more distal catheterisation which may be required to diagnose and cross the aneurysm or

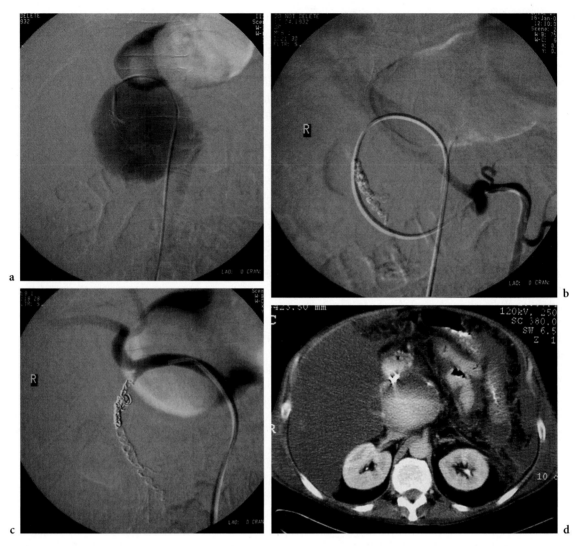

Fig. 7.5a–d. A 76-year-old man with acute on chronic pancreatitis secondary to alcohol abuse was admitted with abdominal pain. Abdominal examination suggested a pulsatile epigastric mass confirmed by CECT and angiography to be a large gastroduodenal artery pseudoaneurysm (**a**). It was clear that this had eroded into the inferior and superior mesenteric veins with a patent portal vein (**a,b**). The Gastroduodenal and inferior pancreaticoduodenal arteries were coil embolized (**c**) with a good result confirmed by a 24-h CT scan which also demonstrated patency of the mesenteric and portal veins. Note the persistent layered contrast in the pseudoaneurysm sac which should not be mistaken for persistent patency (**d**)

pseudoaneurysm. If it is very peripheral, proves difficult due to tortuosity or is stenosed or in spasm, a co-axial system will almost always do so. The CECT scan should indicate the origin of the aneurysm and selective catheterization of the appropriate artery may immediately confirm the CT findings. If the CT scan is not specific for origin, then start with the celiac trunk and follow with the SMA. Coil embolization should be proximal and distal with tightly packed coils (Figs. 7.1, 7.2, 7.4, 7.5, 7.7). If the aneurysm is not seen on either of these selective examinations then superselective catheterization should

be performed according to the CT approximation of site in the following order:

a. Splenic artery
b. Hepatic artery
c. Gastroduodenal artery
d. Gastroepiploic artery
e. Superior pancreaticoduodenal artery
f. Dorsal pancreatic and pancreatica magna arteries
g. Left gastric artery
h. Right and left hepatic arteries
i. Inferior pancreaticoduodenal artery
j. Jejunal arcade

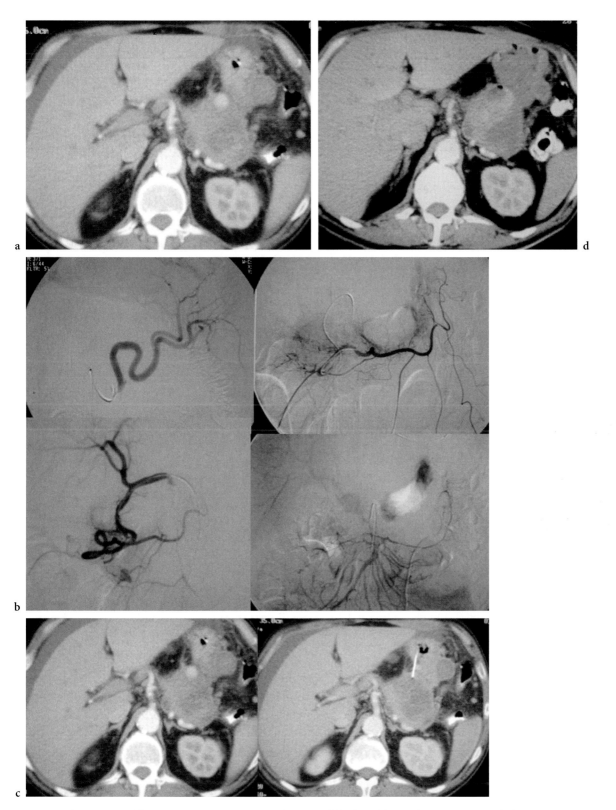

Fig. 7.6a–d. A 48-year-old man with chronic pancreatitis developed further abdominal pain. CECT revealed a pseudoaneurysm in his lesser sac (**a**). Selective and super selective angiography failed to demonstrate any source for the pseudoaneurysm (**b**). It was therefore percutaneously punctured with a 21-Gauge needle (**c**) and thrombosed with 2000 units of autologous thrombin. CECT at 1 week demonstrated occlusion of the pseudoaneurysm (**d**)

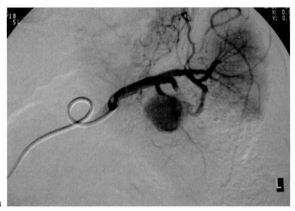

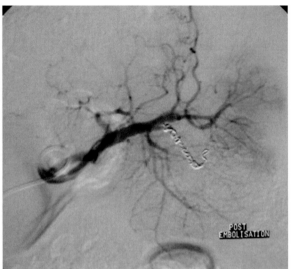

Fig. 7.7a,b. Front and back door embolization of a splenic artery pseudoaneurysm (**a**) secondary to acute on chronic pancreatitis with a good result (**b**). This patient is alive and well with no recurrence at 52 months

If after this, an aneurysm, diagnosed at CT, is not found or fills slowly from no named artery at superselective angiography, do not assume that that the CT scan is incorrect, that the aneurysm does not exist or is unimportant! Check the angiogram for areas of arterial spasm (Fig. 7.2) and if not found, consider percutaneous CT or ultrasound guided autologous thrombin injection.

Post embolization, immediate check angiography is indicated. It is important to perform pre and post contrast enhanced CT initially as the aneurysm will still contain contrast from the initial embolization for up to 4 weeks post procedure (Fig. 7.5d). Further CECT scans at 24 h, 1 week, 1 month and 3 months are indicated. CECT should also be performed anytime where there is recurrent pain or haematemesis.

If the aneurysm does recur, repeat angiography and embolization is indicated if there is still access and recanalization or recruitment of other arteries has occurred. CT guided percutaneous thrombin may also be used but it may be that open surgery is the only alternative. See Table 7.1 for details of technical requirements.

7.3.3
Endovascular Management and Results

There is still some controversy in this area. There are some who believe that "there are several situations in which angiographic management is appropriate. However, because the pseudoaneurysm may be supplied by collaterals which would form rapidly after embolization, a definitive operation should be performed as soon as possible" [23]. However, the literature would suggest that embolization is an effective treatment in its own right (Fig. 7.7). Critics would argue that the bulk of the literature consists of case reports and small case series. In the largest published series of 104 cases, compiled by postal survey, Boudghene described positive angiography in 90 cases of which 32 were embolized [8]. Angiography was therefore negative in 14 cases and there is no explanation as to why embolization was not performed in the other 68 cases. Of the 32 cases that were embolized 12 re-bled and five died. The results published by Boudghene are therefore almost as bad as the published surgical results. The question that needs answering is why some patients rebleed after apparently effective embolization or surgery?

This author's experience over a 3-year period is of 16 patients all of whom had a definitive diagnosis of visceral pseudoaneurysm at CECT but where the aneurysm was only imaged by selective or super selective angiography in nine cases. All nine were embolized using coils and there was no re-bleed or reformation of the aneurysm at between 6 months and 5 years. However, in seven cases pseudoaneurysms could not be seen at angiography (Fig. 7.6) or filled very slowly at super selective catheterisation. All seven of these pseudoaneurysms were within cysts in the omental bursa. In only one of these seven cases was endovascular embolization attempted. In this particular case though embolization was clearly initially effective the pseudoaneurysm reformed within 7 days. A second embolization was again effective but again the aneurysm reformed (Fig. 7.8). Subsequent embolization was not possible, as all the

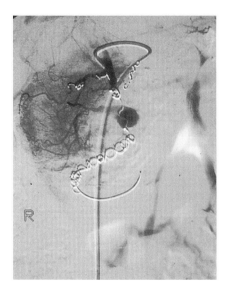

Fig. 7.8. Gastroduodenal arteriogram in a patient who had undergone two previous coil embolizations for a slow filling pseudoaneurysm that filled from small GDA and pancreaticoduodenal branches. In this late phase the pseudoaneurysm has recurred from numerous small duodenal collaterals. Further embolization was not possible

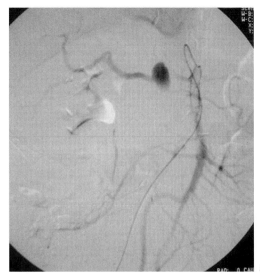

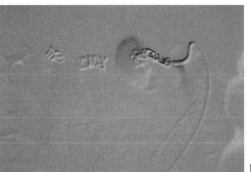

Fig. 7.9a,b. A 52-year-old woman with a recent history of gall stone pancreatitis was admitted with further abdominal pain. A CECT scan suggested an aneurysm of uncertain origin. Angiography revealed a true (Type 1a) aneurysm of an aberrant right hepatic artery (**a**). CECT had revealed a patent portal vein and so proximal and distal coil embolization was performed (**b**). There were no further complications and the patient is alive and well at 36 months

main arterial access points had been embolized. This patient subsequently died at surgery.

It would appear therefore that two different types of visceral aneurysms are possible in the patient with pancreatitis. The first is a true aneurysm (Type 1a) (Fig. 7.9) or a pseudoaneurysm (Type 1b) (Fig. 7.7) arising directly from an eroded major named artery. These can be treated by embolotherapy with coils. The second type of pseudoaneurysm (Type 2) (Figs. 7.6 and 7.8) cannot be seen at angiography or fills very slowly with no major named arterial source. Such aneurysms occur within the omental bursa and are probably formed by the erosion of the arteriolar and capillary bed possibly with a venous contribution. It is possible that such aneurysms account for the rebleeding encountered after surgery and embolotherapy in a significant number of patients. Attempts at embolizing these are likely to fail and a different strategy is necessary. The other six such pseudoaneurysms, described above, were treated by percutaneous thrombin injections under CT guidance.

7.3.4
Percutaneous Ultrasound or CT Guided Embolization or Thrombin Injection

The direct puncture percutaneous approach to pancreatic aneurysm embolization was first described by in 1992 by CAPEK et al. who used coils after puncturing an aneurysm within a pancreatic phlegmon at open surgery [23]. There have been other descriptions of the technique to treat non pancreatitis associated visceral aneurysms [24]. Subsequently LEE et al. described the use of thrombin to occlude an iatrogenic aneurysm caused by a percutaneously inserted drainage catheter [25]. This lead to reports of its use to treat true pancreatitis associated pseudoaneurysms [26, 27].

The author has used percutaneous CT guided thrombin injection in six patients where pancreatitis associated aneurysms could not be seen at selective angiography. The technique is relatively simple, the aneurysm being punctured with a 21-Gauge saline flushed needle under CT guidance and 1000–5000 units of thrombin injected down the needle until resistance is felt. It is important not to aspirate blood into the needle and to rely on the CT image for position. If there is uncertainty about tip position, and aspiration of blood necessary, then the needle must be re-flushed with saline prior to thrombin injection.

Initially human thrombin obtained from the blood transfusion service was used. However, although immediate thrombosis of the aneurysms was observed, recurrence occurred at follow up CECT (Fig. 7.10). This is not surprising in patients with on going pancreatitis. Repeat thrombin injections were required – in one case on three separate occasions. Though eventually permanent occlusion was obtained and the patients are still alive and well, subsequent patients were treated with autologous thrombin prepared from 50 cc of their own venous blood. This was done to avoid potential anaphylaxis,

which has been recorded with repeated human or bovine thrombin injections. The technique for preparing autologous thrombin is described in the literature [28]. The results have been good in all six patients with permanent occlusion of the aneurysm confirmed by subsequent contrast enhanced CT at 6–18 months. However four patients have required one repeat procedure and two patients two, within the first 3 months. Such patients may previously have accounted for the rebleed and death rate post embolization or surgery.

There is one further indication for thrombin occlusion of pancreatitis associated visceral aneurysms. Where the portal vein has occluded as a complication and the patient has a proximal splenic or gastroduodenal aneurysm, the proximal and distal coil embolization of which could compromise the hepatic arterial supply to the liver causing liver infarction, thrombin injection may be a safer technique [29].

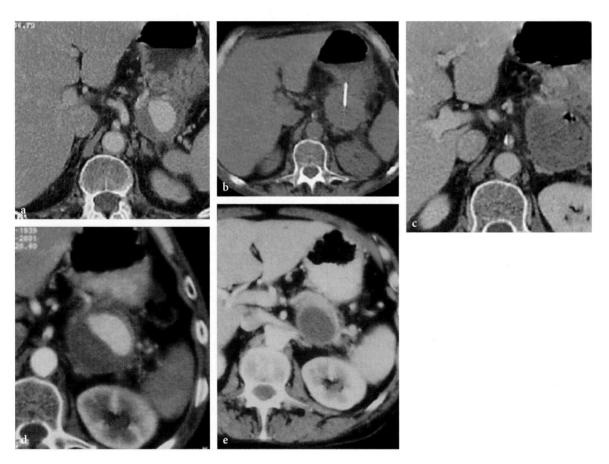

Fig. 7.10a–e. A 36-year-old woman with an occult lesser sac pseudoaneurysm diagnosed at CECT after an acute on chronic episode of pancreatitis (**a**). Angiography revealed a slow filling pseudoaneurysm in pancreaticoduodenal territory but it was not filling from any major artery. It was therefore punctured percutaneously under CT guidance with a 21-gauge needle (**b**) and thrombosed with 3500 units of autologous thrombin with a good result at 24 h (**c**). However, the aneurysm had recurred at 1 month follow-up CECT (**d**) and the procedure was repeated. CECT at 3 months demonstrated thrombosis of the aneurysm (**e**) and the patient is well with no recurrence at 9 months

7.3.5
Complications

The complications of embolization for pancreatitis associated visceral pseudoaneurysms are the same as for the treatment of haemobilia. In addition and as mentioned the repeated use of bovine or human thrombin can lead to anaphylaxis and though rare, autologous thrombin is recommended.

7.3.6
Summary

Aneurysms and pseudoaneurysms causing haemobilia or associated with pancreatitis are potentially fatal. Imaging, particularly CECT, is vital to their diagnosis. Conservative therapy is a poor option and treatment, which was formally via open surgery, is now best carried out by angiography and percutaneous coil embolization in haemobilia and for Type 1a and b pancreatitis associated pseudoaneurysms. Percutaneous CT guided thrombin therapy is indicated for Type 2 aneurysms.

References

1. Sandblom P (1948) Haemorrhage in to the biliary tract following trauma: 'traumatic haemobilia'. Surgery 24:571–86
2. Green MHA, Duell RM, Johnson CD, Jamieson NV (2001) Haemobilia. Br J Surg 88:773–786
3. Nicholson A, Travis S, Ettles DF et al (1999) Hepatic artery angiography and embolization for haemobilia following laparoscopic cholecystectomy. CVIR 22:42–47
4. Kiviluto T, Kivisaari L, Kivilaakso E (1989) Pseudocysts in chronic pancreatitis: surgical results in 102 consecutive patients. Arch Surg 124:204–243
5. Canakkalelioglu L, Gurkan A (1996) The management of bleeding from a pancreatic pseudocyst: a case report. Hepato Gastroenterology 43:278–281
6. Woods MS, Traverso LW, Kozarek RA et al (1995) Successful treatment of bleeding pseudo aneurysms of chronic pancreatitis. Pancreas 10:22–30
7. Van Langenhove P, Defreyne L, Kunnen M (1999) Spontaneous thrombosis of a pseudoaneurysm complicated pancreatitis. Abdominal Imaging 24:491–493
8. Boudghene F, L'Hermine C, Bigot GM (1993) Arterial complications of pancreatitis: diagnostic and therapeutic aspects in 104 cases. J Vasc Interv Radiol 4:551–558
9. Woods MS, Traverso LW, El Hamel A, Parc R, Adda G (1991) Bleeding pseudocysts and pseudoaneurysms in chronic pancreatitis. Br J Surg 78:1059–1063
10. Woods MS, Balthezar EG, Fisher LA (2001) Haemorrhagic complications of pancreatitis: radiological evaluation with emphasis on CT imaging. Pancreatology 1:306–313
11. Frey CF (1975) Pancreatic pseudocyst-operative strategy. Ann Surg 1978, 188:652–662, Ankarins. Br J Surg 62:37
12. Uflacker R, Diehl JC (1982) Successful embolisation of a bleeding splenic artery pseudoaneurysm secondary to necrotising pancreatitis. Gastrointest Radiol 7:379–382
13. Huizinga WK, Kalideen JM, Bryer JV (1984) Control of major haemorrhage associated with pancreatic pseudocysts by transcatheter arterial embolisation. Br J Surg 71:133–136
14. Morita R, Muto N, Konagayer M et al (1991) Successful transcatheter embolisationof pseudoaneurysm associated with pancreatic pseudocyst. Am J Gastroenterol 86:1264–1267
15. Savastano S, Feltrin GP, Antonio T et al (1993) Arterial complications of pancreatitis:diagnostic and therapeutic role for radiology. Pancreas 8:687–692
16. Rai R, Rose J, Manas D (2003) Potentially fatal haemobilia due to inappropriate use of an expanding biliary stent. World J Gastroenterol 9:2377–2378
17. Cardella JF, Vujic I, Tadavarthy SM et al (1997) Vasoactive drugs and embolotherapy in the management of gastrointestinal bleeding. In: Castenada-Zuniga WR (ed) Interventional radiology, 3rd edn, chap 5. Williams and Wilkins, Baltimore, p 243
18. Yamaguchi H, Wakiguchi S, Murakami G (2001) Blood supply to the duodenal papilla and the communicating artery between the anterior and posterior pancreaticoduodenal arterial arcades. J Hepato Biliary Pancreatic Surg 8:238–244
19. Savader SJ, Trerotola SO, Merine DS et al (1992) Haemobilia after transhepatic biliary drainage: treatment with transcatheter embolotherapy. JVIR 3:345–352
20. Stabile BE, Wison SE, Debas HT (1983) Reduced mortality from bleeding pseudocysts and pseudoaneurysm caused by pancreatitis. Arch Surg 118:115
21. Gadcz TR, Trunkey D, Kiefferr F Jr (1978) Visceral vessel erosion associated with pancreatitis. Arch Surg 113:1438
22. Block S, Miae RW, Bittener R et al (1986) Identification of pancreas necrosis in severe acute pancreatitis imaging procedures verses clinical staging. Gut 27:1035–1042
23. Capek P, Rocco M, McGahan J et al (1992) Direct aneurysm puncture and coil occlusion: a new approach to paripancreatic arterial pseudoaneurysms. JVIR 3:653–656
24. Araoz PA, Andrews JC (2000) Direct percutaneous embolization of visceral artery aneurysms: techniques and pitfalls. JVIR 11:1195–1200
25. Lee MJ, Saini S, Geller SC, Warshaw AL, Mueller PR (1991) Pancreatitis with pseudoaneurysm formation: a pitfall for the interventional radiologist. AJR 156:97–98
26. Puri S, Nicholson AA, Breen DJ (2003) Percutaneous thrombin injection for the treatment of a post-pancreatitis pseudoaneurysm. Eur Radiol 13:L79–L82
27. Armstrong EM, Edwards A, Kingsnorth AN et al (2003) Ultrasound guided thrombin injection to treat a pseudoaneurysm secondary to chronic pancreatitis. Eur J Vasc Endovasc Surg 26:448–449
28. Quarmby JW, Engelke C, Chitolie A et al (2002) Autologous thrombin for treatment of pseudoaneurysms. Lancet 359:946–947
29. Sparrow P, Asquith J, Chalmers N (2003) Ultrasonic-guided percutaneous injection of pancreatic pseudoaneurysm with thrombin. Cardiovasc Intervent Radiol 26:312–315

8 Balloon-occluded Retrograde Transvenous Obliteration of Gastric Varices in Portal Hypertension

Koji Takahashi and Shiliang Sun

CONTENTS

8.1 Introduction

The major aims of interventional procedures for portal hypertension are prophylactic and emergent treatment of variceal bleeding, control of hepatic encephalopathy, and treatment of refractory ascites. Hypersplenism associated with hematological disorder is an additional clinical problem in patients with portal hypertension. At present, the main primary embolotherapies available for portal hypertension are balloon-occluded retrograde transvenous obliteration (BRTO) and partial splenic embolization (PSE). In Japan, BRTO has recently been applied for gastric varices instead of either endoscopic treatment or transhepatic intrahepatic portosystemic shunt (TIPS) procedure, and numerous studies have reported that this method has an excellent success rate. Its efficacy for control of hepatic encephalopathy has also been demonstrated.

K. Takahashi, MD
Department of Radiology, Asahikawa Medical College, 2-1-1-1 Midorigaoka, Asahikawa, 078-8510, Japan
S. Sun, MD
Associate Professor of Radiology, University of Iowa Hospitals and Clinics, 200 Hawkins Drive, 3957 JPP, Iowa City, Iowa 52242, USA

8.2 Balloon-occluded Retrograde Transvenous Obliteration

8.2.1 Clinical Consideration and Pathophysiology of Gastric Varices

Gastric varices are seen in approximately 30% of patients with portal hypertension. Although the risk of bleeding from gastric varices has been reported as relatively low, it differs depending on the site of the varices, being much higher in gastric fundal varices (nearly 80%) than in cardiac varices (nearly 10%–40%) [4]. Generally, control of gastric varices is more difficult than control of esophageal varices, and the mortality rate of ruptured gastric varices is as high as 45%–55% [3]. There are several treatment options for gastric varices, including endoscopic sclerotherapy, endoscopic ligation, surgery, and TIPS. However, in gastric fundal varices, endoscopic injection sclerotherapy is not effective due to their fast blood flow, and endoscopic ligation is technically difficult due to their large size. Poor hepatic functional reserve prohibits surgery in most patients with gastric varices. TIPS is a widely accepted procedure for refractory varices bleeding in portal hypertension. Although its success rate in gastric varices has been reported as 90%, the rebleeding rate is approximately 30% [1, 2]. Aggravation of hepatic encephalopathy is seen in 20% of patients after TIPS, and poor primary shunt patency is also a problem in patients undergoing this procedure.

Recently, BRTO as an alternative has been widely applied for the treatment of gastric varices in Japan, and favorable results – i.e., a success rate of greater than 90% and recurrence rate of less than 10% – have been reported. BRTO can be performed in patients with poor hepatic function reserve or hemorrhagic disorders. And because it is less invasive than other procedures, BRTO is expected to get more acceptances for treatment of gastric varices in the future.

The major inflow vessels of gastric varices are the short gastric and posterior gastric veins. Gastric fundal varices in particular receive a large portion of their blood supply from these veins, while the left gastric vein supplies cardiac varices. Gastric varices drain into the gastrorenal shunt in 80%–85% of cases, and drain into the inferior phrenic vein, which joins with the inferior vena cava (IVC) just below the diaphragm (gastro-caval shunt), in 10%–15% of cases. The inferior phrenic vein also joins with the pericardiacophrenic vein or intercostals vein. In rare cases, gastric varices have both gastrorenal and gastrocaval outflow shunts [8] (Fig. 8.1).

8.2.2
Technique of BRTO

Prior to the BRTO procedure, we obtain a contrast enhanced CT image with 3-to 5-mm slice thickness to evaluate the location and extent of gastric varices and their feeding and draining veins. Gastrorenal and/or gastrocaval shunt vessels can be well demonstrated on serial axial CT images with appropriate contrast enhancement. We can also evaluate the size and tortuosity of these shunt vessels. The sclerosant agent consists of a mixture of the same dose of 10% ethanolamine oleate (Oldamin; Mochida Pharmaceutical, Tokyo, Japan) and 300–350 mgI/ ml non-ionic contrast medium. The amounts vary depending on the size and number of varices. Before and during the procedure, 4,000 units of human haptoglobin (Green Cross, Osaka, Japan) are administered to prevent hemolysis and subsequent acute renal failure.

A 6-F balloon catheter (Clinical Supply, Gifu, Japan) is inserted from either the right internal jugular vein or the right femoral vein. The catheter is advanced via left adrenal vein into the gastrorenal shunt vessel and wedged into place by inflating the balloon. Then, a retrograde left adrenal venogram is obtained to evaluate the volume and collateral vessels of gastric varices. Hirota classified gastric varices into five grades according to the degree of progression and the number of collateral veins [4]. The presence of collateral veins may interfere with the complete filling of gastric varices with sclerosant and result in inadequate embolization. Collateral veins that are small and few in number are thrombosed during retrograde injection of sclerosant through the wedged balloon catheter, but those that are medium-to-large in size require selective embolization by an embolic coil or ethanol using

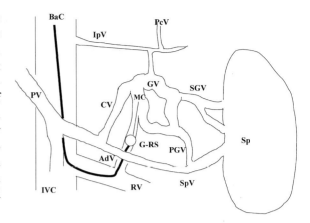

Fig. 8.1. Diagram of anatomy of the gastric varices and collateral vessels. *AdV*, adrenal vein; *BaC*, balloon catheter; *CV*, coronary vein; *IpV*, inferior phrenic vein; *IVC*, inferior vena cava; *G-RS*, gastro-renal shunt; *GV*, gastric varices; *MC*, microcatheter; *PcV*, pericardiacophrenic vein; *PGV*, posterior gastric vein; *PV*, portal vein; *RV*, renal vein; *SGV*, short gastric vein; *Sp*, spleen; *SpV*, splenic vein

a 2.9-F microcatheter system. The sclerosant agent is injected slowly or in a stepwise fashion through either a microcatheter [12] or a balloon catheter until the varices are completely filled, and then is left in the varices for 1–2 h. After the procedure, residual sclerosant is withdrawn through either a microcatheter or a balloon catheter. To evaluate the effect of the treatment, contrast-enhanced CT is performed 1 or 2 weeks after the procedure. In cases with inadequate thrombosis of varices, a second or third procedure is generally needed within an interval of a few weeks. Multiple procedures are more commonly needed in cases with many large collateral veins or a very large gastrorenal shunt with rapid blood flow (Fig. 8.2; Table 8.1).

8.2.3
Results of BRTO

Excellent initial success rates of BRTO of 90%– 100% and low recurrence rates of 0%–10 % have been reported [4, 5, 9]. Complete thrombosis of gastric varices has been identified on the follow-up CT scan. In addition to prophylactic treatment for gastric varices at high risk of bleeding, a high success rate of 82% has also been obtained in gastric varices with bleeding [7]. Some authors have reported an improvement of hepatic function and hepatic encephalopathy after BRTO [3, 6, 10]. However, additional, longer-term studies will be needed to clarify the efficacy of BRTO on hepatic function

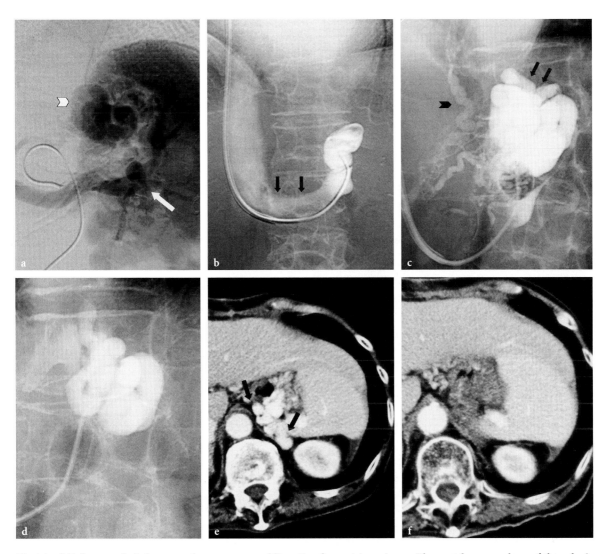

Fig. 8.2a–f. Balloon-occluded retrograde transvenous obliteration for gastric varices. **a** The portal venous phase of the splenic arteriogram shows gastric varices supplied by posterior (*arrow*) and short gastric (*arrowhead*) veins. **b** A left adrenal venogram obtained without balloon occlusion shows antegrade flow to the left renal vein (*arrows*) and inferior vena cava (*arrowheads*). **c** A left adrenal venogram obtained under balloon occlusion shows gastric varices (*arrows*), a few small collateral vessels, and esophageal varices (*arrowhead*). **d** Sclerosant is injected into the gastric varices through a microcatheter. **e** A contrast-enhanced CT image before BRTO shows tortuous gastric fundal varices (*arrows*). **f** A contrast-enhanced CT image obtained 10 days after B-RTO shows thrombosis of the gastric varices

and hepatic encephalopathy. BRTO has also been used successfully to treat ruptured duodenal varices [11] (Fig. 8.3).

Hemoglobinuria is seen after the procedure in nearly all cases, but usually disappears within a few days. Renal dysfunction is rare. One article reported a transient increase in serum creatinine level in 13% of cases, which returned to baseline within one week [7]. Minor symptoms such as mild fever and epigastric pain usually appear after the procedure but resolve within a few days or 1 week. Rare but significant complications, such as anaphylactic reac-

tion, pulmonary edema, hemothorax and disseminated intravascular coagulation were also reported [4]. Aggravation of esophageal varices is seen in 16%–30% of cases after BRTO due to occlusion of the

Table 8.1. Cookbook: Materials for balloon-occluded retrograde transvenous obliteration

– 7-F, 25-cm Sheath (Terumo)
– 6-F Balloon catheter (clinical supply)
– Glidewire, 0.035–0.038 in. (Terumo)
– Renegade or FAS tracker microcathete, 2.9 F

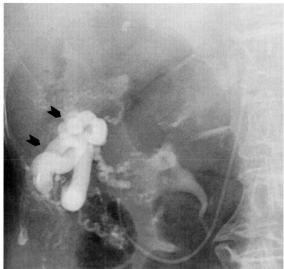

a

Fig. 8.3a–c. Balloon-occluded retrograde transvenous obliteration for duodenal varices. **a** A varicogram obtained by injection of sclerosant through a microcatheter advanced into the pancreaticoduodenal vein shows duodenal varices (*arrowheads*). A balloon catheter is inserted into the right ovarian vein (*arrow*). **b** A contrast-enhanced CT obtained before BRTO shows duodenal varices (*arrow*). **c** A contrast-enhanced CT obtained 7 days after B-RTO shows thrombosis of the duodenal varices

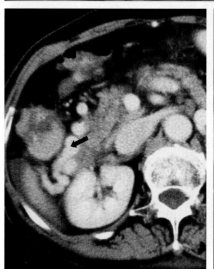

b

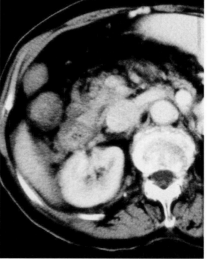

c

outflow tract of varices. This is especially common in patients with preexisting esophageal varices and gastric varices with afferent flow from the left gastric veins. However, these esophageal varices are largely controllable endoscopically.

8.3
Conclusion

BRTO has been proven clinically effective and safe in treatment of isolated gastric varices secondary to portal hypertension. More randomized perspective studies may be necessary to evaluate its usefulness in a worldwide scope and its relationship with other alternatives such as endoscopic therapies and TIPS

in the treatment of complications of portal hypertension.

References

1. Barange K, Peron JM et al. (1999) Transjugular intrahepatic portosystemic shunt in the treatment of refractory bleeding from ruptured gastric varices. Hepatology 30:1139–1143
2. Chau TN, Patch D et al. (1998) "Salvage" transjugular intrahepatic portosystemic shunts: gastric fundal compared with esophageal variceal bleeding. Gastroenterology 114:981–987
3. Fukuda T, Hirota S et al. (2001) Long-term results of balloon-occluded retrograde transvenous obliteration for the treatment of gastric varices and hepatic encephalopathy. J Vasc Interv Radiol 12:327–336

4. Hirota S, Matsumoto S et al. (1999) Retrograde transvenous obliteration of gastric varices. Radiology 211:349–356

5. Kanagawa H, Mima S et al. (1996) Treatment of gastric fundal varices by balloon-occluded retrograde transvenous obliteration. J Gastroenterol Hepatol 11:51–58

6. Kato T, Uematsu T et al. (2001) Therapeutic effect of balloon-occluded retrograde transvenous obliteration of portal-systemic encephalopathy in patients with liver cirrhosis. Intern Med 40:688–691

7. Kitamoto M, Imamura M et al. (2002) Balloon-occluded retrograde transvenous obliteration of gastric fundal varices with hemorrhage. AJR Am J Roentgenol 178:1167–1174

8. Kiyosue H, Mori H et al. (2003) Transcatheter obliteration of gastric varices. RadioGraph 23:911–920

9. Koito K, Namieno T et al. (1996) Balloon-occluded retrograde transvenous obliteration for gastric varices with gastrorenal or gastrocaval collaterals. AJR Am J Roentgenol 167:1317–1320

10. Miyamoto Y, Oho K et al. (2003) Balloon-occluded retrograde transvenous obliteration improves liver function in patients with cirrhosis and portal hypertension. J Gastroenterol Hepatol 18:934–942

11. Sonomura T, Horihata K et al. (2002) Ruptured duodenal varices successfully treated with balloon-occluded retrograde transvenous obliteration. AJR Am J Roentgenol 181:725–727

12. Takahashi K, Yamada T et al. (2001) Selective balloon-occluded retrograde sclerosis of gastric varices using a coaxial microcatheter system. AJR Am J Roentgenol 177:1091–1093

Gynecology and Obstetrics

9 Interventional Management of Postpartum Hemorrhage

Hicham T. Abada, Jafar Golzarian, and Shiliang Sun

CONTENTS

9.1 Introduction

Postpartum hemorrhage (PPH) is a severe, life-threatening clinical event. It has been reported that at least 150,000 women per annum bleed massively during or immediately after labor [1]. High obstetric morbidity and mortality secondary to PPH are reported in both developed and developing countries. Indeed, the mortality rate due to PPH ranges from 13% to 40% [1]. In the United States, the mortality rate is 13%; however, France, with 414 deaths reported over a 4-year period has the highest rate of death related to PPH in Europe [2–5]. PPH represents the most common cause of blood transfusion after delivery.

The role of the interventional radiology in the management of PPH has gained wide acceptance in the obstetric-gynecologic community [6, 7]. This management requires a multidisciplinary approach that involves the obstetrician, intensive care physician and interventional radiologist. Selective transcatheter techniques for the treatment of intractable bleeding after delivery was first reported in 1970 by Brown [8, 9]. Despite the fact that several published series have proven the safety and effectiveness of the procedure, it remains an underused modality for PPH compared to uterine artery ligation or hemostatic hysterectomy [10, 11].

This chapter will describe the role of embolotherapy for the control of PPH as an alternative approach to surgery. We will focus on anatomy and on the embolization techniques that are required for safety and optimal outcomes for the procedure. The clinical and physiological aspects are also discussed to provide a better understanding of the potential adverse effects that might complicate such a procedure in otherwise healthy young women.

9.2 Clinical Considerations

9.2.1 Definitions

PPH is defined as blood loss of more than 500 ml after vaginal delivery or 1000 ml after cesarean delivery [12]. This definition is subjective since the quantification of bleeding is generally difficult to

H. T. Abada, MD
Department of Imaging and Interventional Radiology, Centre Hospitalier René Dubos, 6 Avenue de l'Ile de France, 95303 Cergy-Pontoise, France
J. Golzarian, MD
Professor of Radiology, Director, Vascular and Interventional Radiology, University of Iowa, Department of Radiology, 200 Hawkins Drive, 3957 JPP, Iowa City, IA 52242, USA
S. Sun, MD
Associate Professor of Radiology, University of Iowa Hospitals and Clinics, 200 Hawkins Drive, Iowa City, IA 52242, USA

determine. Another approach to estimating blood loss is 10% or more drops in hematocrit value [13]. The concept of massive postpartum hemorrhage was recently defined to include blood loss (more than 1500 ml), a drop in hemoglobin concentration (≥4 g/dl), and an active massive transfusion (≥4 units of blood) [11].

Blood loss that occurs during the first 24 h is known as primary PPH; secondary PPH is characterized by blood loss occurring 24 h to 6 weeks after delivery.

9.2.2
Clinical Evaluation

PPH diagnosis is often obvious when bleeding is visible and generally correlates with symptoms of hypovolemic shock. On the other hand, a clinical underestimation of visible blood loss is possible by as much as 50%. In addition, most pregnant women are healthy, and this physiologic condition can compensate for the blood loss. Hypovolemic shock occurs after a deep depletion of blood volume [14].

Early diagnosis of PPH is crucial for initiating appropriate management as early as possible. Management includes restoration of the blood volume and identification of the underlying cause. Delay and inappropriate management are the leading causes of maternal death after delivery.

9.3
Pathophysiology

Pregnancy causes an increase in maternal blood volume by approximately 50%, reaching a volume of 4–6 l. The main benefit of this increase is to allow the body to respond to perfusion intake of the low resistance uteroplacental unit in order to handle the blood loss that occurs at delivery [13].

The uterus retains its proper physiological control of postpartum bleeding. Contraction of the myometrium induces compression of spiral arteries resulting in hemostasis. The condition that predisposes and worsens intractable bleeding after delivery is uterine atony, which inhibits the mechanical process of hemostasis. In such circumstances, bleeding might alter hemostatic status, leading to hemorrhagic shock. Endothelial damage resulting from the shock causes disseminated intravascular coagulation (DIC) [15].

One of the most catastrophic accidents occurring after delivery is DIC related to amniotic fluid embolism (AFE). This condition manifests with an acute onset of respiratory failure, circulatory collapse, shock, and thrombohemorrhagic syndrome. In the United States, DIC accounts for about 10% of all maternal deaths. Exaggerated uterine contraction caused by oxytocin, caesarean section, uterine rupture or premature separation of the placenta are risk factors for AFE. Pathophysiology of AFE may be related to lacerations on the membrane from the placenta that provides a portal entry for amniotic fluid into the maternal venous sinuses in the uterus [16].

9.4
Anatomy

9.4.1
Normal Anatomy

A thorough knowledge of vascular anatomy of the pelvis is essential to ensure the safety and effectiveness of embolization in overcoming the intractable bleeding. The main pelvic blood supply during PPH is the uterine artery that arises from internal iliac artery (IIA) (please refer to Chap. 10.3 for more details). The IIA divides into an anterior and posterior branch. The anterior division gives rise to the visceral branches. The uterine artery generally originates from the medial aspect of the anterior trunk. Other branches include the superior vesical, middle hemorrhoidal, inferior hemorrhoidal and vaginal arteries. The arcuate arteries are branches of the uterine artery that extend inward into the myometrium, and also have a circumferential course around the myometrium. The arcuate arteries give rise to radial arteries that are directed toward the uterine cavity to become the spiral arteries in the endometrium (Fig. 9.1). The venous plexus runs parallel to the arteries. It is generally seen on the late phase of angiograms. Its recognition is important and should not be misdiagnosed with contrast media extravasation. The vascular network of the female pelvis in pregnancy is extensive and provides numerous communications between the right and left IIAs. There are also many anastomoses communicating with the branches of the IIA, such as the inferior mesenteric artery, lumbar and iliolumbar, and sacral arteries. A collateral pathway from the external iliac

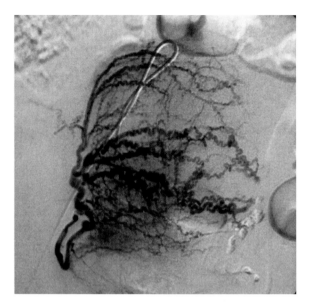

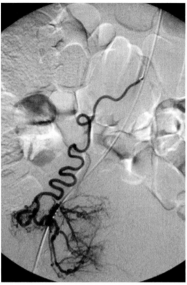

Fig. 9.1. Angiogram of the right uterine artery demonstrating spiral arteries

Fig. 9.2. Selective angiogram of right ovarian artery feeding the right side of the uterus

artery provides anastomosis with iliolumbar and gluteal arteries. An unusual case of massive bleeding originating from the epigastric artery, which was responsible for embolization failure after the occlusion of both internal iliac arteries following cesarean delivery, was reported [17].

9.4.2
Variants

Apart from the classic pattern in which the uterine artery arises from the medial aspect of IIA, there are many other variants that have been identified (please see Chap. 10.3). It may also arise from its anterior or lateral aspect of the IIA [18]. The origin of the uterine artery from the main IIA itself or from the aorta has also been described [18]. A common trunk between the uterine artery and vesical artery is another important variant that might lead to inadvertent vesical ischemia in cases of non-targeted embolization [19]. The uterine artery may also duplicate as illustrated by Redlich et al. [20]. The ovarian artery represents the second main vessel for PPH [21, 22]. The ovarian artery that participates in uterine blood supply could represent the major feeding vessel to the uterus as demonstrated in UFE literature [23] (Fig. 9.2). Recently, Saraiya et al. illustrated uterine artery replacement by the round ligament artery during embolization for leio-

myomata [24]. The role of this artery in PPH was previously documented during angiography [25] (Fig. 9.3).

A personal case of anatomic variant was found during postpartum hemorrhage embolization in which the inferior mesenteric artery was the feeding vessel to the uterus (Fig. 9.4).

9.5
Etiology and Risk Factors

9.5.1
Vaginal Delivery

A recent randomized trial in the US highlighted the increased risk of PPH in patients with labor induction and augmentation, higher birth-weight, chorioamnionitis, and magnesium sulphate use [26].

A report of 37,497 women who delivered in the UK in 1988 showed that in addition to the well-known risk factors to major PPH, other potential risks were obesity, a large baby, and a retained placenta in women classified initially as "low risk" [27]. The most common cause of PPH is uterine atony. It occurs in 2%–5% of deliveries. However, the majority is managed by conservative measures. Other causes of PPH are retained products of conception,

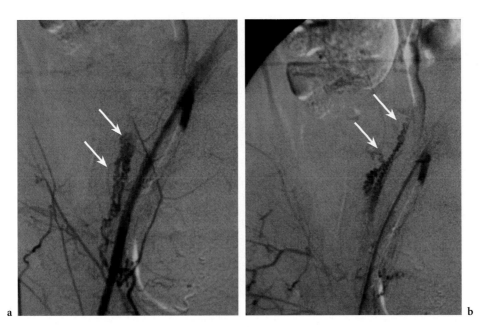

Fig. 9.3a,b. Right iliac angiogram showed collateral pathways from the artery supplying the round ligament after embolization of both right internal iliac and uterine arteries

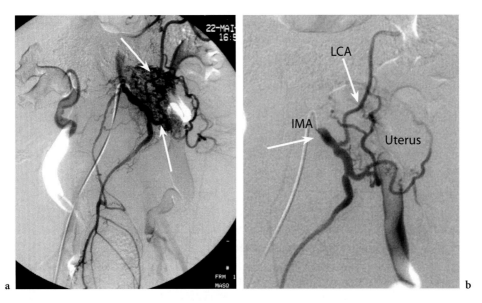

Fig. 9.4a,b. A 31-year-old woman with PPH (**a**). Selective angiogram of the inferior mesenteric artery (*IMA*) showed the left colic artery supplying the uterus (*arrows*). **b** Early phase of selective angiogram of the IMA shows that the second left division feeds exclusively the uterus (*arrow*). (Courtesy of Patrick Garance)

placental abnormalities, uterine rupture, lower genital tract laceration and coagulopathies. In a study of 763 pregnant women who died of hemorrhage, 19% had placental abruption, 16% uterine rupture, 15% uterine atony, 14% coagulopathies, 7% placenta praevia, 6% placenta accreta, 6% uterine bleeding, 4% retained placenta, and 10% other or unknown causes [28].

9.5.2
Cesarean Delivery

A case-controlled study for risk factors of PPH following cesarean among 3052 cesarean deliveries was performed by Combs et al. [29]. The major factor was found to be related to general anesthesia (OR 2.94), followed by amniotitis (OR 2.69), preeclampsia (OR 2.18), protracted active phase of labor (OR 2.40), and second (OR 1.90).

On the other hand, maternal age represents an independent risk factor of blood loss irrespective of the mode of delivery. Indeed, a maternal age equal or superior to 35 years had an OR of 1.6–1.8 [30].

9.6
Treatment

Postpartum hemorrhage is an emergent clinical scenario and requires immediate medical attention. Multidisciplinary collaboration among the intensive care physician, obstetrician and interventional radiologist is crucial for optimal management. Interventional radiologists play a significant role in the treatment of massive or intractable bleeding. In the setting of ongoing bleeding after the delivery, conservative management is the first approach. Measures include vaginal packing, uterine massage, intravenous administration of uterotonic medications such as oxytocin or methylergonovine, curettage of retained placenta, fluid replacement and blood transfusion. These measures successfully control the bleeding in most situations. Embolotherapy should be considered when these measures fail.

9.6.1
Blood Transfusion

Blood transfusion represents a major component during the medical management of severe postpartum hemorrhage. A transfusion may be initiated in patients who continue bleeding, developing shock despite aggressive medical management. However, blood transfusion constitutes a risk of contamination by human immunodeficiency virus or hepatitis B and C [31]. The contemporary obstetrician's practice is to develop measures to reduce blood transfusion. Indeed, blood transfusions dropped from 4.6% in 1976 to 0.9% in 1990. In a recent study, REYAL et al. confirmed these data with a transfusion rate of 0.23% on a cohort of 19,138 deliveries over a 7-year period [32].

Our unpublished data in a retrospective study showed that embolization following PPH might prevent blood transfusion when close medical management and rapid evaluation of the emergency status is performed. These findings probably highlighted an additional advantage of embolization procedures after delivery.

9.6.2
Embolization Procedure

9.6.2.1
Angiography and Embolization

When embolotherapy is indicated, the patient is transferred to an angiographic suite. Intensive care physicians should be present during the procedure. Right femoral artery access is obtained, and a 4- or 5-F sheath is inserted. Additionally, left femoral venous access may be obtained to be used by the intensive care physician if no other central access is available for supportive therapy.

Catheterization of bilateral uterine arteries is mandatory. A cobra-shaped catheter is the best catheter to use for easy insertion into uterine arteries. The cobra catheter is available in three different types, each according to the degree of opening of the curve. The medium sized catheter (C2) is the one most commonly used. When using a 4-F catheter, one should make sure that the lumen of the catheter is able to accept 0.038-in. guidewire for possible microcatheter use. The contralateral internal iliac artery is catheterized first and can be reached by pushing the cobra. In some difficult cases, a curved catheter, such as SOS or sidewinder, could be handy to cross the aortic bifurcation.

The ipsilateral uterine artery access is obtained using the Waltman loop. When the angle of aortic bifurcation is too tight, again the use of a sidewinder allows for easy catheterization.

Angiography can detect contrast medium extravasation; however, this is not seen in the majority of cases. Contrast media extravasations were observed in 18% of patients in a recent study [33]. Even without extravasation, bilateral uterine artery embolization needs to be performed.

The preferred embolic agent is a material that is resorbable. The one most widely used is Gelfoam. Gelfoam can be cut into different sizes depending on the target vessel diameter. The Gelfoam can also be cut in torpedo and inserted into a 1-ml syringe.

Finally, an aortogram is performed to demonstrate the effectiveness of the procedure and the course of ovarian arteries that might be embolized secondarily in cases of rebleeding (Fig. 9.5). One must pay attention to collaterals from ovarian arteries during such embolization procedures because they may be responsible for delayed bleeding. Even though we routinely perform abdominal aortogram after embolization, we never embolize ovarian arteries to prevent possible delayed rebleeding. While we

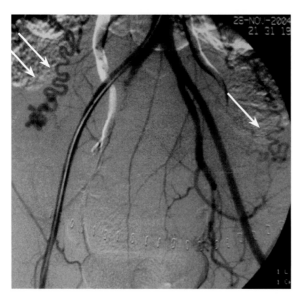

Fig. 9.5. Final aortogram showed complete occlusion of uterine arteries. The patent ovarian arteries were demonstrated (*arrows*)

did not observe contrast extravasations from ovarian arteries during the abdominal aortogram in our data, one must be aware that it could happen. Indeed, Oei et al. demonstrated persistent bleeding following hysterectomy for intractable PPH related to a left ovarian artery that was embolized secondarily [34].

The patient leaves the angiographic suite with the sheath sutured in place in case there is a need for a second embolization session.

9.6.2.2
Personal Technique

As previously mentioned, medical management of obstetric bleeding after delivery is conducted by using drugs such as uterotonic drugs (oxytocin) and prostaglandin E_2 agonist. The latter has a vaso-constrictor effect and thus causes arterial spasm (Fig. 9.6).

For this reason, when an embolotherapy is planned we recommend immediate cessation of prostaglandin E_2 agonist infusion. In case of arterial spasm at the ostium of the uterine artery, the use of a coaxial system with a microcatheter is then required. It is possible to successfully catheterize the distal part of the uterine artery in most cases. In these circumstances, the preferred embolic agent is the one that can be easily delivered through a microcatheter, such as PVA (Polyvinyl alcohol) or Embospheres. We prefer to use particles with larger diameters, such as Embospheres 700–900 mμ. Even if these particles are used for the above-mentioned reasons, additional Gelfoam embolization of internal iliac arteries is performed because of the extensive collateral pathways of the female pelvis.

In the absence of arterial spasm, embolization with Gelfoam pledge of both uterine and internal iliac arteries is always performed in order to obtain a bilateral proximal and distal embolization to prevent rebleeding. Even with Gelfoam pledge, we always use large-cut sizes to prevent embolization that is too distal. Embolization with coils is not per-

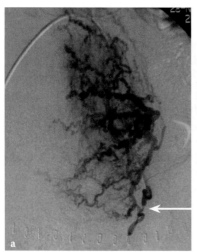 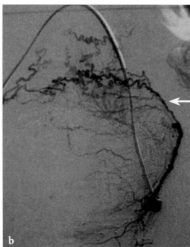 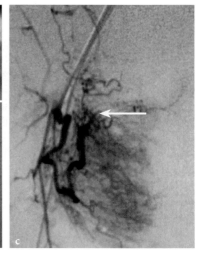

Fig. 9.6a–c. Spasm of uterine artery involving proximal segment (**a**), and distal segments (**b,c**). Spasm induced a complete occlusion of the distal artery in (**c**) (*arrows*)

formed for two reasons: first, it attempts the proximal occlusion that might be less effective; secondly, it could "burn the bridge" for a subsequent embolization in cases of rebleeding. However, microcoils have the potential to stop a bleed from a small vessel as shown in Fig. 9.7.

9.6.2.3
Surgical Treatments

Bilateral internal iliac ligation and hysterectomy are the two surgical treatments that unfortunately are still very commonly used to control PPH. The aim of hypogastric ligation is to reduce the blood flow, allowing normal coagulation to control the bleeding. However, ligation is associated with a high failure rate since it is proximal, and the bleeding may continue through collateral vessels. Moreover, ligation will make the embolization procedure much more challenging. Hysterectomy is the other surgical treatment that is widely used. This surgery is a high-risk procedure in patients with DIC and hemodynamic impairment, and hysterectomy will

not treat the cervicovaginal laceration (Fig. 9.8). Finally, the infertility associated with hysterectomy is an important issue in this young population group. Although this surgical procedure is the only treatment available to control a PPH in some conditions, it should, however, be only used as the last resort.

9.7
Results

Since the first embolization of PPH performed by BROWN in 1979, the reported success rate in 138 patients over a 20-year period was as high as 94.4% [35–43]. To date, 160 patients have been treated at our institution (the first author's institution) by selective uterine and/or internal iliac arteries embolization for intractable bleeding following delivery. Despite the variety of the etiologies and risk factors in our series, no maternal deaths were observed. The main cause of hemorrhage was related to uterine atony, with an incidence of 75%. Cesarean delivery

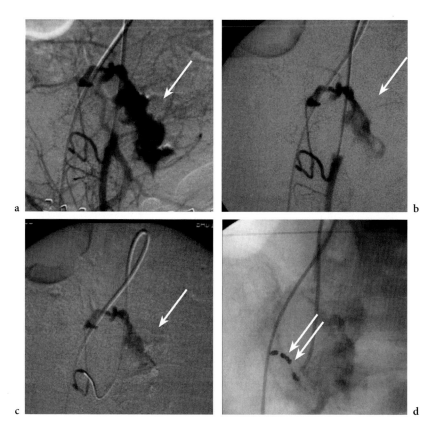

a   b   c   d

Fig. 9.7a–d. Angiogram of right internal iliac artery demonstrates contrast media extravasation (*double arrow*): superselective catheterization using microcatheter and embolization with microcoils (*arrows*). (Courtesy of Patrice Garance)

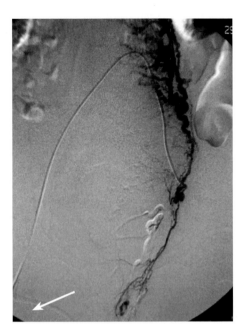

Fig. 9.8. Angiogram of left uterine artery: contrast media extravasation from a vaginal laceration (*arrows*)

was performed in 30% of our population. Lab results and clinical data recorded at the time of the transfer, or at the arrival of the patient in the angiographic suite, showed that a mean drop in hemoglobin was 4.5 g/dl (+/– 9) with a median hemoglobin level of 7.14 (ranging from 3 to 10.2).

A total of 20% of patients received acute massive transfusion, defined as transfusion of 4 or more units of packed red blood cells. Hemodynamic status and blood parameters showed that 30% of patients developed shock, and 50% developed DIC. Hysterectomy was performed in six patients, despite the fact that embolization was initially successful to stop bleeding and improved blood parameters. However, rebleeding occurring at an average of 6 h after embolotherapy justified hysterectomy. No second session of embolization was performed. If we consider that a subsequent hysterectomy represents a failure of the procedure, our success rate was also 94.4%. In our experience, embolization was always effective in the correction of blood parameters and made it possible for gynecologists to perform the hysterectomy, when needed, in a better coagulation and hemodynamic status. On the other hand, shock, DIC, and acute massive transfusion were not the indicators that were able to predict the effectiveness of selective arterial embolization. Indeed, these indicators considered individually or together were not statistically significant in predicting the success of the

procedure. However, despite the latter statement, hysterectomies were all performed in the group of patients with shock, DIC, or acute massive transfusion. We did not find any relationship between contrast media extravasations observed during the procedure and patients' clinical and hemodynamic statuses (Figs. 9.9, 9.10). In all, 71 patients were referred from other hospitals where embolization was not available due to the absence of an interventional radiology unit. The median transfer time was 5.48 h, and this concurred with the time reported in the literature [44]. The transfer itself did not represent a major risk factor [44]. What was critical was to offer the optimal medical managements prior to and during the transfer.

In our experiences, abnormal placentation did not affect the effectiveness of the procedure, concurring with the findings of Descargues et al. [43]. However, Vandelet et al. observed in a series of 29 patients that when an emergency postpartum embolotherapy is attempted, obstetrical history constitute a major risk factor and, furthermore, that transfer increases the morbidity rate [45].

Embolization can also be successful however more challenging after failure of bilateral IIA ligation for primary PPH [46]. The failure was related to the extensive development of pelvic collateral pathways following internal iliac ligation. The bleeding artery was a branch from the epigastric artery. The cases described above may imply that the transcatheter embolization should be the first line of therapeutic approach when patients are hemodynamically stable. It also emphasizes the importance of thorough knowledge of possible collateral pathways post-surgical ligation of internal iliac arteries, and the physiological condition of pregnant women.

9.8
Fertility and Pregnancy

Even though the first goal of embolization following PPH is to achieve hemostasis and overcome a life-threatening condition, this technique clearly helps the patient to avoid hysterectomy, thus preserving fertility.

Evaluation of the fertility in these patients is somewhat difficult because of the lack of information on patient desire for future pregnancy. This information is difficult to obtain if it was not previously indicated in the record during the period of clinical monitoring of the pregnancy. Stancato et

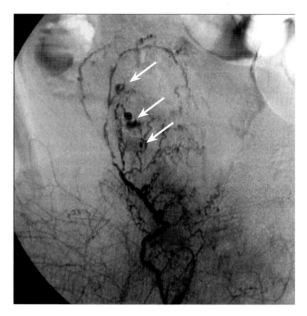

Fig. 9.9. Angiogram of right uterine artery showing contrast media extravasation (*arrows*)

al. reported three pregnancies in 12 women treated by embolization for PPH. Moreover, three full-term pregnancies resulted from the three women in the series who desired to conceive [47]. The same fertility rate following PPH embolization was observed by ORNAN et al., with six pregnancies occurring after a long-term follow-up of 11.7 years (+/– 6.9) [48]. SALOMON et al. followed 17 women between 12 and 80 months after pelvic embolization for PPH. They observed six pregnancies in five women [49]. In the these series, four women with history of PPH developed a new PPH in their following pregnancy.

Causes of PPH, in this study, were related to the placenta in all cases. Nevertheless, in two patients who underwent hysterectomy to stop bleeding, no pathological evidence indicated precisely the causes of these recurrences of bleeding.

Finally, fetal growth retardation (FGR) is reported to occur in patients after uterine artery embolization; this was reported in one case by CORDONNIER et al. [50].

While the technique, embolic agents and clinical conditions of patients with PPH and fibroid embolization (UFE) are different; UFE is also associated with term pregnancy. In a series of 139 patients treated for fibroids, 17 pregnancies were achieved in 14 women who desired to conceive [51]. The incidence of FGR seems higher in the series by GOLDBERG [52]. However, in a recent large cohort study following 671 patients who had UAE for symptomatic fibroids, CARPENTER et al. found 26 completed pregnancies in which only one case of FGR was recorded, supporting the evidence of normal placentation [53] also documented in the RAVINA series [54]. CARPENTER et al. also found that first- and second-term bleeding occurred in 40% and 33%, respectively, miscarriage was found in 27% and primary PPH was observed in 20% [53].

9.9 Prophylactic Approach

PPH in patients with a diagnosis of abnormal placentation (placenta accreta, increta and percreta) is

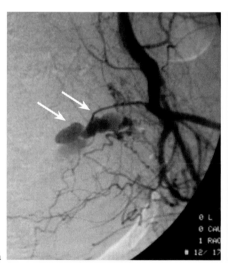
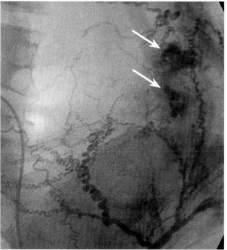

Fig. 9.10a,b. Late phase uterine artery angiograms shows contrast media extravasations (*arrows*)

higher than in other patients. This supported the idea of temporarily limiting the blood flow to the uterus in this high-risk patient population. The so-called prophylactic approach is achieved by selective catheterization of internal iliac arteries using femoral puncture, which is followed by the introduction of balloon catheters in each internal iliac artery. The balloon is inflated prior to the delivery. KIDNEY et al. performed this technique in five patients who were gravida 4 to 5 and para 1 to 4 before hysterectomies for sterilization [55]. The clear goal of such a procedure is to decrease blood loss and potentially prevent blood transfusion and surgical mortality. In case of concern for bleeding in patients with abnormal placentation, some authors use balloon occlusion as a first step to reduce flow in internal iliac arteries followed by internal artery embolization [31].

Our approach to patients with abnormal placentation is to selectively embolize bilateral uterine and internal iliac arteries as soon as possible after delivery. Using the embolization technique, we obtained results similar to that of the prophylactic in controlling PPH, but without the risk of radiation to the fetus.

9.10 Complications

A complication rate of 8.7% was reported in the literature [56–59]. This includes contrast-induced, puncture and embolization related complications. The reported complications related to the embolization include foot ischemia, bladder necrosis, rectal wall necrosis, nerve injury and uterine necrosis. These complications are caused by non-targeted vessel embolization.

Uterine necrosis after arterial embolization was reported in one patient where the PVA particles of 150 μ–250 μ were used. It seems clear that this complication occurred due to the small size of the particles, causing distal embolization that led to myometrium ischemia [59]. We have been using PVA or Embosphere particles with a size range of 500–700 μ and 700–900 μ. No complications have occurred in our latest 21 patients. Recently, a case of both uterus and bladder necrosis was reported when using Gelfoam. The complication became evident 3 weeks after embolization [60]. The embolic agent was obtained by scraping the Gelfoam with a surgical blade, and the resulting product was then injected into the vessel. Deep embolization with smaller particles obtained in this way is the cause of this adverse event.

9.11 Conclusion

The selective transcatheter technique for embolization of uterine and/or internal iliac arteries in the management of intractable bleeding after delivery is safe and effective. In order to create the best hemodynamic and clinical conditions for this therapy, a strong multidisciplinary collaboration is essential to optimize clinical outcomes.

References

1. El-Rafey, Rodeck C (2003) Post partum hemorrhage: definitions, medical and surgical management. A time for change. Br Med Bull 67:205–217
2. Chichakli LO, Atrash HK, Mackay AP, Musani AS, Berg BJ (1999) Pregnancy-related mortality in the United Stats due to hemorrhage: 1979–1992. Obstet Gynecol 94:721
3. World Health Organization (1989) Preventing maternal deaths. WHO, Geneva, pp 107–136
4. World Health Organization (1991) Maternal mortality. A global fact book. WHO, Geneva pp 3–16
5. Levy G (2001) Rapport national du comité d'experts sur la mortalité maternelle 1995–2001. Ministère de la santé, May 2001
6. Velling TE, Brennan FJ, Hall LD, Watabe JT (2000) Role of the interventional radiologist in treating obstetric-gynecologic pathology. AJR Am J Roentgenol 175:1273–1278
7. Abada HT, Golzarian J, Richecoeur J, Muray JM, Garance P (2003) The role of interventional radiology in obstetric and gynecology (Abstract). Am J Roentgenol Vol 180(3):104
8. Brown BJ, Heaston DK, Poulson A et al. (1979) Uncontrollable postpartum bleeding: a new approach to hemostasis through angiographic arterial embolization. Obstet Gynecol 54:361–365
9. Heaston DK, Mineau DE, Brown BJ, Miller FJ jr. (1979) Transcatheter arterial embolization for control of persistent massive puerperal hemorrhage after bilateral surgical hypogastric artery ligation. AJR Am J Roentgenol 133:152–154
10. Vedantham S, Goodwin SC, McLucas B, Mohr G (1997) Uterine artery embolization: an underused method of controlling pelvic hemorrhage. Am J Obstet Gynecol 176:938–948
11. Waterstone M, Bewley S, Wolfe C (2001) Incidence and predictors of severe obstetric morbidity: case-control study. Br Med J 322:1089–1094
12. Baskett TF (1999) Complications of the third stage of labour. In: Essential Management of Obstetrical Emergencies, 3rd ed. Clinical Press, Bristol, England 196–201
13. Cunningham FG, Gant NF, Leveno KJ et al. (eds) (2001) Conduct of normal labor and delivery. In: Williams Obstetrics, 21st ed. McGraw-Hill, New York, pp 320–325
14. Schuurmans N, MacKinnon K, Lane C, Etches D (2000) Prevention and management of postpartum haemorrhage. J Soc Obstet Gynaecol Can 22:271–281
15. Bick RL (2000) Syndromes of disseminated intravascular coagulation in obstetrics, pregnancy, and gynecology.

Objective criteria for diagnosis and management. Hematol Oncol Clin of North Am 14:999–1043

16. Sperry K (1986) Amniotic fluid embolism: to understand enigma. JAMA 255:2183

17. Ko SF, Lin H, Ng SH, Lee TY, Wan YL (2002) Postpartum hemorrhage with concurrent massive inferior epigastric artery bleeding after cesarean delivery. Am J Obstet Gynecol 187:243–244

18. Worthington-Kirsch RL (2000) Anatomy of the uterine artery. AJR Am J Roentgenol 174:258

19. Pelage J, LeDref O, Soyer P et al. (1999) Arterial anatomy of the female genital tract: variation and relevance to transcatheter embolization of the uterus. AJR Am J Roentgenol 172:989–994

20. Redlich A (1909) Die verwendung der x-strahlen fur das studium des arteriellen systems der inneren weiblichen genitalien. Arch Anat u Physiol 33:357

21. Clemente CD (ed.) (1985) Anatomy of the human body (Gray's anatomy), 30th American ed. Lea & Febiger, Philadelphia, p 752

22. Levi CS, Holt SC, Lyons EA, Lindsay DJ, Dashefsky SM (2000) Normal anatomy of the female pelvis. In: Callen PW (ed) Ultrasonography in obstetrics and gynecology, 4th ed. Saunders, Philadelphia, pp 781–813

23. Razavi MK, Wolanske KA, Hwang GL, Sze DY, Kee ST, Dake MD (2002) Angiographic classification of ovarian artery-to-uterine artery anastomoses: initial observations in uterine fibroid embolization. Radiology 224:707–712

24. Saraiya PV, Chang TC, Pelage JP, Spies JB (2002) Uterine artery replacement by the round ligament artery: an anatomic variant discovered during uterine artery embolization for leiomyomata. J Vasc Interv Radiol 13:939–941

25. LeDref O, Pelage J, Kardache M et al. (2000) Superselective embolization of ovarian and round ligament arteries in the management of obstetric menorrhea. Cardiovasc Intervent Radiol 23:103

26. Jackson KW Jr, Allbert JR, Schemmer GK, Elliot M, Humphrey A, Taylor J (2001) A randomized controlled trial comparing oxytocin administration before and after placental delivery in the prevention of postpartum hemorrhage. Am J Obstet Gynecol 185:873–877

27. Stones RW, Paterson CM, Saunders NJ (1993) Risk factors for major obstetric haemorrhage. Eur J Obstet Gynecol Reprod Biol 48:15–18

28. Chichakli LO, Atrash HK, MacKay AP, Musani AS, Berg CJ (1999) Pregnancy-related mortality in the United States due to hemorrhage: 1979–1992. Obstet Gynecol 94:721–725

29. Combs CA, Murphy EL, Laros RK jr (1991) Factors associated with hemorrhage in cesarean deliveries. Obstet Gynecol 77:77–82

30. Ohkuchi A, Onagawa T, Usui R et al. (2003) Effect of maternal age on blood loss during parturition: a retrospective multivariate analysis 10,053 cases. J Perinat Med 31:209–215

31. Dubois J, Garel L, Grignon A, Lemay M, Leduc L (1997) Placenta percreta: balloon occlusion and embolization of the internal iliac arteries to reduce intraoperative blood losses. Am J Obstet Gynecol 176:723–726

32. Reyal F, Sibony O, Oury JF, Luton D, Bang J, Blot P (2004) Criteria for transfusion in severe postpartum hemorrhage: analysis of practice and risk factors. Eur J Obstet Gynecol Reprod Biol 112:61–64

33. Abada HT, Sapoval MR, Richecoeur J, Muray JM, Garance P (2002) Management by embolotherapy of intractable bleeding after delivery: the experience of two centers. Radiology 225:306–307

34. Oei PL, Chua S, Tan L, Ratnan, SS, Arulkumaran S (1998) Arterial embolization for bleeding following hysterectomy for intractable post partum hemorrjage. J Gynecol Obstet 62:83–86

35. Badawi SZ, Etman A, Singh M, Murphy K, Mayelli T, Philadelphia M (2001) Uterine artery embolization: the role in obstetric and gynecology. Clin Imaging 25:288–295

36. Greenwood LH, Glickman MG, Schwartz PE, Morse SS, Denny DF (1987) Obstetric and nonmalignant gynecologic bleeding: treatment with angiographic embolization. Radiology 164:155–159

37. Gilbert WM, Moore TR, Resnik R, Doemeny J, Chin H, Bookstein JJ (1992) Angiographic embolization in the management of hemorrhagic complications of pregnancy. Am J Obstet Gynecol 166:493–497

38. Mitty HA, Sterling KM, Alvarez M, Gendler R (1993) Obstetric hemorrhage: prophylactic and emergency arterial catheterization and embolotherapy. Radiology 188:183–187

39. Yamashita Y, Takahashi M, Ito M, Okamura H (1991) Transcatheter arterial embolization in the management of postpartum hemorrhage due to genital tract injury. Obstet Gynecol 77:160–163

40. Merland JJ, Houdart E, Herbreteau D et al. (1996) Place of emergency arterial embolisation in obstetric haemorrhage about 16 personal cases. Eur J Obstet Gynecol Reprod Biol 65:141–143

41. Pelage JP, Le Dref O, Mateo J et al. (1998) Life-threatening primary postpartum hemorrhage: treatment with emergency selective arterial embolization. Radiology 208:359–362

42. Deux JF, Bazot M, Le Blanche AF, Tassart M, Khalil A, Berkane N, Uzan S, Boudghene F (2001) Is selective embolization of uterine arteries a safe alternative to hysterectomy in patients with postpartum hemorrhage? AJR Am J Roentgenol 177:145–149

43. Descargues G, Douvrin F, Degre S et al. (2001) Abnormal placentation and selective embolization of the uterine arteries. J Obstet Gynecol Reprod Biol 99:47–52

44. Karpati PC, Rossignol M, Pirot M, Cholley B, Vicaut E, Henry P, Kevorkian JP, Schurando P, Peynet J, Jacob D, Payen D, Mebazaa A (2004) High incidence of myocardial ischemia during postpartum hemorrhage. Anesthesiology 100:30–36; discussion 5A

45. Vandelet P, Gilles R, Pease S et al. (2001) Limits to arterial embolization in the management of severe post partum hemorrhage. Ann Fr Anesth Reanim 4:317–324

46. Collins CD, Jackson JE (1995) Pelvic arterial embolization following hysterectomy and bilateral internal iliac artery ligation for intractable primary post partum hemorrhage. Clin Radiol 50:710–713

47. Stancato-Pasik A, Mitty HA, Richard HM 3rd, Eshkar N (1997) Obstetric embolotherapy: effect on menses and pregnancy. Radiology 204:791–3

48. Ornan D, White R, Pollack J, Tal M (2003) Pelvic embolization for intractable post partum hemorrhage: long term follow-up and implication for fertility. Obstet Gynecol 102:904–10

49. Salomon LJ, deTayrac R, Castaigne-Meary et al. (2003)

Fertility and pregnancy outcome following pelvic arterial embolization for severe post-partum haemorrhage. A cohort study. Hum Reprod 18:849–852

50. Cordonnier C, Ha Vien DE, Richard HM et al. (2002) Foetal growth restriction in the next pregnancy after uterine artery embolization for post partum hemorrhage. Eur J Obstet Gynecol Reprod Biol 103:183–184

51. McLucas B, Goodwin S, Adler L, Rappaport A, Reed R, Perrella R (2001) Pregnancy following uterine fibroid embolization. Int J Gynaecol Obstet 74:1–7

52. Goldberg J, Pereira L, Bergghella V (2002) Pregnancy after uterine embolization. Obstet Gynecol 100:869–872

53. Carpenter TT, Walker WJ (2005) Pregnancy following uterine artery embolization for symptomatic fibroids: a series of 26 completed pregnancies. BJOG 112:321–325

54. Ravina JH, Ciraru-Vigneron, Aymard A, Le Dreff O, Merland JJ (2000) Pregnancy after embolization of uterine myoma: report of 12 cases. Ferti Steril 73:1241–1243

55. Kidney D, Nguyen MA, Ahdoot D, Bickmore D, Deutsch LS, Majors C (2001) Prophylactic perioperative hypogastric artery balloon occlusion in abnormal placentation. AJR Am J Roentgenol 176:1521–1524

56. Sherman SJ, Greenspoon JS, Nelson JM, Paul RH (1992) Identifying the obstetric patient at high risk of multiple-unit blood transfusions. J Reprod Med 37:649–652

57. Hare WS, Holland CJ (1983) Paresis following internal iliac artery embolization. Radiology 146:47–51

58. Sieber PR (1994) Bladder necrosis secondary to pelvic artery embolization: case report and literature review. J Urol 151:422

59. Cottier JP, Fignon A, Tranquart F, Herbreteau D (2002) Uterine necrosis after arterial embolization for postpartum hemorrhage. Obstet Gynecol 100:1074–1077

60. Porcu G, Roger V, Jacquier A et al. (2005) Uterus and bladder necrosis after uterine artery embolisation for postpartum haemorrhage. BJOG 112:122–123

10 Fibroids

Gary P. Siskin, Jeffrey J. Wong, Anne C. Roberts, Jean Pierre Pelage,
Arnaud Fauconnier, Pascal Lacombe, Alexandre Laurent, and Jafar Golzarian

10.1 Uterine Fibroid Embolization: Practice Development

Gary Siskin

The practice model for interventional radiology is changing and nowhere is that more evident than in the care surrounding patients undergoing the uterine artery embolization procedure for symptomatic uterine fibroids. For many years, interventional radiologists have had it good. The techniques that we have worked to develop given our skill set and expertise have often been some of the most interesting and cutting-edge procedures performed within all of medicine. Given the minimally invasive nature of our specialty, physicians referred patients to us and relied on our expertise to deliver this state-of-the-art care to their patients. Problems arose when it became evident that we accepted very little responsibility towards delivering the pre-procedure and post-procedure care associated with these procedures and the disease processes bringing these patients to our attention. Physicians from a variety of specialties have learned that it is within their skill set to perform these procedures, and are doing so for obvious economic reasons but also because they have the infrastructure, training, and desire to follow these patients throughout an entire episode of care.

Interventional radiologists now understand that this practice model can no longer continue. Instead, interventionalists must accept a number of responsibilities, including generating referrals, providing the expertise to evaluate and prepare patients for our procedures, and caring for patients as they recover from our procedures.

Uterine fibroid embolization (UFE) represents one of the best examples of a procedure that can only become a successful part of an interventional practice if that practice is willing to take on the responsibilities inherent to this new model. In fact, generating referrals and providing pre- and post-

G. Siskin, MD
Associate Professor of Radiology and Obstetrics and Gynecology, Albany Medical Center, 47 New Scotland Avenue, MC-113, Albany, NY 12208–3479, USA

procedure care are mandatory components of a UFE practice. While most interventional radiologists would quickly state that this is not a radical departure for them and their style of practice, it is not until one becomes immersed in the nuances of this procedure and this patient population that the enormous nature of this commitment and the demands on one's time that are required for it to succeed can be understood.

The patients potentially served by UFE are different to those often seen within an interventional radiology practice because they are healthy people with a lifestyle-altering problem. Because these patients are electively choosing to seek medical care, they make demands on health-care providers that patients with greater morbidity often do not. In addition, this often represents the first time that these patients are seeking treatment for a medical problem. In today's world, with so much medical information available to patients on television, in newspapers, and on the internet, it is no wonder that these patients tend to present for their consultations already armed with a large amount of information regarding UFE and other treatment options for fibroids. In addition, women in general are known to be active participants in the decision-making process surrounding their health care and these patients are certainly no exception.

Interventionalists also have to become prepared to work with gynecologists since they are often the primary care providers for this patient population. Typically, gynecology patients do not require the services offered by interventional radiology. Therefore, gynecologists are not accustomed to referring patients to us. More importantly, they are not accustomed to having another specialty offer an effective treatment for a classic "female problem" that only they have treated in the past. It is clear that their first impression, as a specialty, has been to view UFE with skepticism and even as a threat to their practice. Therefore, gynecologists have not often been immediately forthcoming with referrals although recent acknowledgment by the American College of Obstetrics and Gynecology of the effectiveness or potential for effectiveness of this procedure has been indicative of the growing level of acceptance of this treatment option within the OB-GYN community.

Taking these characteristics into account, one can see that a potential conflict exists between well-informed patients desiring an active role in their own health-care, and gynecologists perceiving UFE as a threat to their practice and therefore not providing their patients with information about this procedure. This conflict forms the basis for the requirement that interventional radiologists participate in generating referrals for UFE because gynecologists are not, in general, going to help start a UFE service. However, it has been our experience that in time, once many UFE procedures have been performed at an institution with outcomes consistent with those reported nationally and internationally, gynecologists begin referring patients and contributing to the continued success of this service. This does take time and in our case, several years have passed between our first cases, when all patients were self-referred, and now, when the majority of cases are referred from our local and regional gynecologists. This trust was earned and grew largely from our ability to understand the above-stated conflict and to find ways to reach out directly to patients while at the same time educating gynecologists and assuring them that UFE will not lead to the demise of their practice.

The cornerstone of our practice development effort was the belief that the long-term success of a UFE service relies on cooperation from gynecologists. We do believe that patients are more informed than they have ever been about matters concerning health care and that they are indeed directing health care decisions. However, it must be acknowledged that most patients still receive their health-care information from their physicians. The relationship between a patient and her gynecologist is often one of trust and, therefore, patients still rely heavily on their advice. It is probably reasonable to assume that direct and aggressive patient advertising will almost certainly lead to a short-term increase in the number of UFE procedures performed by an interventional radiologist. Ultimately, however, it is our belief that gynecologists will not appreciate attempts at working around them and they will likely hurt your UFE practice by simply not supporting it.

With this in mind, we utilized several strategies for generating referrals to our UFE program: (1) education directed at gynecologists and patients regarding UFE; (2) education directed at ourselves regarding fibroids and treatment options for fibroids; (3) consistent support of the relationship between patients and their gynecologists; (4) care which meets the expectations of our patients and their gynecologists; and (5) accessibility for patients and gynecologists to the providers of this service. With this approach, we have earned referrals from local and regional gynecologists that are strongly supported by patient interest and positive word-of-mouth from patients going through UFE at our institution.

Our first task was to educate gynecologists about UFE. Interventional radiologists working within an academic institution may have an advantage here since they are more regularly exposed to educational activities. Offering lectures to medical students and residents concerning interventional radiology and its role in the care of OB-GYN patients is a first step that will likely lead to participation in journal clubs and departmental grand rounds. Our focus on educating students and residents was done with a clear understanding that educating students and residents will lead to future gynecologists that have a good understanding of the role of our services. This has a good chance of translating into long-term success since it is well known that after graduation, residents often remain in the region near where they have trained. Education efforts, however, were not just directed at trainees. Staff and community gynecologists often attend these meetings, providing us with an opportunity to make these physicians aware of what we can do for their patients. We also extended offers to provide lectures to physician groups in surrounding community hospitals in order to increase their awareness of this procedure as well and found that monthly staff meetings or grand rounds at community hospitals make an excellent forum for this type of presentation or discussion.

Once physicians became more informed about UFE, we recognized the importance of informing patients about this treatment option. Keeping the cornerstone of our practice development philosophy in mind, we recognized the challenge to increase patient knowledge without directly advertising and therefore inviting the perception that we do not need gynecology. We utilized the public relations department in our own hospital to help us with this. Once we had just a few patients who had a successful outcome after UFE, our hospital PR department brought these patients to the attention of our local news media. Every local newspaper and local television station has health reporters looking for stories of new and exciting breakthroughs in medical care and our community was no exception. Once we had patients with good stories to tell, these success stories were printed in newspapers and were made the subject of television news reports. It was our belief that these informative reports regarding this new procedure were not "direct advertising" yet had the same desired effect in reaching out to potential patients, making them aware of this option. Our efforts to educate our local gynecologists also enabled us to participate in patient-directed programs at community hospitals. Ultimately, we were able to meet our early goal to provide patients with the information necessary to ask their gynecologists questions regarding UFE, and to provide the information to gynecologists enabling them to answer those questions.

Efforts to educate both gynecologists and patients, however, are not enough. The final step in the education process involved the need to educate ourselves about uterine fibroids and the treatment options available to patients with fibroids. As relationships are established with gynecologists and patients suffering from symptomatic fibroids, it will become clear that knowledge about embolization is not enough. It is impossible to become an expert on UFE without knowing and understanding uterine fibroids and where UFE potentially fits into the management of these patients. Patients will undoubtedly ask you questions about the "other" options and they expect you to know the answers. Therefore, attending conferences and reading books and articles about fibroids will be an important part of a practice development strategy. Reading should not be limited to medical journals and textbooks. Books written for the lay population should also represent mandatory reading because these are the books that your patients are reading. Similarly, familiarity with commonly visited web-sites and chat groups is necessary because this is where patients today are often receiving their medical information.

While education has always been an important component of our efforts to develop this part of our practice, providing care that meets and exceeds the expectations of our patients and our referring physicians is arguably more important for the long-term success of a UFE service. Acceptable outcomes and future referrals are dependent on our ability to provide excellent patient care and we strive to reach that goal at every step of the process. That is because good outcomes speak for themselves.

Meeting the expectations of referring gynecologists is fairly straightforward. Gynecologists expect that UFE will be offered to patients with the highest probability of success and that we will achieve the success that we claim can be expected with this procedure. Therefore, familiarity with expected outcomes is mandatory for interventional radiologists as is a fair assessment of a patient's probability of success with this procedure. Gynecologists also expect that their patients will be comfortable during the procedure and that these procedures are performed with an appropriate level of expertise. We have therefore encouraged all gynecologists to observe procedures performed on their patients. Every gynecologist who has taken us up on that offer has consistently referred patients to us. Gynecologists also expect reliable communication with our office so that they are aware when a patient is considering this procedure, has undergone the procedure, and has demonstrated clinical improvement.

When gynecologists refer patients to interventional radiology for UFE, they are doing so with the understanding that everything surrounding the UFE procedure will be managed by the interventionalists, including insurance pre-approval, hospital admission, pain management, and initial assessment in the event of a complication. There is no reason why any interventional radiologist cannot observe a patient overnight (if necessary) and provide pain management services during a patient's recovery from UFE. It is perfectly acceptable to consult anesthesia as pain management protocols are developed but it is not acceptable to perform this procedure and then rely on gynecologists to manage the pain experienced during recovery. No, we cannot perform a hysterectomy in the event of a complication requiring that procedure. We can, however, assess that patient, communicate with their gynecologist if we suspect a complication, and maintain an appropriate level of involvement in that patient's care during the management of that complication (facilitating imaging and researching questions that arise during these episodes). By taking on these responsibilities, we will earn our place as legitimate providers of this service. If an interventional radiologist is not willing to take on these responsibilities, then it is unreasonable to expect referrals since most of the hard work still rests on the shoulders of the gynecologist.

In our experience, meeting the expectations of the patients has been more challenging. As a result, we have changed a lot about the way we practice and have carried these changes over to virtually all aspects of our interventional radiology practice. Patients expect to be seen by a physician in consultation before any management decisions are made and any procedures are performed. For decades, interventional radiologists were performing procedures that are essentially equivalent to surgery without ever meeting their patient outside of a brief pre-procedure visit immediately before the procedure started. Today, this cannot be tolerated and patients being considered for UFE must be seen in consultation first and we believe that this is best performed in a true outpatient clinic setting in order to meet the expectations of our patients.

In order to effectively participate in clinical patient management, interventionalists require an infrastructure within their practice to manage patients in both the inpatient and outpatient setting. One would be hard-pressed to find a clinical specialty that does not consider space designed exclusively for establishing, maintaining, and fostering the physician–patient relationship a priority for their clinical practice. Most radiologists, however, work within hospital departments or outpatient imaging centers that are not optimized for "non-imaging" outpatient consultations. Therefore, interventional radiologists seeking to develop this type of outpatient practice will need to overcome this obstacle by finding appropriate space either within or outside the hospital setting in order to evaluate patients in a true outpatient office.

An equally important expectation held by patients is the need for both expertise and compassion from their physician and the team making up an interventional practice. Attention must be paid to establishing rapport and communicating honestly and effectively with patients since this will form the basis of a successful doctor–patient relationship. Creating a good rapport with patients in an outpatient clinic setting will increase their comfort, enhancing the discussions about their medical history and treatment options. As technology has improved, most physicians often focus on diagnosing and treating the disease causing the patient to seek treatment. While this is of course a necessary component of any medical treatment, time should be set aside to understand how best to treat both the disease and the way that the disease has affected the patient's quality of life. As medical knowledge and technology have improved, most physicians, and perhaps interventionalists in particular, have become focused on diagnosing and treating disease. An interventionalist skilled at diagnosing and treating complex medical problems but understanding that disease and the procedures used to diagnose and treat disease have implications on a patient's quality of life, will have the insight necessary to successfully contribute to the overall care of their patients.

We have found it to be very helpful for our patients to make sure they have the opportunity to speak with a female nurse who is familiar with all aspects of this procedure and we have devoted the resources necessary to support nurse practitioners and a nurse clinician who are themselves experts in UFE and in the care of UFE patients. Nursing support is critical to success with UFE because it enables more patients to confide in our team regarding the true nature of their symptoms and as a result, the true nature of their expectations. Once these non-physician providers are integrated into a practice, the physicians must respect their role as the patient advocate within the practice and support them in the eyes of the patient so the patient is comfortable in their dealings with them and has confidence in utilizing all of the personnel resources within a cohesive practice.

It is also important to be accessible to patients to be willing to address their concerns before and after their UFE procedure. This requires a commitment on the part of an interventional radiology service because these patients do ask questions and do make demands on staff. There is no doubt that nursing staff dedicated to providing this type of care to these patients is critical for success. We have always tried to anticipate the needs and concerns of our patients and make it a rule to proactively call patients individually at defined times during the recovery period in order that they know we are there for them. In addition, a willingness on our part to address concerns via e-mail added a level of convenience not experienced by most patients and, in truth, is easier for us since focused answers to questions can be provided in very little time. When this part of our service runs smoothly, patients are almost uniformly impressed and very satisfied, which often leads to positive feedback to their gynecologist, family, and friends (all potential sources of future referrals).

By taking the "education" and "service" approach to practice development, we have been successfully moving towards our initial goal of having local and regional gynecologists mention UFE in the list of possible treatment options for uterine fibroids. It was and still has never been our expectation that every patient with fibroids gets referred for UFE. Including UFE in that list is a big step for most gynecologists but by no means assures you of referrals. It does, however, assure that patients will ask questions and gynecologists will need to provide answers. Even if a gynecologist still recommends hysterectomy for most patients, the mere fact that UFE is listed as an alternative to surgery will provide an option for patients looking for a nonsurgical treatment.

It has also never been our expectation to "take these patients away" from the gynecologist. We understand that nobody controls a patient. In fact, it is our belief that any group claiming to have "control" over a patient or group of patients is doing so because they have established the outpatient based practice that enables them to do so. Being confident in our ability to provide that service, we divert the focus away from "control", support the relationship between a patient and their gynecologist, and do not undermine that relationship in any way. Therefore, we communicate frequently with referring gynecologists and require that every patient be under the care of a gynecologist (preferably their own) before undergoing the UFE procedure. When patients tell us that they are angry with their gynecologist for not discussing UFE, we defend that gynecologist and explain that it takes time for any physician to feel comfortable recommending a new procedure. We would rather not have patients sever their relationship with a gynecologist because of UFE because, again, that does not bode well for the long-term success of our program and, more importantly, is not necessarily in the best interest of our patients. Yes, we are not happy when we hear that, but we look at it as an opportunity to communicate with this gynecologist, educate him or her about UFE, and add to the number of patients from that practice treated successfully with UFE.

We are pleased to report that the referral pattern for UFE has changed with time. As mentioned, most of our referrals now come from gynecologists instead of from the patients themselves. In addition, several practices in our area send almost all patients with fibroids to our office before treatment decisions are made, simply to educate them regarding all available treatment options. This has clearly exceeded our expectations. Most other practices may not be as forthcoming, but they are still willing to refer patients who are interested in nonsurgical alternatives and I believe that represents an achievable goal for any interventional radiologist interested in providing this service. Yes, there are still gynecologists in this area who deny all knowledge of this procedure (even with successful patients in their practice) but the number of physicians discouraging patients from UFE has dropped significantly.

Now, our task is to sustain this level of interest. We continue to provide the above-described level of care to our patients and continue to communicate frequently with referring gynecologists (with copies of letters always sent to primary care practitioners). We regularly participate in local health fairs in order to interact directly with referring physicians and potential patients. In our region, there is a women's health fair sponsored by ACOG and we are regular participants in that event. We believe this demonstrates our commitment to this service to the large number of gynecologists participating in this event and we also like to take advantage of events that will provide us with opportunities to interact with gynecologists face to face. We have also put together a summary of our own experience, which we sent out to all gynecologists in this region, both to continue with our education efforts and to establish ourselves as the experts in this region. We also continue to provide educational lectures to house-staff in gynecology and continue inviting students and residents to our lab to observe procedures. We have clearly not stopped with our efforts to develop this service.

In conclusion, a UFE service requires a level of commitment not typically required for other interventional radiology services. Without that commitment, success is not likely and you will quickly find that all parties participating in the care of these patients, including the patients themselves, expect this level of commitment. This effort, however, is not without its reward. UFE works and has a tremendous impact on both the disease process and the patient's overall quality of life. When you successfully treat a healthy patient with their first significant health problem, you have a high probability of making that patient very happy. This is what makes the effort worth it, especially when you begin noticing that most patients undergoing UFE are satisfied with their results. Gynecologists have already recognized the outcomes that are associated with UFE and making the effort that is described throughout this chapter will cause them to take notice and contribute to the development of a successful UFE practice.

10.2 Pre-op Work-Up and Post-op Care of Uterine Fibroid Embolization

Jeffrey J. Wong and Anne C. Roberts

CONTENTS

10.2.1
Introduction

10.2.1.1
Epidemiology

Uterine leiomyomata, also known as uterine fibroids, are the most commonly occurring pelvic tumor in women, occurring in 20%–40% of women aged 35 or older [51]. The size and prevalence increase with age until menopause, when they often regress in response to the decreasing hormone levels that occur. Women of African heritage not only have a 30% higher prevalence than white women [58], but also experience faster fibroid growth and onset at a younger age. Uterine leiomyomatas' high prevalence and significant symptoms ranging from pelvic bleeding to infertility represent a significant health issue in relatively young women.

J. J. Wong, MB ChB, BMedSc
Senior House Officer, Royal National Orthopaedic Hospital, London, UK
A. C. Roberts, MD
University of California, San Diego Medical Center, Division of Vascular and Interventional Radiology, 200 West Arbor Drive, San Diego, California, 92103-8756, USA

10.2.1.2
Traditional Therapies

Traditionally symptomatic fibroids have been treated either surgically or medically. Surgical treatments include hysterectomy, myomectomy (either by open procedure, laparoscopically or hysteroscopically), myolysis or endometrial ablation.

Hysterectomy is a definitive and curative treatment. In the US, more than 600,000 hysterectomies are performed per year, while in Europe the number varies from 73,000 in the UK to 200,000 in Germany. Over a third of those performed in the US are performed for symptomatic uterine fibroids [34, 56, 74, 107]. Most patients are pleased with the results of this procedure [51, 88] which not only removes the fibroids but also eliminates the potential risk of other uterine malignancies such as endometrial carcinoma. However, hysterectomy exposes the patient to standard anesthetic and surgical risks, a prolonged post-operative inpatient stay (2.3 days vs. 0.83 days for UAE [87]), and an prolonged time to return to work (33 days vs. 11 days [87]) and leaves the patient infertile. The morbidity ranges from 17%–23% [41, 59] dependent upon the approach and mortality of 10–20/1000 [33]. Common long-term complications include abdominal adhesions, sexual dysfunction, vaginal prolapse and urinary incontinence associated with laxity of pelvic musculature. Myomectomy involves surgically resecting the leiomyomata from the uterus, retaining potential for fertility. Myomectomy can be performed laparoscopically or hysteroscopically if the offending fibroid is on either the serosal or mucosal surfaces. It is, however, associated with excessive blood loss [53], a significant complication rate (25% vs. 11% for UAE [72]), a prolonged hospital stay (2.9 days vs. 0 days following UAE [72]) and a longer time to return to normal activities (36 days vs. 8 days following UAE [72]). It can be technically challenging and conversion to a more "invasive procedure" occurs in 5.4% of patients [93]. Myomectomy carries additional risks of rupture of the pregnant uterus and recurrence of the fibroids [28] (43% [30]).

Myolysis involves coagulating the serosal or submucosal fibroid through the use of hysteroscopically or laparoscopically placed probes that apply an electric current or laser directly to the fibroid, inducing shrinkage. This procedure does not carry the risks of an open laparotomy and can be done as a same-day surgery. Cryomyolysis is based on a similar concept only the fibroid is instead frozen with liquid nitrogen. Both procedures result in a loss of fertility.

The medical alternative involves hormonal manipulations with a variety of pharmaceuticals. Types of medications include oral contraceptives, NSAIDs and gonadotrophin releasing hormone (GnRH) analogues. The most common of these is Lupron, which is a GnRH analogue and blocks estrogen production artificially, creating a state of menopause. A woman initiated on a GnRH agonist has shrinkage of the fibroids, and a decrease in symptoms; however, after stopping the GnRH agonist the fibroids re-grow and the symptoms tend to recur. Therefore, GnRH agonists are usually reserved for those women nearing menopause or with planned surgery to aid intraoperatively. However, it has been shown that pre-treatment with a GnRH agonist has no significant effect on intraoperative blood loss [102].

MRI-guided focused ultrasound fibroid ablation is the newest of the non-invasive techniques and is still in the experimental stages. The ultrasound waves are directed from a transducer into a small focal volume. The tissue at the focal point receives condensed energy and increases in temperature, causing protein denaturation, cell death and coagulative necrosis. While a commercial device is available, long term data on this procedure does not yet exist [45].

The first report of uterine artery embolization (UAE) was in 1979 when embolization was used to stop postpartum bleeding [44, 63]. Since then, embolization in the setting of pelvic trauma, post-obstetric bleeding, ectopic pregnancy and AV malformations has been well documented. In 1994, RAVINA et al. [69] described pre-operative UAE prior to scheduled myomectomy for symptomatic fibroids with the intention of reducing intraoperative blood loss. However, reduction in patients' fibroid-related symptoms led to a number of patients deciding to forego surgery and the group then began to evaluate UAE as a definitive therapy. UAE is now a recognized alternative to traditional therapies and with the continued publication of high quality research demonstrating successful outcomes, UAE has become an alternative to the more traditional the uterus-sparing therapies for treating uterine fibroids.

10.2.2
Pathophysiology of Fibroids

Leiomyomata are benign neoplasms consisting of smooth muscle cells. Although the pathogenesis of fibroids is not well understood, several predisposing factors have been identified, including age (late reproductive years), African-American ethnicity, nulliparity, and obesity. The genetic basis for the strong predisposition to African-American women has yet to be mapped, but non-random tumor-specific cytogenetic abnormalities have been found in 25%–40% of pathological specimens [75]. Estrogen receptors are found on leiomyomata in a higher concentration than normal myometrial tissue [108] causing the fibroids to be responsive to the female sex hormones. Thus, with pregnancy, fibroids may enlarge [14, 57, 89] by up to 25% [2] and in the postmenopausal state, when estrogen levels fall, leiomyomata will decrease in size due to the reduced hormonal stimulation. Progesterone receptors have also been found in elevated levels in leiomyomata compared with myometrium [12, 81, 95, 108] and studies suggest a growth promoting effect [15, 32, 49]. Androgens may have a role in leiomyomata growth; 5-α androgens have been found in myoma biopsies, suggesting sensitivity to the hormone [73]. Clinical improvement is frequently seen when androgenic therapies such as danazol and gestrinone are used [22, 25], further supporting this theory.

Leiomyomata are vascular tumors and angiogenesis is vital to their growth. They have been shown to have more veins and arteries and greater vessel caliber than normal myometrium [29, 31]. One of these angiogenic growth factors, basic fibroblastic growth factor (bFGF), has been found in increased concentrations in the extracellular matrix of leiomyomatous tissues when compared with normal myometrium [60]. bFGF has been shown to stimulate mitogenic activity on both myometrial and leiomyomatous smooth muscle cells [54], while the receptor for bFGF has been found to be dysregulated in the leiomyomatous uterus [7].

Leiomyomas originate within the uterine wall, but can extend into the uterine cavity from the submucosal surface (see Fig. 10.2.1) and into the abdominal cavity from the subserosal surface. Like

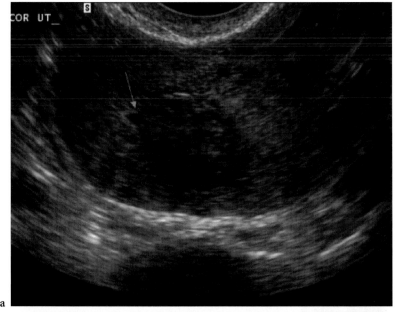

a

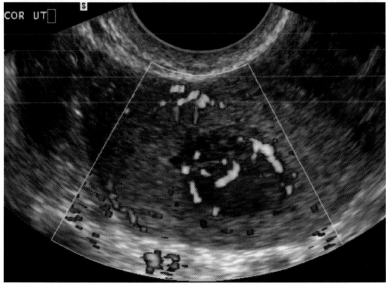

b

Fig. 10.2.1a,b. Sonographic appearance of a submucosal fibroid. **a** A well circumscribed hypoechoic round mass with some internal heterogeneity is characteristic of a leiomyoma. **b** Doppler can be used to show the hypervascularity of this benign tumor

polyps, these tumors can be flat or pedunculated (Fig. 10.2.2). Vascular supply comes primarily from the uterine arteries, a branch of the anterior division of the internal iliac artery, but collateral supply can arise from the ovarian arteries and the vesicovaginal arteries [61].

The mechanism by which fibroids cause abnormal uterine bleeding is not known. However, there have been several theories proposed. One theory claims that the increase in size of the endometrial surface area causes the bleeding and is therefore most pertinent to submucosal fibroids [91]. The increased vascularity and vascular flow to the uterus as a result of fibroids has also been held responsible

[91]. JHA et al. chose to measure vascularity as an indicator of success. They found that hypervascular tumors were more susceptible to UAE than hypovascular tumors [47]. Fibroid cellularity was studied by DESOUZA et al. who found that leiomyomas that were high in signal intensity on T2-weighted images prior to embolization showed a significantly greater reduction in volume at 4 months, compared with the leiomyomas that were low in signal intensity [27].

Another theory describes the ulceration of a submucosal fibroid into the endometrial surface [91]. The fibroids may compress the venous plexus within the myometrium which may lead to uterine engorgement and greater bleeding [91]. The latest

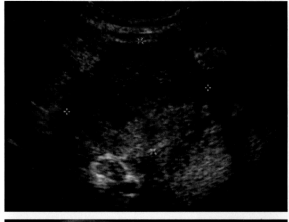

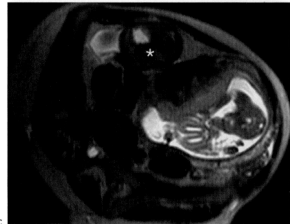

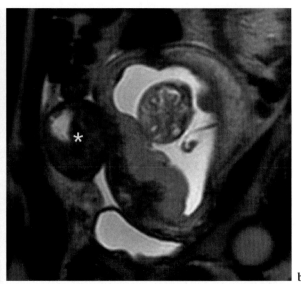

Fig. 10.2.2a–c. An 18-year-old female who is 17 weeks pregnant. Patient presents with right lower quadrant abdominal pain. **a** Ultrasound demonstrates a large heterogeneous mass. **b,c** Sagittal and axial views on MR demonstrate a pedunculated subserosal fibroid (*asterisk*). Regions of high attenuation within the fibroid indicate a degree of necrotic degeneration and torsion of the fibroid stalk was suspected. The patient was taken to the operating room at which time, a purple, torsed, pedunculated fibroid was found. The fibroid was torsed 360°

theory proposes that the dysregulation of several angiogenic growth factors or their receptors may be responsible for vascular abnormalities that lead to dysregulation of the vascular structures in the uterus and cause menorrhagia [90]. In a recent study that evaluated premenopausal women with and without abnormal bleeding, women with abnormal bleeding were significantly more likely to have either an intramural (58% vs. 13%) or submucosal leiomyoma (21% vs. 1%) when compared with asymptomatic women [19].

10.2.3
Symptoms (and Signs) of Fibroids (Including What Symptoms Should Prompt Treatment)

The most common symptom of uterine fibroids is abnormal uterine bleeding occurring in 30% of women with fibroids [16], which commonly causes anemia and is associated with fibroids located in the submucosa. The two abnormal bleeding patterns that are most commonly associated with uterine leiomyomas are an increase in the amount of blood loss per month, menorrhagia, and prolonged (>7 days) vaginal bleeding, otherwise known as metrorrhagia. Many women will experience both heavy and prolonged vaginal bleeding, commonly referred to as menometrorrhagia. Exceptionally heavy flow and the passage of clots is colloquially known as 'flooding'. Clinically, it is defined as total blood loss exceeding 80 ml per cycle or menses lasting longer than 7 days.

When large in volume, fibroids exert a mass effect on other pelvic structures such as the bladder, bowel and the lumbosacral plexus giving rise to symptoms of urinary frequency, abdominal distension, constipation, bloating, and back and leg pain. Gynecological symptoms include pelvic pain, miscarriages, menstrual cramps (subserosal and/or intramural tumors predominantly disturb uterine contractility), infertility, and dyspareunia. Unlike menorrhagia, fibroids must be large to cause this class/subset of symptoms. Therefore, patients who do not present with bleeding tend to have subserosal or intramural fibroids instead of submucosal fibroids. Studies have shown no difference in complication rate post-UAE in patients with large uteri (>780 cm³) or large fibroids (>10 cm diameter) compared with smaller uteri or fibroids [48, 68]. Control of menorrhagia post-UAE has also shown to be independent of initial uterine size or fibroid size [37, 48, 85]. There are a few studies that contradict this trend. JHA et al. observed that larger pre-treatment uterine volumes showed worse outcome. For every 100 cm³ increment in volume, they noticed volume reduction after UAE decreased by 20% [11]. Conversely, BRADLEY et al. noted good volume reductions in patients with particularly large fibroids [83].

Initial studies have shown that UAE can improve menorrhagia in 90% of patients at 1 year after therapy and pelvic pressure symptoms by 91% at 1 year after therapy [83]. On average, the volume of the fibroids decrease by 30%–60% and the associated symptoms (of mass effect) are successfully treated in 71% of patients [72]. A study comparing myomectomy to UAE suggests myomectomy is superior in treating symptoms relating to the pelvic mass effect while UAE is superior for treating menorrhagia [38].

Although fibroids are extremely common in the female population over 30 years of age, approximately 20%–40% of women with fibroids are symptomatic [16]. If the woman is asymptomatic no therapy would be warranted. If the woman is symptomatic, the options for treatment should be explained and the decision left to her.

10.2.4
Differential Diagnosis of Fibroids

It is imperative that other causes for presenting symptoms are excluded prior to decision to proceed with UAE. For menorrhagia, the differential diagnosis includes adenomyosis (Fig. 10.2.3) and a range of endometrial disorders. Endometrial carcinoma is an absolute contraindication to UAE (Fig. 10.2.4) and all women with endometrial bleeding should be investigated with endometrial biopsy to try and exclude endometrial cancer. Endometrial polyps are benign nodular protrusions of the endometrial surface that are a common cause of dysfunctional uterine bleeding and abnormal endometrial thickening, a sonographic feature shared with endometrial carcinoma. MRI or hysteroscopy have been shown to

be more specific at distinguishing between these two diagnoses [39].

Adenomyosis causes similar symptomatology as fibroids with menorrhagia, enlargement of the uterus and pelvic pain. Characterized by the ectopic growth of endometrial tissue in the myometrium, adenomyosis causes diffuse enlargement of the uterus [64] and has been suggested to predispose the patient to clinical failure after UAE [55, 65]. However, SISKIN et al. [80] showed symptomatic improvement in 12 of 13 patients (92.3%) who underwent UAE for adenomyosis. They also noticed significant reductions in the median uterine volume (42%), median fibroid volume (71%), and mean junctional zone thickness (33%) [80]. In our practice, we have seen clinical improvement in a patient with concurrent adenomyosis (Fig. 10.2.5) and leiomyomas. Endovaginal ultrasound can be used to detect thickening of the endometrial stripe and the ill-defined hypoechoic areas characteristic of adenomyosis, unless performed meticulously, can be inaccurate and MRI is the imaging modality of choice to make this diagnosis.

The symptoms of mass effect may be caused by other processes that should be excluded. The first symptoms of ovarian carcinoma, another contraindication to UAE, are usually a result of its significant mass effect. As such a large tumor size is required before symptoms are evident, ovarian carcinomas tend to be in the advanced stages on presentation.

Leiomyosarcomas are malignant tumors of the uterus with an incidence of less than 0.3% in fibroid uteri [42], and present with similar symptoms and radiologic presentations to that of benign disease

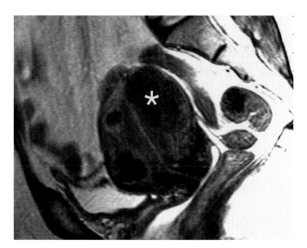

Fig. 10.2.3. T2-weighted sagittal non-breath hold image of the pelvis shows a 53-year-old female with focal adenomyoma (*asterisk*) and concurrent fibroids

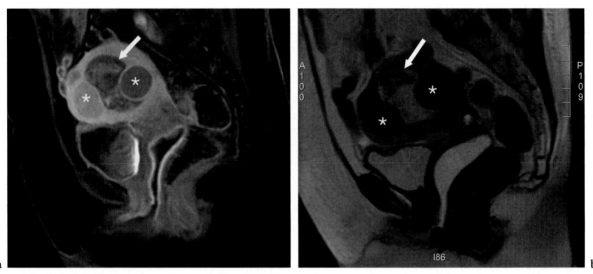

Fig. 10.2.4a,b. A 70-year-old female with endometrial carcinoma and fibroids. **a** Delayed post-gadolinium T1-weighted sagittal image of the pelvis. The *asterisks* indicate two submucosal fibroids. Note the difference in signal intensity between them. The higher signal indicates greater vascularity, while the reduced signal intensity necrosis. An endometrial carcinoma is seen at the fundus of the uterus (*arrow*). **b** T2-weighted sagittal fast-spin echo non-breath hold image of the pelvis. Two submucosal fibroids are seen adjacent to the uterine cavity. The tumor margins of the endometrial carcinoma (*arrow*) are more clearly seen with the distinct increase in signal intensity at the uterine cavity

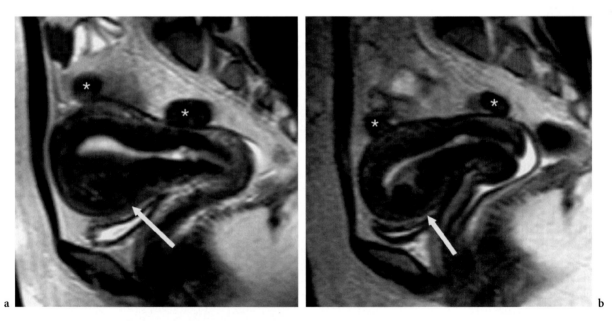

Fig. 10.2.5a,b. These sagittal T2-weighted images demonstrate diffuse adenomyosis with two subserosal fibroids. **a** Pre UAE, the characteristic punctuate markings seen in diffuse adenomyosis (*white arrow*) can be seen with two fibroids (*asterisks*). **b** Post UAE, the adenomyosis has decreased in size

[43]. Unfortunately, it is currently impossible to distinguish these tumors from benign leiomyomata without pathologic examination. One paper has suggested that Doppler US shows higher peak systolic velocity within leiomyosarcoma as compared to leiomyomata [5, 21] while there are several reports of using MRI to distinguish between benign and malig-

nant disease [77]. As current literature suggests that leiomyosarcomas do not respond to embolotherapy [40] and metastasize early with a poor prognosis (20% 5-year survival with any extra-uterine spread) [109], this undetectable malignant diagnosis is an understandable concern. However, one must consider the low prevalence in comparison to the mortality of hysterectomy for benign disease excluding pregnancy (1:1600) [78]. Continued fibroid growth after the cessation of estrogen stimulation (e.g. menopause) should raise suspicion of leiomyosarcoma and should be investigated with needle biopsy [13, 47]. Likewise, if rapid interval growth is seen following UAE, the suspicion of malignancy should be raised.

The differential diagnosis of pelvic pain is wide and includes ovarian vein varices, pelvic infection and endometriosis. Untreated pelvic infections are an absolute contraindication to UAE. They are a known cause of a hydrosalpinx a collection of fluid in the fallopian tube and a recognized cause of infertility. This diagnosis is best established on hysterosalpingography.

Evaluating patients with symptoms of fibroids can be challenging and is best approached by working in conjunction with the patient's gynecologist. A good working relationship with gynecologists is important for the work-up of patients and ensures UAE is an appropriate choice of treatment.

10.2.6
Pre-procedure Evaluation

The first step in the interventionalist's evaluation of a woman with fibroids is a detailed patient history. The patient should have a gynecologic examination, either prior to seeing the interventionalist or should be referred to a healthcare professional with expertise in gynecologic care. Patients should have had a recent Papanicolaou smear of the cervix and if menorrhagia is a presenting symptom, then an endometrial biopsy should be performed to rule out neoplasm. Baseline laboratory tests should include CBC and renal function. The pre-procedure assay of follicle stimulating hormone (FSH) levels may be pertinent, but is not currently routine practice.

The role of imaging in uterine fibroids is not only to characterize the number, type and size of the tumors, but also to screen for other causes of the presenting symptoms. Ultrasound is typically the initial imaging modality used in the work-up of uterine fibroids, but it is subject to operator variability and therefore lacks reproducibility (Fig. 10.2.2). Ultrasound is best suited as a screening test for fibroids and to exclude any obvious pelvic pathology. MRI not only provides the consistency required for post-procedure comparisons [13, 26], but also reliably excludes adenomyosis and all but stage I carcinomas of the endometrium [13]. At our institution the same MR sequences are used pre and post UAE and are described in Table 10.2.1.

Some investigators have assessed the arterial supply to the uterus with dynamic gadolinium-enhanced three-dimensional fast imaging with steady-state precession MR angiography [47]. It is clear that imaging aids not only with diagnosis, but also provides information that can be used to predict outcome of UAE.

One of the first details noted is the location of the fibroid. A 31-patient study showed that submucosal fibroids displayed 30%–40% greater reduc-

Table 10.2.1. MR imaging sequences pre and post uterine artery embolization

Coronal haste from the mid kidneys to the symphysis pubis
Sagittal T2 turbo spin echo (TSE) BH – 6 mm skip zero
Sagittal T2 TSE non-BH – 6 mm skip zero
Axial oblique T1 2D FLASH. BH DE IP and OP (perpendicular to the endometrial stripe) – 6 mm skip zero
Axial oblique T2 BH (same slice thickness and angle as oblique T1) – 6 mm skip zero
Straight axial T2 BH – 8 mm skip zero
Following hand injection of 20 ml gadolinium via butterfly needle
Sagittal T1 2D FLASH BH IP FS as above.
Axial oblique T1 2D FLASH BH IP FS (perpendicular to the endometrial stripe)
Straight axial T1 2D FLASH BH FS (for easier communication)
For those who do not respond to uterine artery embolization:
Same sequences as above, except with MRA+MRV ensuring gonadal arteries are included using 40 mls of gadolinium
Coronal 3D FLASH BH 2 mm skip zero. Arterial, portal venous, delayed phases
Post-processing using subtractions and MIPS
BH, breath hold; DE, double echo; IP, in phase; OP, out of phase; FS, fat saturation.

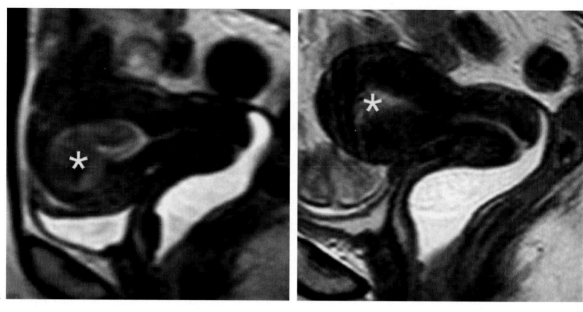

Fig. 10.2.6a,b. A 35-year-old female with a submucosal fibroid. **a** T2-weighted sagittal image of the pelvis shows a submucosal fibroid (*asterisk*) enlarging the endometrial cavity. Note the low signal intensity on T2-weighted images as well as the broad base on the endometrial wall. This was taken just prior to UAE. **b** T2-weighted sagittal image of the pelvis performed 1 year later post UAE. Note the fibroid previously seen has virtually disappeared

tion in volume when compared with intramural or subserosal fibroids [47] (Fig. 10.2.6). This could be explained by the vascular anatomy of the fibroid which favors distribution of the embolization particles to the inner aspect of the uterus, i.e. the submucosal surface [8]. However, their close proximity to pathogens in the uterine cavity has been hypothesized to account for their increased incidence of infective complications [97].

BURN et al. [13] studied the relationship between signal intensity characteristics on MR and total percentage volume reduction in 17 post-UAE patients. They noted that, on T1-weighted images, tumors showing signal intensity brighter than that of myometrium compared with those of lower intensity than myometrium showed poor response to UAE ($p=0.008$), also reported by JHA et al. [47]. This MR characteristic is thought to result from hemorrhagic necrosis and the presence of blood breakdown products. Therefore, if seen in a fibroid pre-UAE, it likely has already undergone degeneration and loss of vascular supply and will not respond well to embolization.

Meanwhile, on T2-weighted images, tumor intensity brighter than that of skeletal muscle compared to those equal to or lower than that of skeletal muscle was predictive of good response ($p=0.007$), echoed also by DESOUZA and WILLIAMS [27]. High

signal on T2-weighted images was presumed to be due to increased fibroid cellularity and/or vascularity [13].

The indications and contraindications for UAE are summarized in Table 10.2.2.

Table 10.2.2. A summary of the contraindications to UAE

Absolute contraindications	Relative contraindications
Asymptomatic fibroids	Coagulopathy
Pregnancy	Immunocompromised
Pelvic active infection	Contrast allergy
	Renal impairment

10.2.7
What is the Place of Embolization in Patients Desiring Pregnancy?

Currently, UAE is not recommended as the first line of therapy in patients with infertility presumed to be caused by fibroids. Patients in whom fibroids are not symptomatic but who are infertile, should be evaluated for other causes of infertility and, if fibroids are the cause, the potential for myomectomy. In patients who are symptomatic from the fibroids (menorrhagia, bulk symptoms) and whom myomectomy is not an option, UAE should be attempted before proceeding with a hysterectomy as UAE may adversely affect fertility.

Vascular anastomotic communications between the uterine and ovarian arteries provide a route by which embolization materials can affect the ovarian blood supply and ovarian function, either permanently or temporarily [71]. One case report describes embolic microspheres found within the ovarian arterial vasculature of a pathological specimen following uneventful UAE [66]. Unintentional embolization of the ovarian arteries is theorized to cause ovarian failure. However, the incidence of ovarian failure post UAE is no different to hysterectomy [100]. In fact, it is not clear whether UAE has any effect on ovarian function at all. There are studies that support its lack of effect [3, 17, 99, 100] and a few case reports that document transient or permanent amenorrhea [92, 98].

It is thought that the ovarian arteries shrink with age leading to increased ovarian dependence upon uterine-tubal anastomoses [9]. This may explain an increased chance (from 0% incidence compared with 21%) of ovarian failure post UAE in patients aged 45 years or older [18]. A similar study looking at basal FSH after UAE showed a significantly increased risk of perimenopausal FSH levels in patients older than 45 years [84]. Thus, older women appear to be more at risk of losing their ovarian function than younger women.

Uterine devascularization is another proposed mechanism. Devascularization has been reported in one case [98] to cause endometrial atrophy resulting in persistent amenorrhea. Endometritis secondary to a perivascular necrotizing arteritis has been seen following UAE with gold-colored gelatin microspheres, however, as an eosinophilic component was seen in this patient, a hypersensitivity reaction to the gold could have been the cause [76]. It has been theorized that a devascularized endometrial lining may not be able to support a term pregnancy [23], however, there are two reports of twins pregnancies delivered at term [35, 70] where the endometrial vascular reserve would have been tested.

A paper published in 2004 quoted 53 published pregnancies worldwide following UAE [36] and concluded that compared with those with prior laparoscopic myomectomy, pregnancies following UAE were at increased risk for preterm delivery and malpresentation (Table 10.2.3). However, an earlier paper by the same authors comparing pregnancies following UAE to those of the normal obstetric population concluded the miscarriage and complication rate was higher following UAE [35], but noted that the UAE population is not directly comparable, not least due to the older average age, a similar difference also seen in the laparoscopic myomectomy group. In fact, one study showed no difference at all [79]. Other smaller studies have not demonstrated a difference in obstetric complications.

If left untreated, pregnancies in women with known leiomyoma have higher caesarian section rates (39%) and antepartum hemorrhage (>500 ml) rates (48%) [52]. One study has shown the incidences of preterm delivery (less than 37 weeks), preterm premature rupture of membranes, in utero growth retardation (less than 5th percentile), placental abruptio, placenta previa, postpartum hemorrhage (more than 500 cc), and retained placenta are not significantly increased in women with myomas compared with the general population [103]. However, in this study cesarean sections were significantly more common in women with myomas (23% vs. 12%).

Table 10.2.3. Prevalence of obstetric complications seen in the general population, those following UAE and those following laparoscopic myomectomy

Complication	General population (%)	UAE (n/N)		LM (n/N)		Odds ratio	95% Cl	p Value
Spontaneous abortion	10–15	12/51	(24%)	20/133	(15%)	1.7	0.8–3.9	0.175
Postpartum hemorrhagea	4–6	2/35	(6%)	1/104	(1%)	6.3	0.6–71.8	0.093
Preterm deliverya	5–10	5/32b	(16%)	3/104	(3%)	6.2	1.4–27.7	0.008
Cesarean deliverya	22	22/35	(63%)	61/104	(59%)	1.2	0.5–2.6	0.662
Small for gestational agea	10	1/22c	(5%)	8/95c	(8%)	0.5	0.1–4.4	0.541
Malpresentationa	5	4/35	(11%)	3/104	(3%)	4.3	1.0–20.5	0.046

It must be remembered that the presence of normal hormonal assays and normal menstruation are not the only factors that assure a successful pregnancy. Further studies must be performed before UAE can be regarded as a safe procedure for women desiring future fertility.

10.2.8
Consent

When obtaining consent for UAE, we cover the potential sequelae listed in Table 10.2.4.

Table 10.2.4. Complications discussed when obtaining consent for UAE

1. Complications associated with placing catheters
Bleeding
Hematoma
Infection of catheter site
2. Complications associated with angiographic procedure
Contrast reaction
Exacerbation of renal insufficiency
3. Complications associated with embolization procedure
Damage vessels requiring surgery (dissection, plaque disruption, extravasation)
Embolization of structures other than uterus – lead to bowel ischemia, bladder ischemia, nerve or muscle ischemia, skin
Ovarian failure
4. Infection of uterus requiring hysterectomy
5. Failure of procedure to correct symptoms

10.2.9
Post-procedure Care of Patient

The post-procedure period consists of hospitalization and the outpatient follow-up. Inpatient stays typically are less than 24 h, so the majority of the patient care will be on an outpatient basis. There have been some reports of patients being successfully treated on an outpatient basis [86]; however, in most practices a short hospitalization seems to be preferred by most patients. Using a study of 400 patients Spies et al. reported a comprehensive list of complications, some of which are shown in Table 10.2.5 [20].

Crampy pelvic pain commonly occurs within the first 24 h of UAE and is usually controlled with a patient controlled analgesia (PCA) pump using morphine or another narcotic. Patients should be placed on an anti-inflammatory prior to the embolization and while in the hospital. Toradol intravenously prior to the embolization and during the hospitalization appears to be very effective. It is reasonable to develop a set of standard orders that the patient will receive to cover the most common eventualities.

Patients should be warned pain is the most common reason for re-admission [105]. On discharge, analgesia is switched to oral medications, consisting of non-steroidal anti-inflammatories (NSAIDs) and narcotics. The NSAIDs should be taken around the clock for approximately 10 days with narcotics used as needed. The peak of the pain usually occurs during the first 8–12 h although once they are discharged from the hospital, their pain may be more troublesome for the first day home and will gradually resolve within the next week. If, after improvement of the initial post-procedure pain, the patient develops recurrence of pain, she should immediately report back to the interventionalist since this can represent infection or possibly fibroid expulsion.

Nausea is also a common side effect of UAE and can be accentuated by the narcotic analgesia. Antiemetic medication should therefore be routinely prescribed. Transdermal scopolamine placed behind the ear prior to beginning the procedure may be helpful in decreasing the amount of nausea.

Post-embolization syndrome should be expected in all patients post UAE and consists of low-grade fever, malaise, nausea and leukocytosis. It can occur

Table 10.2.5. Complications seen in UAE

Complication	Percentage (%) prevalence
Leiomyoma passage	10
Recurrent/prolonged pain	5
Urinary tract infection	4
Endometritis	2
Femoral nerve injury	3
Arterial injury	3
Urinary retention	2
Vaginal discharge	4
Hematoma	1
Deep vein thrombosis	1
Pulmonary embolism	1

anytime after the procedure from a few hours to a few days and requires only symptomatic treatment. This can lead to a diagnostic dilemma as uterine infection, a complication that may lead to hysterectomy, also presents with a fever. If a sudden rise in temperature to greater than 38.5° occurs with increasing pain, one should suspect infectious etiology and admit the patient for further investigations and possible antibiotic therapy and appropriate interventions [24, 101]. Two patients have died from fatal pelvic sepsis post UAE [104]. The common findings between these cases were a symptom-free period after UAE and presentation with a 24 h history of gastrointestinal symptoms. Antibiotic therapy was too late to prevent overwhelming sepsis. The source of the infection in these cases was a necrotic uterus.

Like hormonal treatments for fibroids, UAE has also been known to cause amenorrhea. Two studies totaling 650 patients showed that at 12–16 months post UAE, between 94% [86] and 98% [6, 82] had normal menses, respectively. There has also been reported transient episodes of amenorrhea and menopausal symptoms [86].

Thromboembolic complications including pulmonary embolism, deep vein thrombosis and arterial thrombosis [67] have been reported. There have been two deaths from pulmonary embolism [62]. One study chronicled blood coagulation markers post-UAE [1, 10]. This showed that prothrombin fragment 1.2, plasmin-α_2-antiplasmin complex and thrombin-antithrombin complex increased as a result of UAE, suggesting that a prothrombotic state may result after the procedure. Prophylactic treatment with anticoagulation or venous compression devices may be appropriate for patients thought to be at higher risk for thromboembolic complications, such as exogenous sources of oestrogen or a history of thromboembolic events. In most patients early ambulation and NSAIDs are probably sufficient to prevent thromboembolic complications.

In some patients a chronic vaginal discharge lasting longer than 2 months and described as a "major irritant" occurs following UAE. This has been reported by WALKER and PELAGE [104] to occur in 4% of patients. In another report WALKER et al. [106] describes this vaginal discharge to be caused by a persisting sinus that connected a superficial necrotic excavation within the fibroid to the endometrial cavity through a perforation in the endometrium. This results in a slow persistent drainage of necrotic material into the uterus and subsequently the vagina [106]. There were 16 patients with a chronic vaginal discharge that were treated with hysteroscopic opening of the sinus and resection of the necrotic tissue. Following the procedure 94% of the women were either completely cured or had a very mild discharge [106].

The passage of leiomyoma tissue commonly occurs with those fibroids in contact with the endometrial surface. This phenomenon has been seen up to 12 months after the UAE procedure. This symptom is associated with significant pain, bleeding and most importantly, infection [86]. In cases of suspected fibroid expulsion, MRI should be performed as many fibroids do not pass through the cervix spontaneously or remain attached to the uterine wall and therefore require dilatation and curettage.

Once discharged, between 3.5% [20] and 10% [86] of patients return to the emergency department, with between 4% [20] and 6% [72] requiring re-admission. If a patient is re-admitted, it is essential that someone from the interventional team be available by telephone or pager during their stay. Current literature quotes between 8 days [20, 83, 104] and 17 days [87] time required from work/time to recovery [20] (see Table 10.2.6).

Table 10.2.6. Hospital stay, returns, and re-admissions after embolization [27]

Hospital stay (nights)[a]	Number of patients (%)[b]
0	12 (2)
1	438 (80)
2	70 (13)
≥3	28 (5)
Mean hospital stay (range)	1.3 nights (0–11)
Inadequate length of hospital stay	66 (12)
Indications for LOS >1 night	98 (18)
Pain/nausea/vomiting	75 (14)
Pain/fever	16 (3)
Hypertension	3 (0.6)
Respiratory depression	1 (0.1)
Aspiration pneumonia	1 (0.1)
Pulmonary edema	1 (0.1)
Seizure	1 (0.1)
Dissatisfaction with interventional care	17 (3)
Dissatisfaction with ward care	70 (13)

[a] Those staying 3 nights or longer: 17 for 3 nights, four for 4 nights, three for 5 nights, two for 6 nights, one for 7 nights and one for 11 nights.

[b] Values in parentheses are percentages unless otherwise indicated.

As a routine, patients should be followed-up either by phone or in clinic at 24–48 h and 1–3 weeks after discharge to monitor symptom control and screen for early complications.

10.2.10
Unusual Complications in Individual Case Reports

There are a few unique complications reported following UAE. One case describes a 27-year-old woman who, 3.5 years post UAE presents with recurrence of dysmenorrhea and menorrhagia which was thought to be due to retained fragments of calcified fibroids seen on ultrasound [96]. Passage of these fragments resulted in resolution of her recurrent symptoms.

Another case features a transient necrotic-appearing area on the right labium minus 5 days post UAE in a 38-year-old woman [110]. This was thought to be due to non-target labial embolization during UAE, perhaps of the internal pudendal artery. Spontaneous resolution occurred during the ensuing 4 weeks.

Generalized oedema of the face, body and extremities was a complication seen in one 41-year-old patient 24 h following UAE [94]. In this case, a transient spike in vascular endothelial growth factor (VEGF) level was seen to coincide with the oedema. VEGF has permeability-increasing activity for vascular endothelial cells [46] and was hypothesized to have been released by the hypoxic fibroids.

One 48-year-old patient required an emergency hysterectomy following massive vaginal hemorrhage 1 month following UAE [50]. Histological examination of the bleeding uterus did not provide definitive answers, but it was hypothesized that the bleeding originated from partially infracted myometrial tissue, adjacent to the treated fibroid, in which several large blood vessels were noted.

10.2.11
Post-procedure Imaging

The best imaging to evaluate the perfusion and size/volume of the fibroids following the procedure is MR. The timing of the imaging is not standardized. In our practice we typically image at 6 months which gives a chance for the fibroids to have changed in volume and offers the patient an opportunity to visualize the decrease in size of the fibroids. However, perfusion changes (as measured by immediate reduction in maximal leiomyoma enhancement as seen on MR) immediately after the procedure have been shown to be predictors of clinical response at 12 months (as measured by length, blood loss, and associated pain of menses) [27].

The MR characteristics post embolization have been well documented. One should expect an increase in signal intensity on T1-weighted images [27, 47] immediately following UAE and a reduction in signal intensity on T2-weighted images after the first month [4]. DeSouza et al. [27] demonstrated that reduction in leiomyoma perfusion (as measured by maximal gadolinium enhancement on T1-weighted images) immediately after UAE correlated with a clinical response after 12 months. Unlike the fibroids themselves, the myometrium tends to reperfuse to normal levels during that time and thus once again appear bright on contrast-enhanced images.

Long-term follow-up is indicated 3–6 months after the procedure. Pelage et al. [67] have emphasized the use of T1-weighted contrast-enhanced MR to evaluate fibroid perfusion and in turn predict long-term outcome. Areas of complete infarction and partial infarction can co-exist within a given fibroid tumor and are clearly demarcated as areas of dark or bright signal, respectively. This study showed that fibroids that had homogenously complete infarction at 3-months post procedure had 100% infarction at 3 years. If the fibroid was incompletely infarcted at 3 months, then only 40% of the fibroids were completely infarcted at 3 years. However, the volume reduction was similar between these two groups. They observed that areas of incomplete infarction (viable fibroid tissue) were more likely to re-grow and to potentially cause relapse of symptoms. Their conclusion was that the success of the procedure may be better measured by the achievement of complete infarction, as opposed to absolute volume reduction [38].

It is important to evaluate the uterine and fibroid volumes as patients that show poor reductions in uterine volume post embolization may be more likely to require hysterectomy [4]. MR not only provides easily understood images that can be shown to patients, but also information that can be used to predict future fibroid shrinkage or to predict regrowth and possible further therapy.

Post-operative knowledge of the fibroid vasculature is of particular interest when UAE results in negligible shrinkage and persistent symptoms as it may suggest possible sources of alternate blood supply, such as ovarian or vesicovaginal arteries. In this scenario, MR angiography is indicated to evaluate the status of the ovarian vasculature.

Using transvaginal ultrasonography, one can visualize the thrombosed uterine arteries represented by tortuous, brightly echogenic tubular structures in the adnexal region. This radiographic sign has been named the 'white snake' sign and its persistence 6 months after UAE has been shown to correlate with more favorable symptomatic outcome.

10.2.12
Conclusion

Uterine artery embolization has become a recognized alternative to traditional surgical therapies for uterine fibroids. It has also become the procedure that has forced interventional radiologists out of the role of simply performing a procedure and into the role of a true clinical consultant and physician directly caring for patients. The actual procedure of UAE is by and large straightforward. It is the consultation with the patient prior to the procedure, educating her about the options for treating her fibroids, and the possible complications and alternatives that has become important. The care of the patient following the procedure is the most challenging part of the interventionalist's job. There always seems to be a new situation or problem that arises no matter how experienced the interventionalist is. This field continues to undergo tremendous knowledge growth, and there will be many more clinical aspects of UAE that will be elucidated in the months and years ahead. It is critically important to try and stay abreast of the information being reported on the clinical aspects of UAE in order to provide appropriate counsel and care for patients with uterine fibroids.

References

1. Abbara S, Spies JB et al (1999) Transcervical expulsion of a fibroid as a result of uterine artery embolization for leiomyomata. J Vasc Interv Radiol 10:409–411
2. Aharoni A, Reiter A et al (1988) Patterns of growth of uterine leiomyomas during pregnancy. A prospective longitudinal study. Br J Obstet Gynaecol 95:510–513
3. Ahmad A, Qadan L et al (2002) Uterine artery embolization treatment of uterine fibroids: effect on ovarian function in younger women. J Vasc Interv Radiol 13:1017–20
4. Ahmad I, Ray CE Jr et al (2003) Transvaginal sonographic appearance of thrombosed uterine arteries after uterine artery embolization: the "white snake" sign. J Clin Ultrasound 31:401–406
5. Al-Badr A, Faught W (2001) Uterine artery embolization in an undiagnosed uterine sarcoma. Obstet Gynecol 97:836–837
6. Amato P, Roberts AC (2001) Transient ovarian failure: a complication of uterine artery embolization. Fertil Steril 75:438–439
7. Anania CA, Stewart EA et al (1997) Expression of the fibroblast growth factor receptor in women with leiomyomas and abnormal uterine bleeding. Mol Hum Reprod 3:685–691
8. Aziz A, Petrucco OM et al (1998) Transarterial embolization of the uterine arteries: patient reactions and effects on uterine vasculature. Acta Obstet Gynecol Scand 77:334–340
9. Beavis EL, Brown JB et al (1969) Ovarian function after hysterectomy with conservation of the ovaries in premenopausal women. J Obstet Gynaecol Br Commonw 76:969–978
10. Berkowitz RP, Hutchins FL Jr et al (1999) Vaginal expulsion of submucosal fibroids after uterine artery embolization. A report of three cases. J Reprod Med 44:373–376
11. Bradley EA, Reidy JF et al (1998) Transcatheter uterine artery embolisation to treat large uterine fibroids. Br J Obstet Gynaecol 105:235–240
12. Brandon DD, Bethea CL et al (1993) Progesterone receptor messenger ribonucleic acid and protein are overexpressed in human uterine leiomyomas. Am J Obstet Gynecol 169:78–85
13. Burn PR, McCall JM et al (2000) Uterine fibroleiomyoma: MR imaging appearances before and after embolization of uterine arteries. Radiology 214:729–734
14. Buttram VC Jr, Reiter RC (1981) Uterine leiomyomata: etiology, symptomatology, and management. Fertil Steril 36:433–445
15. Carr BR, Marshburn PB et al (1993) An evaluation of the effect of gonadotropin-releasing hormone analogs and medroxyprogesterone acetate on uterine leiomyomata volume by magnetic resonance imaging: a prospective, randomized, double blind, placebo-controlled, crossover trial. J Clin Endocrinol Metab 76:1217–1223
16. Chavez NF, Stewart EA (2001) Medical treatment of uterine fibroids. Clin Obstet Gynecol 44:372–384
17. Chiu CY, Wong WK et al (2001) Uterine artery embolisation for treatment of fibroids: experience in Chinese women. Singapore Med J 42:148–154
18. Chrisman HB, Saker MB et al (2000) The impact of uterine fibroid embolization on resumption of menses and ovarian function. J Vasc Interv Radiol 11:699–703
19. Clevenger-Hoeft M, Syrop CH et al (1999) Sonohysterography in premenopausal women with and without abnormal bleeding. Obstet Gynecol 94:516–520
20. Colgan TJ, Pron G et al (2003) Pathologic features of uteri and leiomyomas following uterine artery embolization for leiomyomas. Am J Surg Pathol 27:167–177
21. Common AA, Mocarski EJ et al (2001) Therapeutic failure of uterine fibroid embolization caused by underlying leiomyosarcoma. J Vasc Interv Radiol 12:1449–1452
22. Coutinho EM, Goncalves MT (1989) Long-term treatment of leiomyomas with gestrinone. Fertil Steril 51:939–946

23. D'Angelo A, Amso NN et al (2003) Spontaneous multiple pregnancy after uterine artery embolization for uterine fibroid: case report. Eur J Obstet Gynecol Reprod Biol 110:245–246

24. De Blok S, de Vries C et al (2003) Fatal sepsis after uterine artery embolization with microspheres. J Vasc Interv Radiol 14:779–783

25. De Leo V, la Marca A et al (1999) Short-term treatment of uterine fibromyomas with danazol. Gynecol Obstet Invest 47:258–262

26. Dequesne JSN (1998) Laser hysteroscopic resection of fibroids. In: Sutton DM (ed) Endoscopic surgery for gynecologists. Saunders, London, UK, pp 534–539

27. deSouza NM, Williams AD (2002) Uterine arterial embolization for leiomyomas: perfusion and volume changes at MR imaging and relation to clinical outcome. Radiology 222:367–374

28. Falcone T, Bedaiwy MA (2002) Minimally invasive management of uterine fibroids. Curr Opin Obstet Gynecol 14:401–407

29. Farrer-Brown G, Beilby JO et al (1971) Venous changes in the endometrium of myomatous uteri. Obstet Gynecol 38:743–751

30. Fedele L, Parazzini F et al (1995) Recurrence of fibroids after myomectomy: a transvaginal ultrasonographic study. Hum Reprod 10:1795–1796

31. Folkman J (1995) Angiogenesis inhibitors generated by tumors. Mol Med 1:120–122

32. Friedman AJ, Barbieri RL et al (1988) A randomized, double-blind trial of a gonadotropin releasing-hormone agonist (leuprolide) with or without medroxyprogesterone acetate in the treatment of leiomyomata uteri. Fertil Steril 49:404–409

33. Geller SE, Bernstein SJ et al (1997) The decision-making process for the treatment of abnormal uterine bleeding. J Womens Health 6:559–567

34. Gimbel H, Ottesen B et al (2002) Danish gynecologists' opinion about hysterectomy on benign indication: results of a survey. Acta Obstet Gynecol Scand 81:1123–1131

35. Goldberg J, Pereira L et al (2002) Pregnancy after uterine artery embolization. Obstet Gynecol 100:869–872

36. Goldberg J, Pereira L et al (2004) Pregnancy outcomes after treatment for fibromyomata: uterine artery embolization versus laparoscopic myomectomy. Am J Obstet Gynecol 191:18–21

37. Golzarian JLP, Walker WJ, Lampmann L, Pelage JP (2003) Uterine fibroid embolization for large symptomatic fibroids. J Vasc Interv Radiol 14:(S38)

38. Goodwin SC, McLucas B et al (1999) Uterine artery embolization for the treatment of uterine leiomyomata midterm results. J Vasc Interv Radiol 10:1159–1165

39. Grasel RP, Outwater EK et al (2000) Endometrial polyps: MR imaging features and distinction from endometrial carcinoma. Radiology 214:47–52

40. Hannigan EV, Gomez LG (1979) Uterine leiomyosarcoma. Am J Obstet Gynecol 134:557–564

41. Harkki-Siren P, Kurki T (1997) A nationwide analysis of laparoscopic complications. Obstet Gynecol 89:108–112

42. Harlow BL, Weiss NS et al (1986) The epidemiology of sarcomas of the uterus. J Natl Cancer Inst 76:399–402

43. Hata K, Hata T et al (1997) Uterine sarcoma: can it be differentiated from uterine leiomyoma with Doppler ultrasonography? A preliminary report." Ultrasound Obstet Gynecol 9:101–104

44. Heaston DK, Mineau DE et al (1979) Transcatheter arterial embolization for control of persistent massive puerperal hemorrhage after bilateral surgical hypogastric artery ligation. AJR Am J Roentgenol 133:152–154

45. Jaaskelainen J (2003) Non-invasive transcranial high intensity focused ultrasound (HIFUS) under MRI thermometry and guidance in the treatment of brain lesions. Acta Neurochir (Wien) [Suppl] 88:57–60

46. Jelkmann W (2001) Pitfalls in the measurement of circulating vascular endothelial growth factor. Clin Chem 47:617–623

47. Jha RC, Ascher SM et al (2000) Symptomatic fibroleiomyomata: MR imaging of the uterus before and after uterine arterial embolization. Radiology 217:228–235

48. Katsumori T, Nakajima K et al (2003) Is a large fibroid a high-risk factor for uterine artery embolization? AJR Am J Roentgenol 181:1309–1314

49. Kawaguchi K, Fujii S et al (1989) Mitotic activity in uterine leiomyomas during the menstrual cycle. Am J Obstet Gynecol 160:637–641

50. Kerlan RK Jr, Coffey JO et al (2003) Massive vaginal hemorrhage after uterine fibroid embolization. J Vasc Interv Radiol 14:1465–1467

51. Kjerulff KH, Langenberg PW et al (2000) Effectiveness of hysterectomy. Obstet Gynecol 95:319–326

52. Koike T, Minakami H et al (1999) Uterine leiomyoma in pregnancy: its influence on obstetric performance. J Obstet Gynaecol Res 25:309–313

53. LaMorte AI, Lalwani S et al (1993) Morbidity associated with abdominal myomectomy. Obstet Gynecol 82:897–900

54. Lee BS, Stewart EA et al (1998) Interferon-alpha is a potent inhibitor of basic fibroblast growth factor-stimulated cell proliferation in human uterine cells. Am J Reprod Immunol 40:19–25

55. Leibsohn S, d'Ablaing G et al (1990) Leiomyosarcoma in a series of hysterectomies performed for presumed uterine leiomyomas. Am J Obstet Gynecol 162:968–974; discussion 974–976

56. Lepine LA, Hillis SD et al (1997) Hysterectomy surveillance – United States, 1980–1993. MMWR CDC Surveill Summ 46:1–15

57. Lev-Toaff AS, Coleman BG et al (1987) Leiomyomas in pregnancy: sonographic study. Radiology 164:375–380

58. Ligon AH, Morton CC (2000) Genetics of uterine leiomyomata. Genes Chromosomes Cancer 28:235–245

59. Makinen J, Johansson J et al (2001) Morbidity of 10 110 hysterectomies by type of approach. Hum Reprod 16:1473–1478

60. Mangrulkar RS, Ono M et al (1995) Isolation and characterization of heparin-binding growth factors in human leiomyomas and normal myometrium. Biol Reprod 53:636–646

61. Nikolic B, Spies JB et al (1999) Ovarian artery supply of uterine fibroids as a cause of treatment failure after uterine artery embolization: a case report. J Vasc Interv Radiol 10:1167–1170

62. Nikolic B, Kessler CM et al (2003) Changes in blood coagulation markers associated with uterine artery embolization for leiomyomata. J Vasc Interv Radiol 14:1147–1153

63. Oliver JA Jr, Lance JS (1979) Selective embolization to con-

trol massive hemorrhage following pelvic surgery. Am J Obstet Gynecol 135:431–432

64. Ota H, Igarashi S et al (1998) Morphometric evaluation of stromal vascularization in the endometrium in adenomyosis. Hum Reprod 13:715–719

65. Parker WH, Fu YS et al (1994) Uterine sarcoma in patients operated on for presumed leiomyoma and rapidly growing leiomyoma. Obstet Gynecol 83:414–418

66. Payne JF, Robboy SJ et al (2002) Embolic microspheres within ovarian arterial vasculature after uterine artery embolization. Obstet Gynecol 100:883–886

67. Pelage JP, Jacob D et al (2004) Re: fatal sepsis after uterine artery embolization with microspheres. J Vasc Interv Radiol 15:405–406; author reply 406

68. Prollius A, de Vries C et al (2004) Uterine artery embolisation for symptomatic fibroids: the effect of the large uterus on outcome. BJOG 111:239–242

69. Ravina JH, Merland JJ et al (1994) Preoperative embolization of uterine fibroma. Preliminary results (10 cases). Presse Med 23:1540

70. Ravina JH, Vigneron NC et al (2000) Pregnancy after embolization of uterine myoma: report of 12 cases. Fertil Steril 73:1241–1243

71. Razavi MK, Wolanske K. A et al (2002) Angiographic classification of ovarian artery-to-uterine artery anastomoses: initial observations in uterine fibroid embolization. Radiology 224:707–712

72. Razavi MK, Hwang G et al (2003) Abdominal myomectomy versus uterine fibroid embolization in the treatment of symptomatic uterine leiomyomas. AJR Am J Roentgenol 180:1571–1575

73. Reddy VV, Rose LI (1979) delta 4-3-Ketosteroid 5 alpha-oxidoreductase in human uterine leiomyoma. Am J Obstet Gynecol 135:415–418

74. Reidy JF, Bradley EA (1998) Uterine artery embolization for fibroid disease. Cardiovasc Intervent Radiol 21:357–360

75. Rein MS, Friedman AJ et al (1991) Cytogenetic abnormalities in uterine leiomyomata. Obstet Gynecol 77:923–926

76. Richard HM 3rd, Siskin GP et al (2004) Endometritis after uterine artery embolization with gold-colored gelatin microspheres. J Vasc Interv Radiol 15:406–407

77. Schwartz LB, Zawin M et al (1998) Does pelvic magnetic resonance imaging differentiate among the histologic subtypes of uterine leiomyomata? Fertil Steril 70:580–587

78. Shibata S, Kawamura N et al (2000) Diagnostic accuracy of needle biopsy of uterine leiomyosarcoma. Oncol Rep 7:595–597

79. Siskin GP, Stainken BF et al (2000) Outpatient uterine artery embolization for symptomatic uterine fibroids: experience in 49 patients. J Vasc Interv Radiol 11:305–311

80. Siskin GP, Tublin ME et al (2001) Uterine artery embolization for the treatment of adenomyosis: clinical response and evaluation with MR imaging. AJR Am J Roentgenol 177:297–302

81. Soules MR, McCarty KS Jr (1982) Leiomyomas: steroid receptor content. Variation within normal menstrual cycles. Am J Obstet Gynecol 143:6–11

82. Spies JB, Scialli A. R et al (1999) Initial results from uterine fibroid embolization for symptomatic leiomyomata. J Vasc Interv Radiol 10:1149–1157

83. Spies JB, Ascher SA et al (2001a) Uterine artery embolization for leiomyomata. Obstet Gynecol 98:29–34

84. Spies JB, Roth AR et al (2001b) Ovarian function after uterine artery embolization for leiomyomata: assessment with use of serum follicle stimulating hormone assay. J Vasc Interv Radiol 12:437–442

85. Spies JB, Roth AR et al (2002a) Leiomyomata treated with uterine artery embolization: factors associated with successful symptom and imaging outcome. Radiology 222:45–52

86. Spies JB, Spector A et al (2002b) Complications after uterine artery embolization for leiomyomas. Obstet Gynecol 100:873–880

87. Spies JB, Cooper JM et al (2004) Outcome of uterine embolization and hysterectomy for leiomyomas: results of a multicenter study. Am J Obstet Gynecol 191:22–31

88. Stewart EA (2001) Uterine fibroids. Lancet 357:293–298

89. Stewart EA, Friedman AJ (1992) Steroidal treatment of myomas: preoperative and long-term medical therapy. Thieme, New York

90. Stewart EA, Nowak RA (1996) Leiomyoma-related bleeding: a classic hypothesis updated for the molecular era. Hum Reprod Update 2:295–306

91. Stovall DW (2001) Clinical symptomatology of uterine leiomyomas. Clin Obstet Gynecol 44:364–371

92. Stringer NH, Grant T et al (2000) Ovarian failure after uterine artery embolization for treatment of myomas. J Am Assoc Gynecol Laparosc 7:395–400

93. Subramanian S, Clark MA et al (2001) Outcome and resource use associated with myomectomy. Obstet Gynecol 98:583–587

94. Takeda T, Osuga K et al (2004) A case of generalised oedema secondary to uterine artery embolisation for leiomyomata. BJOG 111:179–180

95. Tamaya T, Motoyama T et al (1979) Estradiol-17 beta-, progesterone and 5 alpha-dihydrotestosterone receptors of uterine myometrium and myoma in the human subject. J Steroid Biochem 10:615–622

96. Tan TL, Rafla N (2004) Retained calcified fibroid fragments after uterine artery embolization for fibroids. Fertil Steril 81:1145–1147

97. Togashi K, Ozasa H et al (1989) Enlarged uterus: differentiation between adenomyosis and leiomyoma with MR imaging. Radiology 171:531–534

98. Tropeano G, Litwicka K et al (2003) Permanent amenorrhea associated with endometrial atrophy after uterine artery embolization for symptomatic uterine fibroids. Fertil Steril 79:132–135

99. Tropeano G, di Stasi C et al (2004) Uterine artery embolization for fibroids does not have adverse effects on ovarian reserve in regularly cycling women younger than 40 years. Fertil Steril 81:1055–1061

100. Tulandi T, Sammour A et al (2002) Ovarian reserve after uterine artery embolization for leiomyomata. Fertil Steril 78:197–198

101. Vashisht A, Studd J et al (1999) Fatal septicaemia after fibroid embolisation. Lancet 354:307–308

102. Vercellini P, Trespidi L et al (2003) Gonadotropin-releasing hormone agonist treatment before abdominal myomectomy: a controlled trial. Fertil Steril 79:1390–1395

103. Vergani P, Ghidini A et al (1994) Do uterine leiomyomas influence pregnancy outcome? Am J Perinatol 11:356–358

104. Walker WJ, Pelage JP (2002) Uterine artery embolisation for symptomatic fibroids: clinical results in 400 women with imaging follow up. BJOG 109:1262–1272

105. Walker WJ, Pelage JP et al (2002) Fibroid embolization. Clin Radiol 57:325–331

106. Walker WJ, Carpenter TT et al (2004) Persistent vaginal discharge after uterine artery embolization for fibroid tumors: cause of the condition, magnetic resonance imaging appearance, and surgical treatment. Am J Obstet Gynecol 190:1230–1233

107. Wilcox LS, Koonin LM et al (1994) Hysterectomy in the United States, 1988-1990. Obstet Gynecol 83:549–555

108. Wilson EA, Yang F et al (1980) Estradiol and progesterone binding in uterine leiomyomata and in normal uterine tissues. Obstet Gynecol 55:20–24

109. Wingo PA, Huezo CM et al (1985) The mortality risk associated with hysterectomy. Am J Obstet Gynecol 152:803–808

110. Yeagley TJ, Goldberg J et al (2002) Labial necrosis after uterine artery embolization for leiomyomata. Obstet Gynecol 100:881–882

10.3 Fibroid Embolization: Anatomy and Technical Considerations

ANNE C. ROBERTS

CONTENTS

10.3.1
Introduction

The anatomy of uterine fibroids and uterine artery embolization (UAE) consists of the fibroids, their position in the uterus, and the vasculature associated with the uterus. The vasculature of the ovarian arteries is also important because of the potential for collateral blood flow from the ovarian arteries supplying the fibroids. Communication between the uterine arteries and the ovarian arteries are also important because of the risk of embolization of the ovaries through uterine-ovarian anastomoses.

A. C. ROBERTS, MD
University of California, San Diego Medical Center, Division of Vascular and Interventional Radiology, 200 West Arbor Drive, San Diego, California 92103-8756, USA

10.3.2
Anatomy

10.3.2.1
Fibroids

Fibroids are classified by their position in the uterus. Serosal fibroids are found in the outer layer of the uterus and expand outward. They usually do not affect bleeding during the menstrual period, but may cause symptoms due to their size and pressure on other pelvic organs such as the bladder and bowel. Intramural fibroids develop within the substance of the uterus. They enlarge the uterus and can cause both bleeding and pressure symptoms. Submucosal fibroids involve the inner layer of the uterus, and cause the most problems with heavy and prolonged periods and sometimes gushing bleeding also described as flooding. Submucosal and serosal fibroids may be pedunculated, protruding from the uterine wall, sometimes with long stalks.

The size, position, and number of fibroids in the uterus have a bearing on the success of the embolization procedure. The vascular anatomy also has a major impact on the success and complications of the embolization procedure.

10.3.3
Vascular Anatomy and Variants

10.3.3.1
Uterine Arteries

The uterine blood supply is primarily from the uterine arteries. The uterine arteries arise as branches of the internal iliac (hypogastric) arteries. In most cases, the internal iliac artery divides into a posterior division that gives off the iliolumbar, the lateral sacral and the superior gluteal arteries and an anterior division that gives rise to parietal branches (the obturator, inferior gluteal and internal pudendal arteries) and visceral branches (the superior vesical, middle hemorrhoidal, uterine and vaginal arteries) [1]. However, the anatomy is variable and variant vascular patterns occur in about 10%–15% of the population [2]. When the arterial anatomy is studied angiographically, the divisions can be into three branches in 14%, four or more in 3% and one main branch in 4% [3]. The anterior division is particularly variable in terms of its branching pattern.

The uterine artery arises from the anterior division of the internal iliac artery usually close to, or in common with the middle hemorrhoidal or vaginal artery. There are several configurations for the origin of the uterine artery. It can be the first branch of the inferior gluteal artery (Fig. 10.3.1a); a second or third branch of the inferior gluteal artery (Fig. 10.3.1b); a trifurcation of the uterine artery, inferior gluteal artery, and superior gluteal artery (Fig. 10.3.1c); or the first branch of the hypogastric artery (Fig. 10.3.1d) [4]. The most common variants are for the uterine artery to be the first branch of the inferior gluteal, or for it to arise from the trifurcation of the uterine artery, inferior gluteal artery and superior gluteal artery [4]. In some cases no uterine artery is identified.

The uterine artery has a very characteristic U-shaped configuration, with a parietal or descending segment running downward and medially, then

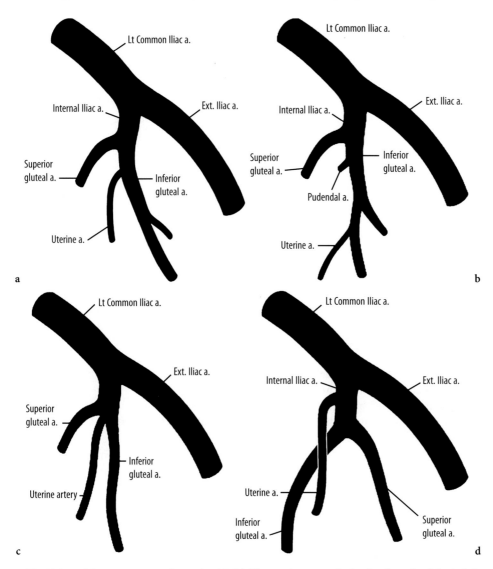

Fig. 10.3.1. a Most common configuration (45%). The uterine artery is the first branch of the inferior gluteal. **b** An uncommon variant (6%) the uterine artery is a second or third branch of the inferior gluteal artery. **c** The second most common configuration (43%). There is a trifurcation of the superior gluteal, inferior gluteal and uterine artery. **d** Another uncommon configuration (6%). The uterine artery is the first branch of the internal iliac, proximal to superior gluteal and inferior gluteal

there is a transverse segment coursing medially, and then an ascending segment, which runs along the side of the uterus. The uterine artery crosses above the urethra, to which it supplies a small branch [5]; it enters the broad ligament and reaches the side of the uterus about 2 cm above the cervix. As it reaches the uterus, it gives off a descending cervical branch, which surrounds the cervix and anastomoses with branches of the vaginal artery [1, 5]. The anastomosis of the uterine artery with the vaginal artery leads to formation of the "azygos arteries", two median parallel arteries located on the anterior and posterior position of the vagina [2, 5]. The main uterine artery courses upward along the lateral side of the uterus, giving rise to intramural branches to the anterior and posterior surfaces of the uterus. These intramural arteries in the uterine muscle are extremely tortuous and are termed "arcuate arteries" [3] or "helicine arteries" [2]. There are anastomoses between the arcuate arteries on either side [3, 4]. The uterine artery terminates in a tubal branch and an ovarian ramus that anastomoses with the ovarian artery [1].

The vaginal artery may arise as a branch from the hypogastric artery directly, from the uterine artery or from the superior vesical artery. In one angiographic study it arose from the anterior division of the internal iliac artery just below the uterine artery in 50% of patients [3]. In a small percentage (9%) it arose from a common trunk formed with the uterine artery. It anastomoses with the descending branches of the uterine artery and forms a network of vessels around the vagina [1]. Only the superior third of the vagina is functionally connected to the uterus via arterial collaterals. The lower third of the vagina receives more blood from the urethral arterial collaterals. The vesicular artery, arises from the anterior division of the internal iliac artery usually above the uterine artery, but in 1% of patients was found to be a common trunk with the uterine artery [3]. Very occasionally the round ligament artery can supply the uterus. This artery arises directly from the external iliac artery or from the proximal epigastric artery and can supply the uterus, which may be important in fibroid embolization [6] or as a cause of recurrent vaginal bleeding after embolization for postpartum hemorrhage [7]. It may be a cause of failure of UAE to infarct the fibroid [8].

The uterine veins parallel the arteries forming the plexuses that end into the internal iliac vein; uterine veins merge with vaginal plexus downward and with the ovarian veins upwards. Venous blood from the upper part of the uterus drains into the ovarian veins, while most of the venous uterine blood is collected into the iliac vein [5].

The anatomy of the uterine artery has relevance to the procedure of UAE. When the uterine artery arises from the anterior division of the internal iliac artery, the contralateral oblique projection gives the best visualization of its origin, allowing for easier catheterization [4, 9]. When the uterine artery is arising from several stems, then the ipsilateral projection is the best for visualization [4, 9].

The most common complications which have been reported with uterine artery embolization are amenorrhea, either permanent or transient presumably secondary to ovarian failure [10–13], or are related to the fibroid, including infection of the fibroid, or fibroid expulsion [12]. However, rarely non-target embolization occurs. This non-target embolization may be due to some of the variant anatomy described above, or may be due to reflux out of the uterine artery into arteries that originate close to the uterine artery. Case reports of labial necrosis [14], vesicouterine fistula [15, 16], necrosis of the cervix and vaginal [16, 17], bladder necrosis [18], buttock necrosis [19, 20], have been reported. Sexual dysfunction after uterine artery embolization has also been reported. It is unclear what is the cause of this dysfunction; however, it is possible that the uterovaginal nerve plexus may have been damaged by the embolization, resulting in an adverse effect on sexual arousal and orgasm [21, 22]. Embolization of the cervicovaginal branch may have an impact on both vaginal and clitoral sensation [21, 22]. Although, these complications appear to be extremely rare, they should raise the awareness of the importance of careful evaluation of the vasculature to look for aberrant vessels, and to avoid reflux of particles into neighboring arteries.

10.3.3.2
Fibroid Vascularity

Intramural fibroids are the most common type of fibroids. Their blood supply comes from one or more nutrient arteries. As the fibroid increases in size, the nutrient artery, and the arcuate artery enlarge [4]. Submucosal fibroids also obtain their blood supply from the nutrient arteries. However, with subserosal fibroids, the fibroid may adhere to other structures, and derive blood supply from those adjacent structures [4], including the ovarian arteries.

10.3.3.3
Ovarian Arteries

The ovarian arteries arise from the ventral surface of the aorta just below the origin of the renal arteries. In 80% of individuals there is a single ovarian artery on each side [2]. In more than 70% of patients, the ovarian arteries originate from the ventral surface of the abdominal aorta a few centimeters below the origin of the renal arteries. The arteries are small normally less than 1 mm [2]. The ovarian arteries course downward and laterally over the psoas muscles and the ureter. They tend to be very tortuous distally, with a characteristic sinuous course. The arteries enter the pelvis, crossing the common iliac artery. They enter the broad ligament at the junction of the superior and lateral border of the broad ligament. The arteries continue beneath the fallopian tube, entering the mesovarium to supply the ovary [1]. Anastomoses occur with the ovarian rami of the uterine arteries, branches also extend to the ampullary and isthmica portions of the tube, the ureter and the round ligament [1]. There is also a branch to the skin of the labia and inguinal area. Proximally there are branches to the ureter, perirenal and periureteric fat.

Variant anatomy of the ovarian arteries includes the gonadal artery originating from the renal artery in about 20% of individuals [2]. Very rarely the artery arises from the adrenal, lumbar, or iliac arteries [2]. In some cases, the right ovarian artery passes behind the cava and over the right renal vein. The left ovarian artery will occasionally also pass over the left renal vein [2]. There is very rarely a common trunk of left and right gonadal arteries, and occasionally there are multiple gonadal arteries.

10.3.3.4
Tubo-ovarian Anastomoses

Communications between the ovarian artery and the uterine artery has two potential adverse outcomes, it may allow continued blood supply to the fibroid, leading to failure of the procedure, and alternatively it can lead to permanent ovarian failure following embolization. Because of these potential problems, there has been considerable interest in how best to evaluate the ovarian arteries. Flush arteriography has been an approach to evaluating the ovarian arteries to determine if there is enlargement of the ovarian artery and supply to the fibroid [23]. In one study [23] of 294 aortograms, 75 ovarian arteries were identified (25%) in 59 women (20%). Bilateral ovarian artery identification was seen in 16 women, and unilateral identification in 43 women. In the bilateral group, there were six enlarged ovarian artery and 11 moderately enlarged arteries, 15 arteries were considered small. When the ovarian artery was enlarged it was supplying fibroids, in most cases these were large fundal fibroids although in some cases there had been previous pelvic or tubo-ovarian surgery [23].

In the majority of patients undergoing UAE, tubo-ovarian anastomoses are not identified. However, when they are seen prior to embolization, menopausal symptoms (amenorrhea, hot flashes) are common although usually transient [4]. RAZAVI et al. [24] have described three main angiographic patterns of anastomoses between uterine and ovarian arteries. Type I anastomoses are divided into type Ia and type Ib. In both types the ovarian arteries are a major source of blood supply to the fibroid, with anastomosis between the ovarian artery and the intramural uterine artery. In type Ia (13%), the flow in the tubal artery is towards the uterus, without evidence of retrograde reflux in the direction of the ovary on selective uterine angiograms. In type Ib (9%), flow in the tubal artery was towards the uterus, but reflux into the ovarian artery is seen on the preembolization selective uterine angiogram. Type II (4%) has direct fibroid supply from the ovarian arteries, with the flow to the fibroids being anatomic independent of the uterine artery. Type III (6%) has flow in the tubal artery towards the ovary on selective uterine angiograms, with an ovarian blush being present. In 8% there were bilateral anastomoses of the Ib or III type, and in 68% there were no anastomoses present [24]. In evaluating for menopausal symptoms, the incidence of menopause following the procedure was 6% overall, 16% in patients over the age of 45, and in patients with bilateral type Ib and/or type III, 50% became menopausal.

CICINELLI et al. [5] described an interesting pattern of collateral flow between the uterine and ovarian arterial supply to the uterus. In doing measurements of blood flow in premenopausal women, this group found there is more blood flow to the uterus from the ovarian artery during the follicular phase, whereas in the luteal phase most of the uterus is supplied from the uterine artery. Whether this change in blood flow patterns is changed in patients with fibroids is not clear. No studies of the effect of the phase of the menstrual cycle on the effectiveness of uterine artery embolization have been performed at this point.

10.3.3.5
Equipment

10.3.3.5.1
Catheters and Microcatheters

10.3.3.5.1.1
Catheters

There are a number of catheters that can be used for uterine artery embolization. If an aortogram is being performed, a standard aortic flush catheter such as a pigtail catheter, or a catheter such as an Omni Flush (Angiodynamics, Inc., Queensbury, NY), or Varrel Contralateral Flush (VCF) (Cook, Inc., Bloomington, IN), is appropriate. For selective catheterization of the internal iliac artery and uterine artery a 4-F or 5-F Cobra 2 (C2) catheter is a standard catheter. The C2 catheter is positioned into the contralateral iliac artery over a standard guidewire; however, an angled Glidewire (Terumo Medical Corporation, Elkton, MD) can be very helpful in performing the subselective catheterization. The uterine artery tends to be prone to spasm and minimizing wire use will help to avoid spasm, which will help to decrease complications such as arterial dissection. To access the ipsilateral internal iliac and uterine artery, the C2 catheter can be formed into a looped configuration, a Waltman loop [25]. This configuration allows for subselective catheterization. The Waltman loop technique was originally described with a larger catheter than is now usually used, and with smaller catheter sizes the looped configuration is more likely to be lost as the catheter is being manipulated. It is very important that a soft

wire be used in a catheter that has been formed into a Waltman loop, otherwise the shape will be lost. An alternative catheter is essentially a preformed Waltman loop; this is a long reversed curve catheter (RUC, Roberts Uterine Catheter, Cook, Inc, Bloomington, IN) (Fig. 10.3.2). The catheter is 5 F tapering to 4 F at the distal end, with a soft, atraumatic, radiopaque tip, there is a small radiopaque marker where the catheter makes a sharp loop or genu and the catheter has excellent torque control. This catheter allows the benefits of the Waltman loop, with less chance of losing the looped configuration during manipulations.

10.3.3.5.1.2
Microcatheters

Initial descriptions of UAE included the routine use of microcatheters; however, many operators reserve these catheters for times when standard catheters are not appropriate. If the artery is small, there is marked spasm, or there are branches such as the cervicovaginal artery that the standard catheter has difficulty getting past, then microcatheters may be very helpful. The small size and the flexibility of these catheters helps to avoid spasm and allows for distal placement of the catheter [26]. A number of microcatheters also have a hydrophilic coating that gives improved trackability, allowing for improved catheterization of tortuous arteries. Use of a high-flow microcatheter is usually the best for embolization since the larger lumen of these catheters helps avoid clogging of the catheter with the embolic material, and allows for a more rapid embolization procedure. Such high-flow catheters include the Renegade Hi-Flo catheter (Boston Scientific, Natick, MA), the MassTransit catheter (Cordis, Miami, FL), and EmboCath (Biosphere, Rockland, MA).

Disadvantages of the microcatheters include the additional, high cost of the catheters. They are also more difficult to see, may require a leading wire which can induce spasm in front of the catheter, and since they are prone to clog, a more dilute suspension of embolic material should be used which increases the time of the procedure, and more importantly tends to increase the fluoroscopy time.

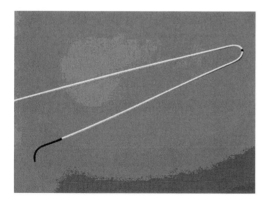

Fig. 10.3.2. A long-reverse curve catheter. Very useful for catheterizations in the pelvis and for uterine artery embolization. Tip is tapered to 4 F. Radiopaque marker at genu of catheter marks the point where the catheter should be positioned over the aortic bifurcation

10.3.3.5.2
Embolization Materials

A variety of embolic materials have been used for treating uterine fibroids. Although there are at least theoretical benefits of using one material compared to others, it is not clear at this time if there are any clinical differences [27]. It is probably most important for the operator to feel comfortable with the material used, and to use it appropriately.

10.3.3.5.2.1
Polyvinyl Alcohol Particles (PVA)

PVA particles probably remain the most common embolic used for uterine fibroids. These particles have been used for many years in a variety of vascular beds and are considered to be safe and effective. PVA is available from a number of manufacturers. It is important to recognize that different manufacturers produce different versions of PVA. Some of the PVA is quite jagged and tends to clump together such as PVA Foam particles (Cook Inc., Bloomington, IN) or Contour PVA particles (Boston Scientific, Natick, MA) (Fig. 10.3.3). It is very important with all types of embolic material to use a solution that allows for the best possible suspension of the particles. Clumping of PVA may be a function of the contrast dilution, and enough contrast should be used to allow the particles to be free floating and not aggregated. With PVA Foam particles, an iodine concentration of 240 mg/mL contrast tends to give the best suspension (Charles Kerber, M.D., personal communication) (Fig. 10.3.4). The irregularly shaped PVA particles were those used in the original description of uterine artery embolization, and a size of 300–500 μm seemed to be the best size for this application. This PVA works well with the 4- to 5-F catheters, but is more likely to jam in the microcatheters [27]. Although the jagged nature of the PVA has been considered by some to be a negative, one could consider that these particles allow interlocking which may make for a more efficient embolization.

Spherical PVA is now available (Contour SE Microspheres; Boston Scientific, Natick, MA), PVA Plus (Angiodynamics, Inc., Queensbury, NY), Bead Block (Terumo) which has a smooth surface and a more uniform size distribution (Fig. 10.3.5). These particles should minimize catheter clogging, and may provide a better matching of the embolic to the vessel size. Because these particles are more homogeneous, it is recommended that the size of the particles should be larger than the irregular PVA particles, so a size of 500–700 μm or 700–900 μm is usually used. There are increasing reports suggesting a higher clinical and imaging failure with spherical PVA.

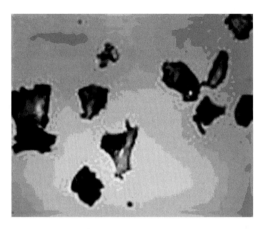

Fig. 10.3.3. Irregular shape of the non-spherical PVA

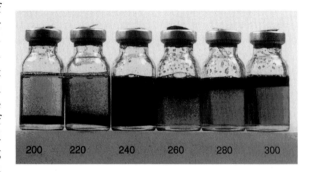

Fig. 10.3.4. Different dilution of contrast changes the suspension of the PVA, when 240 mg/ml is used there is suspension of the PVA in solution. In other dilutions it floats or sinks

10.3.3.5.2.2
Embospheres

A newer embolic which is a tris-acryl collagen-coated microsphere (Embospheres, Biosphere Medical, Rockland, MA) was the first embolic approved by the FDA specifically for fibroid embolization. These particles are hydrophilic and nonabsorbable. They have a very smooth surface, and are softer and more deformable than PVA. They are easily administered through a microcatheter since they have a reduced tendency for clumping and aggregation.

The embolic comes in pre-filled syringes to which the same volume of undiluted contrast is added. It is recommended that several minutes be allowed after adding the contrast so that the microspheres achieve suspension.

Another microsphere also made by Biosphere Medical is EmboGold, the microspheres are manufactured with the addition of gold, which is used to provide coloring. This product is specifically not cleared by the FDA for use in uterine fibroid embolization and has been associated with delayed pain and/or

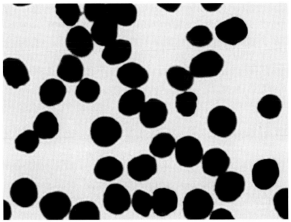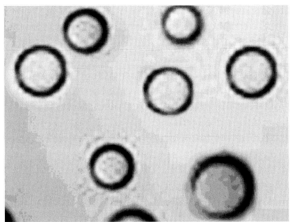

a   b

Fig. 10.3.5. a Spherical PVA are much more uniform and with smoother edges. b Embospheres are very smooth and very uniform in size

rash when used in these procedures (Biosphere Medical Instruction for Use for EmboGold Microspheres). There has been the report of endometritis in seven patients after uterine artery embolization when the EmboGold microspheres were used [28].

10.3.3.5.2.3
Gelfoam

Absorbable gelatin sponge (Gelfoam, Pharmacia & Upjohn Co. Kalamazoo, MI) has been widely used for intraarterial embolization. It is considered a "temporary" agent that may allow recanalization of the embolized artery. Because of the perception that it is a temporary agent its use is suggested for patients who may want to preserve their fertility [29]. Gelfoam causes an acute arteritis of the arterial wall that induces thrombosis [30]. There is resorption of Gelfoam in 6 weeks after embolization with minimal tissue reaction [30]. Whether the artery always recanalizes is not clear [29, 31]. Gelfoam has been used for uterine artery embolization with pathologic verification of coagulation necrosis of the fibroid [32] and essentially the same success rates published for other particle embolizations [33].

Gelfoam can be placed through a microcatheter [33], but it does tend to clog the microcatheter. Very small pieces and careful flushing between pieces can help in avoiding occlusion of the catheter.

10.3.3.5.2.4
General Considerations

The embolic particles are usually delivered using a three-way stopcock to which a syringe containing the particle-contrast mixture is attached. A 1-ml or 3-ml injection syringe is attached to the second port and then the stopcock is attached to the catheter. The particles can be re-suspended by transferring the contents of syringes from one to another, allowing mixing. The injection of the particles should be done using a slow, pulsatile injection, and watching the progress of the contrast into the uterine artery. If there is rapid flow of the particles away from the catheter then fluoroscopic monitoring is not required for the entire 1-ml injection. When the flow begins to slow, then more rigorous monitoring with fluoroscopy is required to avoid over embolization.

Gelfoam can be delivered by cutting the gelatin sponge into small fragments that are placed in a solution of saline and contrast. These are injected through the catheter. The Gelfoam pieces can also be place in a syringe with a saline and contrast solution with a three-way stopcock and macerated by the to-and-fro motion of between the two syringes, making a slurry of the Gelfoam. There is a tendency for Gelfoam to clog microcatheters so very careful technique is required if a microcatheter is being used, and the use of one of the larger lumen microcatheters is recommended.

Since the communications between the uterine artery and the ovarian arteries have been measured at 500 microns, particle sizes larger than 500 µm should help avoid having particles cross the anastomoses to enter the ovaries [9, 30, 34].

10.3.3.5.3
Medications

Most of the medications used in uterine artery embolization are focused on post-procedure pain management. However, these medications are most effective if they are given prior to the development of pain.

Most patients will benefit from a pre-procedure anxiolytic medication. Lorazepam (Ativan) 1 mg given sublingually is an excellent pre-medication. It is preferable to give a medication that can be administered sublingually since this allows the medication to be absorbed much more quickly, and to bypass the first pass through the liver that occurs if the drug is given as a swallowed, oral, medication. A pre-medication that helps control anxiety makes other anti-anxiety and pain medications more effective. During the procedure an anxiolytic such as midazolam (Versed) 0.5–1 mg titrated to patient comfort, and a pain medication such as fentanyl (Sublimaze) 25–50 mg titrated to patient comfort should be given. The patient will ideally be on a PCA pump following the procedure, so starting the PCA (particularly if a low-dose continuous infusion is being prescribed) during the procedure can provide another way of giving pain medication. The pain medication can provoke nausea in some patients. Although intravenous anti-nausea agents can be administered, the prophylactic placement of a scopolamine patch containing 1.5 mg scopolamine (Transderm Scop, Novartis) behind the ear is very effective at decreasing the severity of nausea. It is contraindicated in patients with narrow angle glaucoma.

Anti-inflammatory agents are very important to help in the control of pain. An intravenous nonsteroidal anti-inflammatory should be administrated. Ketorolac (Toradol) is an excellent agent. It has potent analgesic and anti-inflammatory activity; it also inhibits platelet aggregation, which is reversible within 24–48 h following discontinuation of the drug. The first dose should be given prior to beginning the procedure and then it should be continued while the patient is hospitalized. In most young, healthy women, Toradol is given in an intravenous dose of 30 mg every 6 h. The total length of treatment with Toradol cannot be more than 5 days.

The use of prophylactic antibiotics is controversial and there are no studies to determine whether antibiotic prophylaxis reduces the risk of infectious complications [35]. Most practitioners will give a single dose prior to beginning the procedure. Cefazolin (Ancef) 1 gm is a popular agent for prophylaxis but there is no consensus as to which agents should be used [35]. Some practitioners give an antibiotic following the procedure for 5–7 days [36]. Others believe that any potential infectious episodes can be more properly identified and cultured and treated if peri- or postprocedural antibiotics have not masked or disguised the organism responsible [22]. In addition, there is always the concern for selecting out more resistant organisms that may prove more difficult to treat. It is possible that prophylactic antibiotics destroy normal Gram-positive organisms allowing Gram-negative bacteria to proliferate [37].

Spasm is a concern during catheterization, and is relatively easy to induce with a guidewire or catheter. The development of spasm can reduce the efficacy of embolization by limiting the delivery of embolic particles. This can lead to premature closure of the larger uterine artery possibly leaving the distal branches patent [30]. The first strategy should be careful techniques to minimize the development of spasm, use of non-ionic contrast, careful use of guidewires and catheters, and possibly the use of microcatheters. The most common pharmacologic treatment of spasm is the use of intraarterial nitroglycerin (100–200 mcg) via the catheter. Some operators will give this as a routine medication in all patients. Others will give it only in patients when spasm develops. It is not known whether the fibroid vasculature responds to nitroglycerin or if only the normal uterus vasculature responds. If the latter, then the routine use of nitroglycerin may be counter productive since it would only cause vasodilatation of the normal vascularity potentially allowing increased embolization of the normal uterus. Although other vasodilators such as nifedipine have been given for peripheral vascular disease procedures, they are not commonly administered to patients undergoing uterine artery embolization.

10.3.3.5.4
Technique

10.3.3.5.4.1
Arterial access

The right common femoral artery is the most common site for arterial access. It is the most familiar and tends to be the most comfortable for the operator. Usually the entire procedure can be easily performed from a single arterial puncture. The contralateral artery is certainly very easy to approach with a C2 catheter as described above. The ipsilateral artery can be more difficult, particularly if a long, reversed curve catheter is not used. Occasionally the patient's anatomy will require the other femoral artery to be accessed.

Because of the potential difficulty of accessing the ipsilateral artery, some authors have advocated a bilateral common femoral artery approach [38].

The rational for this approach is that the more difficult ipsilateral catheterization is avoided, and injections of contrast can be performed simultaneously decreasing the amount of imaging sequences. There is at least a potential for decreasing the patient's radiation exposure. The concern regarding bilateral femoral artery punctures is that the risk of a puncture site complication is doubled. In addition, the use of bilateral femoral artery sheaths and placement of overlapping catheters in the distal aorta potentially increases the risk of thromboembolic complications [30].

Although an upper extremity approach using a brachial, axillary or radial artery puncture could be used, in actual practice this is almost never performed. It does have the advantage of not requiring the ipsilateral catheterization of the femoral approach, but there are significant disadvantages. The brachial and radial arteries have a very small caliber raising the concern for direct catheter trauma or thrombosis of these arteries. In addition, this approach requires the manipulation of the catheter in the region of the great vessels placing the patient at risk of a cerebral vascular event.

10.3.3.5.4.2
Catheterization Techniques

Whichever access is chosen, a 4- or 5-F sheath depending on the catheter, which is going to be used, is placed into the artery. A sheath is a good idea when embolization is going to be performed, in case there is clogging or damage to the catheter that would prevent a wire from being placed through the catheter to allow an exchange. If there is embolic material in the catheter that would be unsafe to deliver, the catheter can be removed and replaced with a fresh catheter if a sheath is in place. The sheath also facilitates the exchange of catheters and the manipulation of the catheters at the groin, which otherwise might enlarge the puncture site leading to a hematoma.

My technique for embolization of uterine fibroids starts with placing a flush catheter that allows a contralateral approach (VCF or Omni Flush catheter) into the aorta and positioning it just below the level of the renal arteries. The image intensifier is centered over the pelvis and a angiogram is performed which allows for visualization of ovarian artery collaterals, and provides visualization of the iliac anatomy (Fig. 10.3.6a). The flush catheter is then positioned

at the aortic bifurcation with the tip in the contralateral common iliac artery and a wire (most commonly a Glidewire) is advanced into the contralateral common femoral or superficial femoral artery (Fig. 10.3.6b). The flush catheter is removed and the RUC catheter is advance over the wire until the genu of the catheter, with the radiopaque marker, is lying directly on the aortic bifurcation (Fig. 10.3.6c). The wire is then pulled back into the catheter until it is in the ipsilateral portion of the catheter. The catheter is pushed up at the groin, which causes the catheter to form a loop in the aorta (Fig. 10.3.6d). As the catheter is pushed in at the groin, the tip of the catheter moves up in the contralateral artery. Once the tip of the catheter is above the internal iliac artery, the wire is taken out, the catheter is flushed, and a contrast syringe is placed on the catheter. The catheter can then be rotated so that the tip points medially (rotation of the catheter usually will not rotate the tip of the catheter without the catheter being moved either forward or back). With the catheter directed medially it could be pulled down at the groin, advancing the tip into the internal iliac artery (Fig. 10.3.6e,f). Using a small amount of contrast to help visualize the arterial anatomy the catheter can be gently advanced and twisted to select the uterine artery (Fig. 10.3.6g,h). When the uterine artery is catheterized, the catheter can be gently pulled into the artery to approximately the level of the transverse section of the artery. If the artery is very small, then a microcatheter can be used to access the uterine artery. In this event, the RUC catheter is pushed up so that the tip is just at the origin of the uterine artery allowing good blood flow through the artery. Following embolization of the contralateral artery, the catheter is advanced at the groin to allow the tip to disengage from the uterine artery. An injection of contrast can then be performed to verify appropriate embolization.

The catheter is then advanced at the groin until the tip is back in the aorta (Fig. 10.3.6i) and then the catheter is pulled back at the groin and manipulated until the tip of the catheter engages the internal iliac artery (Fig. 10.3.6j,k) the tip is then maneuvered into the uterine artery using small injections of contrast for guidance (Fig 10.3.6l). Once the artery is catheterized, and embolized, the catheter is again advanced at the groin disengaging the tip and the catheter is advanced up into the aorta until the tip of the catheter is above the bifurcation. The catheter is then pulled back using the tip to engage the contralateral iliac artery, and continuous pulling back allows the tip to slide down the contralateral

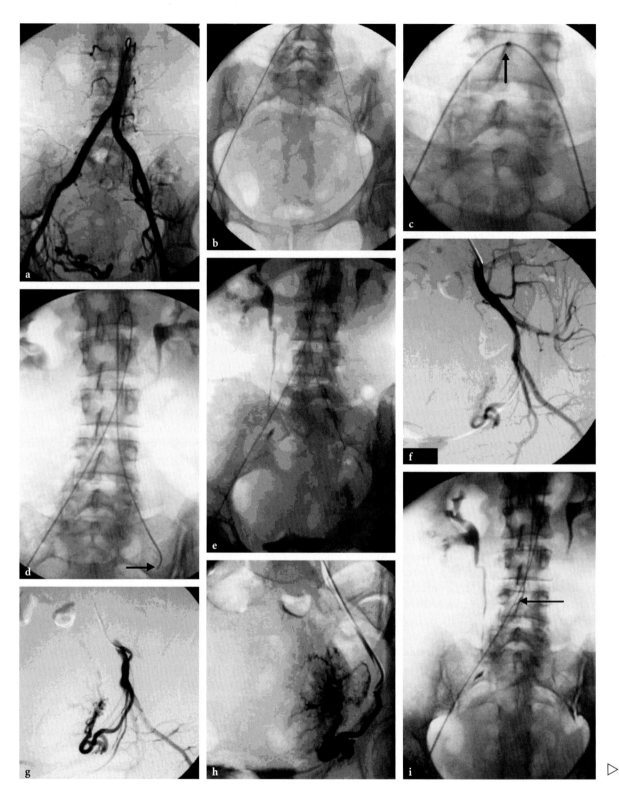

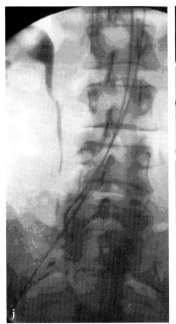
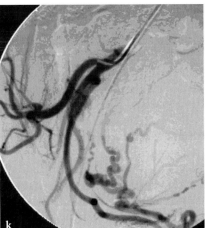
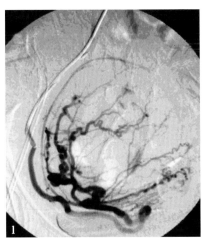

Fig. 10.3.6. a Aortogram demonstrating pelvic anatomy, no uterine arteries identified. **b** Flush catheter used to position a Glide-wire over the bifurcation. **c** The RUC catheter has been positioned over the bifurcation. The radiopaque marker designates the spot where the loop will form (*arrow*), this must lie on the bifurcation. **d** The catheter is being pushed up at the groin and a loop is beginning to form in the aorta. The tip of the catheter (*arrow*) has moved from the region of the common femoral artery towards the internal iliac artery. **e,f** The catheter tip is being advanced above the internal iliac and then with some contrast an injection is pulled down with gentle manipulation until it enters the internal iliac artery. **g,h** The catheter tip is then manipulated and gently pulled down, giving injections of contrast to visualize the uterine artery, it is gently pulled down until appropriately positioned, or if spasm results, then decision made whether to use a microcatheter. **i** Following the embolization of the contralateral uterine artery, the catheter is again advanced at the groin until the tip of the catheter (*arrow*) is above the aortic bifurcation. Then it is pulled down, advancing the catheter tip into the common iliac artery. **j,k** The catheter is pulled down pointed medially until it engages the internal iliac artery, the tip may then be turned slightly to try and catheterize the uterine artery. **l** The catheter is positioned in the uterine artery and if in good position then embolization can proceed

external iliac and into the common femoral artery until the catheter is again settled against the aortic bifurcation. Continued withdrawal of the catheter will allow the catheter to be taken out of the sheath.

The benefit of this type of catheter is that essentially the entire catheterization can be performed without having a guidewire in the internal iliac or uterine artery thus helping to prevent spasm. In addition since the catheter is being maneuvered without a wire in place, injection of the contrast allows for visualization of the vessels and consequently a much faster catheterization with minimal fluoroscopy time.

An alternative way of catheterizing the uterine artery using selective catheters is described by Andrews [30]. Following an aortogram, the flush catheter is used to direct a wire over the iliac bifurcation. A 4-F Berenstein catheter (or another selective catheter such as a C2) is then placed into the contralateral common iliac artery. Repeat imaging

of the internal iliac may be necessary to better visualize the origin of the uterine artery. A guidewire is then placed, and the catheter is advanced in to the internal iliac artery. The wire is used to gently probe for the uterine artery. Road mapping is probably very helpful at this point, although it can increase dose rates relative to conventional fluoroscopy in some angiographic suites [39]. The course of the wire when it is in the uterine artery will be medially directed initially and then will turn cephalad. If the wire does not engage the uterine artery, then the catheter can be advanced distally, beyond the expected point of origin and contrast injected as the catheter is slowly withdrawn. When the uterine artery origin is reached, contrast will be seen, the catheter is held in position and the guidewire reintroduced and again gentle probing is used to try and access the uterine artery. Once the wire is in place, then the catheter is advanced gently into the first 1–2 cm of the artery and a uterine artery angiogram is performed. If there is little or no flow, then it may be necessary to place a microcatheter and withdraw the primary catheter into the internal iliac artery. In any case after the initial uterine artery angiogram some type of catheter needs to be advanced more distally into the uterine artery, ideally into the medial aspect of the horizontal segment, past the cervicovaginal branch, if it is identified. After embolization of the contralateral uterine artery, a Waltman loop is formed using the selective catheter, and the catheter is directed into the ipsilateral uterine artery using the soft end of the Glidewire. Again angiography followed by more selective catheterization and embolization is performed on the ipsilateral side.

This dependence on the guidewire for location of the uterine artery, and advancement of the catheter is much more likely to lead to spasm than used of the long reversed curve catheter. If spasm occurs, then nitroglycerin (100–200 mcg) can be given to help relieve the spasm. Alternatively, slow injection of saline may break the spasm and allow resumption of flow [30].

Very occasionally it is not possible to embolize one of the uterine arteries, despite multiple catheters, guidewires, microcatheters and even alternative access sites. If an artery is difficult to catheterize, the first approach should be to access the other uterine artery and embolize it, prior to spending a great deal of time on the difficult artery. After successful embolization of one artery, a reattempt of the difficult artery should then be tried. In some cases there is flow redistribution which can facilitate the catheterization [40]. After occluding the flow in one uterine artery, there is vasodilatation of the contralateral uterine artery that may make embolization easier [30]. If, despite considerable effort, one is not able to embolize the artery, rather than sending the patient to surgery, it is reasonable to have the patient come back for another attempt in a few weeks or a few months [41]. The fibroids that have been successfully embolized decrease in size, changing the positioning of the uterus, which in turn may change the angulation of the artery allowing for easier catheterization.

10.3.3.5.4.3
Use of Closure Devices

There has been increased use of percutaneous closure devices for closing the femoral artery puncture site. These devices are particularly helpful in patients that are being anticoagulated. There are a number of types of hemostatic devices: hemostatic patches, collagen-mediated devices, and suture

closure devices. There has been a debate regarding the use of these devices in women undergoing uterine artery embolization. The concern is that in young women with essentially normal arteries, manual compression is usually effective in obtaining hemostasis in 15–20 min, and after 4–6 h of bed rest there is a very low incidence of bleeding or other puncture site complication. However, because of the post-embolization pain patients may have more difficulty holding their leg still, particularly if they are getting substantial doses of narcotics. Also, if one wanted to perform the embolization procedure as an outpatient procedure, having an effective arterial closure would be beneficial. Two studies evaluating closure devices in patients undergoing angiographic procedures came to different conclusions. In one evaluation of a percutaneous suture-mediated closure device in 100 patients undergoing angiographic procedures, primarily uterine artery embolization procedures (65 patients), were retrospectively compared with patients not having the closure device [42]. This report described a 5% major complication rate (all in women undergoing UAE). One patient required thromboendarterectomy and patch angioplasty to repair the common femoral occlusion, as well as amputation of a gangrenous toe. There were also two cases of external iliac artery dissection, one with distal embolization.

A second study [43] was a prospective, although not randomized study, evaluating only patients undergoing UAE. This study had 342 patients enrolled, 328 of them received a suture-mediated closure device. There were no major complications. Approximately 21% of the patients complained of anteromedial thigh pain that responded to non-steroidal anti-inflammatory medications. This pain was postulated to result from irritation of the anterior femoral cutaneous nerve and presumably results from the nerve fibers being trapped by the sutures during deployment.

If closure devices are going to be used, then complications can be minimized by adherence to meticulous sterile technique and confirmation of the appropriate indication and anatomy. Whether the potential risk of the closure device is outweighed by patient satisfaction and convenience is not clear at this point.

10.3.3.5.4.4
Radiation Exposure

Since uterine artery embolization is performed in relatively young patients, some of whom are desiring future fertility, it is critical that radiation exposure be minimized. The gonads are among the most radiation-sensitive organs, and the potential for malignant degeneration increases directly with cumulative radiation dose [39]. In order to have the best success rate and the least complications, the angiographic equipment should be of high quality. There must be adjustable collimators, and the capability of serial radiography and digital subtraction [35]. Ideally the unit will be equipped with reduced-dose pulsed fluoroscopy and last image hold. The unit should be able to perform oblique and compound angulation to facilitate selective catheterization. There should be a mechanism for recording patient radiation dose, such as dose-area product or cumulative dose at the interventional reference point or skin entrance dose [35]. Although roadmapping can be useful in subselective catheterizations, the activation of roadmapping can disable the low-dose or pulsed fluoroscopic modes and may cause marked increase in dose rates [30].

There are angiographic techniques that can reduce a patient's radiation exposure. Such variables include minimizing the number of images acquired during the procedure, perhaps electing to record a image from the last fluoroscopic image from each injection of contrast which avoids dedicated DSA runs and increase the number of images acquired during the procedure [39]. Minimizing the amount of image magnification and the degree of imaging obliquity will decrease radiation exposure. Full magnification can increase the dose by 30%–155% [30, 38, 39, 44]. The obliquity of the image intensifier can be changed frequently but with only a slight degree of angulation to avoid one area of the patient getting most of the radiation beam. If an oblique view is required for catheterization, the imaging configuration should be restored to a frontal projection as soon as the catheterization has been achieved [30]. Raising the patient as far from the beam source as practical while simultaneously minimizing the distance between the patient and the image intensifier can decrease the dose for fluoroscopy and imaging by up to 50% [30, 39]. Tight collimation is critical to decrease exposure.

10.3.3.5.5
Endpoints

The angiographic endpoint of uterine artery embolization with non-spherical PVA or Gelfoam is usually until there is stasis or near stasis in the artery [35, 45–49].

There have been studies looking at microspheres in animal models that demonstrate these particles are more effective than PVA particles in achieving target vascular occlusion and tissue necrosis, with a more segmental arterial occlusion [50]. A small study of patients undergoing uterine artery embolization followed by myomectomy demonstrated aggregation of the PVA in vessels in the perifibroid myometrium, and microspheres within the fibroid arteries [51]. These findings seem to confirm the animal studies that microspheres are more likely to penetrate the fibroid vasculature than PVA. Because of this more complete arterial occlusion, the end point of embolization is felt to be different with spherical embolization particle [52]. The particle size should be larger for spherical embolization particles than for non-spherical PVA particles [52]. Non-spherical PVA is usually 300–500 μm in size while spherical particles should be 500–700 or 700–900 μm. The degree of penetration into the vascular system is actually greater with PVA spheres, and they may occlude on an even more distal level than tri-acryl spheres, perhaps because of different compressibility properties [50]. Since a more targeted embolization is possible with calibrated microspheres a limited embolization is preferred. Instead of embolizing until there is complete stasis in the uterine artery, the embolization is stopped when: (1) no residual hypervascularization related to the fibroids is visible, (2) there is flow redistribution with identification of normal myometrial branches, (3) easy reflux into the ovarian artery that was not present earlier, (4) filling of cross-uterine branches, (5) stasis in the distal part of the uterine artery, or (6) reduced flow in the proximal part of the uterine artery [34, 50, 53]. This results in a "pruned tree" appearance of the uterine artery [50, 51].

Although there are theoretical advantages to the use of Embospheres, clinical studies have not shown an advantage over PVA particles [27]. The volume decrease of the fibroids, and the uterine volume reduction is similar between Embospheres and PVA [54]. The volume of microspheres required for an embolization is larger than the volume of PVA required to complete an embolization [27]. In both retrospective and prospective study there does not seem to be a difference in post procedure pain or the use of narcotic use between PVA and microspheres [27, 55].

10.3.3.5.5.1
Ovarian Artery Supply

There is no current consensus regarding the appropriateness and timing of searching for and treating collateral blood supply [35]. Some practitioners obtain an initial aortograms with the catheter at the level of the renal arteries prior to the uterine artery embolization (Fig. 10.3.7) [23, 56]. Others do not evaluate the ovarian supply or perform an angiogram after the embolization [30, 31]. Those who do not evaluate the ovarian supply may wait and evaluate the patient's clinical symptoms. If the symptoms do not respond appropriately, patients can either get an magnetic resonance angiographic (MRA) study to evaluate for ovarian collaterals (Fig. 10.3.8) or undergo another angiogram [30]. If there are large ovarian collaterals found on the initial study, there

is debate about how to handle these arterial collaterals. Some operators will wait to see how the patient responds to the initial uterine artery embolization and if there are continued symptoms will bring the patient back for a repeat angiogram and embolization. Some routinely get consent for embolization of the ovarian arteries prior to the procedure, and if they are large, will embolize the ovarian arteries during the initial procedure [30].

If large ovarian arteries are found, they maybe embolized with relatively large embolic particles, PVA 500–700 μm or spherical embolic particles 700–900 μm (Fig. 10.3.9a,b). Alternatively many

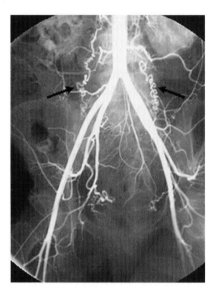

Fig. 10.3.7. Preliminary aortogram demonstrating bilateral enlarged ovarian arteries

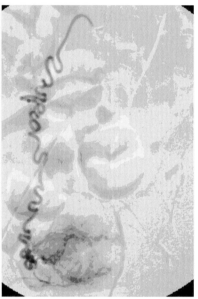

a

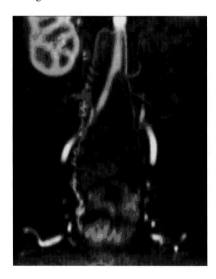

Fig. 10.3.8. Patient with recurrent symptoms following uterine artery embolization. MRA demonstrating large right ovarian artery

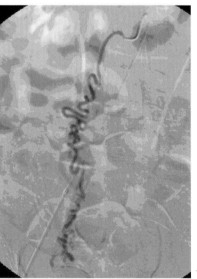

b

Fig. 10.3.9. a Right ovarian artery supplying fibroid. **b** Post embolization, stasis in ovarian artery and no supply to fibroid

operators will use Gelfoam for embolization of the ovarian arteries [30, 31].

In conclusion, the success of uterine artery embolization for uterine fibroids is dependent on an understanding of the anatomy, and particularly an appreciation of the variant anatomy that can be the source of some unusual complications. There are a number of technical considerations that can influence the ease of the procedure, and the safety of the procedure. The operator should be well versed in the variety of catheters that can be used for this procedure, as well as the characteristics of the embolic materials. Attention needs to be paid to radiation safety; there are a number of factors that the operator controls and which can markedly decrease the radiation exposure for both the patient and the operator.

Cookbook:

5-F sheath

Wires
- Bentsen
- 15-J standard wire
- Glidewire

4- to 5-F catheters
- Flush catheter (if planning aortogram)
- Selective catheters
  - C2 catheter
  - Bernstein or Kumpe catheters
  - RUC catheter

Microcatheters
- Hydrophilic, high-flow catheters

Microwires – if using microcatheters
- Hydrophilic

Embolic materials
- Non-spherical PVA (300–500 μm)
- Biospheres 500–700 μm, 700–900 μm

Medications
- Ativan 1 mg sublingual as preop
- Fentanyl
- Versad
- Scopolamine 1.5-mg patch behind ear
- Ancef 1 gm (or other prophylactic antibiotic)
- Nitroglycerin (100–200 mcg aliquots) as needed for spasm, or may be given "prophylactically"
- Toradol 30 mg

References

1. Netter FH (1977) Reproductive system. Summit, N.J., Ciba Pharmaceutical Company
2. Kadir S (1991) Atlas of normal and variant angiographic anatomy. W.B. Saunders, Philadelphia
3. Pelage JP, Soyer P, Le Dref O, et al. (1999) Uterine arteries: bilateral catheterization with a single femoral approach and a single 5-F catheter – technical note. Radiology 210:573–575
4. Gomez-Jorge J, Keyoung A, Levy EB, Spies JB (2003) Uterine artery anatomy relevant to uterine leiomyomata embolization. Cardiovasc Intervent Radiol 26:522–527
5. Cicinelli E, Einer-Jensen N, Galantino P, Alfonso R, Nicoletti R (2004) The vascular cast of the human uterus: from anatomy to physiology. Ann N Y Acad Sci 1034:19–26
6. Saraiya PV, Chang TC, Pelage JP, Spies JB (2002) Uterine artery replacement by the round ligament artery: an anatomic variant discovered during uterine artery embolization for leiomyomata. J Vasc Interv Radiol 13:939–941
7. LeDref O, Pelage JP, Kardache M (2000) Superselective embolization of ovarian and round ligament arteries in the management of obstetric menorrhage. Cardiovasc Intervent Radiol 23[suppl]:103
8. Jones K, Walker WJ, Sutton C (2003) A case of failed fibroid embolisation due to an unusual vascular supply. Bjog 110:782–783
9. Pelage JP, Le Dref O, Soyer P, et al. (1999) Arterial anatomy of the female genital tract: variations and relevance to transcatheter embolization of the uterus. AJR Am J Roentgenol 172:989–994
10. Amato P, Roberts AC (2001) Transient ovarian failure: a complication of uterine artery embolization. Fertil Steril 75:438–439
11. Hascalik S, Celik O, Sarac K, Hascalik M (2004) Transient ovarian failure: a rare complication of uterine fibroid embolization. Acta Obstet Gynecol Scand 83:682–685
12. Hovsepian DM, Siskin GP, Bonn J, et al. (2004) Quality improvement guidelines for uterine artery embolization for symptomatic leiomyomata. Cardiovasc Intervent Radiol 27:307–313
13. Tropeano G, Litwicka K, Di Stasi C, Romano D, Mancuso S (2003) Permanent amenorrhea associated with endometrial atrophy after uterine artery embolization for symptomatic uterine fibroids. Fertil Steril 79:132–135
14. Yeagley TJ, Goldberg J, Klein TA, Bonn J (2002) Labial necrosis after uterine artery embolization for leiomyomata. Obstet Gynecol 100:881–882
15. Sultana CJ, Goldberg J, Aizenman L, Chon JK (2002) Vesicouterine fistula after uterine artery embolization: a case report. Am J Obstet Gynecol 187:1726–1727
16. El-Shalakany AH, Nasr El-Din MH, Wafa GA, Azzam ME, El-Dorry A (2003) Massive vault necrosis with bladder fistula after uterine artery embolisation. Bjog 110:215–216
17. Lowenstein L, Solt I, Siegler E, Raz N, Amit A (2004) Focal cervical and vaginal necrosis following uterine artery embolisation. Eur J Obstet Gynecol Reprod Biol 116:250–251
18. Huang LY, Cheng YF, Huang CC, Chang SY, Kung FT (2003) Incomplete vaginal expulsion of pyoadenomyoma with sepsis and focal bladder necrosis after uterine artery embolization for symptomatic adenomyosis: case report. Hum Reprod 18:167–171
19. Hutchins FL, Jr., Worthington-Kirsch R (2000) Embolo-

therapy for myoma-induced menorrhagia. Obstet Gynecol Clin North Am 27:397–405, viii

20. Dietz DM, Stahlfeld KR, Bansal SK, Christopherson WA (2004) Buttock necrosis after uterine artery embolization. Obstet Gynecol 104:1159–1161

21. Lai AC, Goodwin SC, Bonilla SM, et al. (2000) Sexual dysfunction after uterine artery embolization. J Vasc Interv Radiol 11:755–758

22. Sterling KM, Vogelzang RL, Chrisman HB, et al. (2002) V. Uterine fibroid embolization: management of complications. Tech Vasc Interv Radiol 5:56–66

23. Pelage JP, Walker WJ, Le Dref O, Rymer R (2003) Ovarian artery: angiographic appearance, embolization and relevance to uterine fibroid embolization. Cardiovasc Intervent Radiol 26:227–233

24. Razavi MK, Wolanske KA, Hwang GL, Sze DY, Kee ST, Dake MD (2002) Angiographic classification of ovarian artery-to-uterine artery anastomoses: initial observations in uterine fibroid embolization. Radiology 224:707–712

25. Waltman AC, Courey WR, Athanasoulis C, Baum S (1973) Technique for left gastric artery catheterization. Radiology 109:732–734

26. Spies JB (2003) Uterine artery embolization for fibroids: understanding the technical causes of failure. J Vasc Interv Radiol 14:11–14

27. Spies JB, Allison S, Flick P, et al. (2004) Polyvinyl alcohol particles and tris-acryl gelatin microspheres for uterine artery embolization for leiomyomas: results of a randomized comparative study. J Vasc Interv Radiol 15:793–800

28. Richard HM, 3rd, Siskin GP, Stainken BF (2004) Endometritis after uterine artery embolization with gold-colored gelatin microspheres. J Vasc Interv Radiol 15:406–407

29. Spies JB, Benenati JF, Worthington-Kirsch RL, Pelage JP (2001) Initial experience with use of tris-acryl gelatin microspheres for uterine artery embolization for leiomyomata. J Vasc Interv Radiol 12:1059–1063

30. Worthington-Kirsch RL, Andrews RT, Siskin GP, et al. (2002) II. Uterine fibroid embolization: technical aspects. Tech Vasc Interv Radiol 5:17–34

31. Worthington-Kirsch RL (2004) Uterine artery embolization: state of the art. Semin in Interv Radiology 21:37–42

32. Katsumori T, Bamba M, Kobayashi TK, et al. (2002) Uterine leiomyoma after embolization by means of gelatin sponge particles alone: report of a case with histopathologic features. Ann Diagn Pathol 6:307–311

33. Katsumori T, Nakajima K, Mihara T, Tokuhiro M (2002) Uterine artery embolization using gelatin sponge particles alone for symptomatic uterine fibroids: midterm results. AJR Am J Roentgenol 178:135–139

34. Pelage JP, Le Dref O, Beregi JP, et al. (2003) Limited uterine artery embolization with tris-acryl gelatin microspheres for uterine fibroids. J Vasc Interv Radiol 14:15–20

35. Andrews RT, Spies JB, Sacks D, et al. (2004) Patient care and uterine artery embolization for leiomyomata. J Vasc Interv Radiol 15:115–120

36. Siskin GP, Stainken BF, Dowling K, Meo P, Ahn J, Dolen EG (2000) Outpatient uterine artery embolization for symptomatic uterine fibroids: experience in 49 patients. J Vasc Interv Radiol 11:305–311

37. Mehta H, Sandhu C, Matson M, Belli AM (2002) Review of readmissions due to complications from uterine fibroid embolization. Clin Radiol 57:1122–1124

38. Nikolic B, Abbara S, Levy E, et al. (2000) Influence of radiographic technique and equipment on absorbed ovarian dose associated with uterine artery embolization. J Vasc Interv Radiol 11:1173–1178

39. Andrews RT, Brown PH (2000) Uterine arterial embolization: factors influencing patient radiation exposure. Radiology 217:713–722

40. Worthington-Kirsch RL (1999) Flow redistribution during uterine artery embolization for the management of symptomatic fibroids. J Vasc Interv Radiol 10:237–238

41. McLucas B, Reed RA, Goodwin S, et al. (2002) Outcomes following unilateral uterine artery embolisation. Br J Radiol 75:122–126

42. Wagner SC, Gonsalves CF, Eschelman DJ, Sullivan KL, Bonn J (2003) Complications of a percutaneous suture-mediated closure device versus manual compression for arteriotomy closure: a case-controlled study. J Vasc Interv Radiol 14:735–741

43. Chrisman HB, Liu DM, Bui JT, et al. (2005) The safety and efficacy of a percutaneous closure device in patients undergoing uterine artery embolization. J Vasc Interv Radiol 16:347–350; quiz 351

44. Nikolic B, Spies JB, Lundsten MJ, Abbara S (2000) Patient radiation dose associated with uterine artery embolization. Radiology 214:121–125

45. Goodwin SC, McLucas B, Lee M, et al. (1999) Uterine artery embolization for the treatment of uterine leiomyomata midterm results. J Vasc Interv Radiol 10:1159–1165

46. Goodwin SC, Vedantham S, McLucas B, Forno AE, Perrella R (1997) Preliminary experience with uterine artery embolization for uterine fibroids. J Vasc Interv Radiol 8:517–526

47. Goodwin SC, Walker WJ (1998) Uterine artery embolization for the treatment of uterine fibroids. Curr Opin Obstet Gynecol 10:315–320

48. Walker WJ, Pelage JP (2002) Uterine artery embolisation for symptomatic fibroids: clinical results in 400 women with imaging follow up. Bjog 109:1262–1272

49. Walker WJ, Pelage JP, Sutton C (2002) Fibroid embolization. Clin Radiol 57:325–331

50. Pelage JP (2004) Polyvinyl alcohol particles versus tris-acryl gelatin microspheres for uterine artery embolization for leiomyomas. J Vasc Interv Radiol 15:789–791

51. Chua GC, Wilsher M, Young MP, Manyonda I, Morgan R, Belli AM (2005) Comparison of particle penetration with non-spherical polyvinyl alcohol versus tris-acryl gelatin microspheres in women undergoing premyomectomy uterine artery embolization. Clin Radiol 60:116–122

52. Pelage JP, Jacob D, Le Dref O, Lacombe P, Laurent A (2004) Re: fatal sepsis after uterine artery embolization with microspheres. J Vasc Interv Radiol 15:405–406; author reply 406

53. Joffre F, Tubiana JM, Pelage JP (2004) FEMIC (Fibromes Embolises aux MICrospheres calibrees): uterine fibroid embolization using tris-acryl microspheres. A French multicenter study. Cardiovasc Intervent Radiol 27:600–606

54. Banovac F, Ascher SM, Jones DA, Black MD, Smith JC, Spies JB (2002) Magnetic resonance imaging outcome after uterine artery embolization for leiomyomata with use of tris-acryl gelatin microspheres. J Vasc Interv Radiol 13:681–688

55. Ryu RK, Omary RA, Sichlau MJ, et al. (2003) Comparison of pain after uterine artery embolization using tris-acryl gelatin microspheres versus polyvinyl alcohol particles. Cardiovasc Intervent Radiol 26:375–378

56. Binkert CA, Andrews RT, Kaufman JA (2001) Utility of nonselective abdominal aortography in demonstrating ovarian artery collaterals in patients undergoing uterine artery embolization for fibroids. J Vasc Interv Radiol 12:841–845

10.4 Results and Complications

JEAN-PIERRE PELAGE, ARNAUD FAUCONNIER, and PASCAL LACOMBE

CONTENTS

J.-P. PELAGE, MD, PhD; P. LACOMBE, MD
Department of Radiology Hôpital Ambroise Pare, 9, Avenue
Charles De Gaulle, 92104 Boulogne Cedex, France
A. FAUCONNIER, MD, PhD
Department of Obstetrics and Gynecology, Centre Hospitalier
de Poissy, 10, rue du Champ Gaillard, 78300 Poissy Cedex,
France

10.4.1
Introduction

Since the first reports of its use as a therapeutic option for women with symptomatic uterine fibroids, uterine artery embolization has become increasingly accepted as therapy for this patient population. With the increasing frequency of its use in this setting, a greater understanding of both the advantages and the potential risks of this procedure has occurred.

With the growing popularity of uterine fibroid embolization (UFE), the scientific evidence has also greatly improved. Evaluation of results associated with UFE has included clinical success rate and uterine/fibroid volume reduction. Cost, recovery time, change in quality-of-life and patient acceptance are other important considerations. The associated risks of complications associated with UFE are of paramount importance before offering this procedure to young women interested in future fertility.

There is, however, enough scientific data from the literature to suggest that UFE is a highly effective, minimally invasive alternative to surgery and is now widely accepted for the management of fibroid-related symptoms. This chapter summarizes the published results of UFE with respect to clinical benefits and potential complications, change in health-related quality-of-life measurements, fibroid devascularization and uterine volume reduction, and patient satisfaction. The initial studies comparing embolization to surgical procedures will also be presented and their results discussed.

10.4.2
Technical Success

Technical success has been described as successful embolization of both uterine arteries [1, 2]. The reason is that, except in rare cases, the procedure is unlikely to be successful unless both arteries are treated [2, 3]. In early series, complete occlusion of both uterine arteries to stasis with polyvinyl alcohol (PVA) particles, often supplemented with either gelatin sponge pledgets or coils, was the standard end-point of embolization [4–7]. With the introduction of tris-acryl gelatin microspheres, the appropriate end-point has become a subject of discussion [8]. Limited embolization of the uterine arteries leaving patent the main arterial trunk has been reported [9, 10]. The reported technical success rates range from 84% to 100% with most series reporting more than 95% technically successful procedures [1, 4, 7, 9].

Increasing operator experience will likely improve the technical success and efficiency of the procedure, with concomitant reduction of procedure duration and fluoroscopy time [1, 7].

10.4.3
Clinical Success

Clinical success has been measured by the degree of improvement or the frequency of resolution of symptoms [11]. In most studies, these symptoms include heavy menstrual bleeding, pelvic pain and bulk-related symptoms (pressure, bloating and urinary frequency). In most of the published studies, PVA particles were used as the embolization agent [5–7, 11–15]. Success rates for treating menorrhagia, pelvic pain and bulk-related symptoms ranged from 81% to 96%, 70% to 100% and 46% to 100%, respectively [4–6, 16–19]. In a series of 305 women, HUTCHINS reported control of menorrhagia and bulk-related symptoms in 92% of cases at 12 months [4]. Three prospective studies with more than 200 patients enrolled have been recently published in the gynecological literature [7, 9, 11]. From a cohort of 508 patients undergoing UFE using PVA particles in Canada, significant improvements were reported for menorrhagia (83%), dysmenorrhea (77%) and urinary frequency (86%) at 3 months [11]. Menorrhagia was significantly improved with a reduction in the mean menstrual duration from 7.6 to 5.4 days [11]. WALKER and PELAGE [7] reported on their experience with UFE in 400 women with symptomatic fibroids with a mean clinical follow-up of 16.7 months. Menstrual bleeding improved in 84% of women and pelvic pain was improved in 79%. In a series of 200 women, SPIES reported similar results with improvement of menorrhagia and bulk symptoms in 90% and 91% of cases, respectively at 12 months [9]. Recently, MARRET reported 83.5% overall clinical improvement of symptoms at a mean follow-up of 30 months in 85 patients [20]. With objective measurements of menstrual blood loss, KHAUND et al. [21] reported significant reduction from 162 ml pretreatment to 41 ml at 36–48 months. The results of the largest prospective studies are summarized in Table 10.4.1.

In the short-term, UFE using gelatin sponge pledgets alone seems to show comparable results as those obtained with PVA particles [22]. KATSUMORI reported improvement in menorrhagia and in bulk-related symptoms in 98% and 97% of cases respectively at 4 months after embolization [22].

The initial experience with the use of tris-acryl microspheres mirrors the results obtained with PVA particles [10, 14]. SPIES reported significant reduction of menstrual bleeding and pelvic pain in 92% of treated patients at 3 months [14]. PELAGE

Table 10.4.1. Results of three prospective studies (including more than 200 patients) evaluating uterine fibroid embolization

Study	Number of patients	Mean follow-up in months	Efficacy on menorrhagia	Efficacy on pain	Efficacy on pelvic pressure	Efficacy on urinary frequency	Uterine volume redution (%)	Fibroid volume reduction (%)	Hysterectomy for complication (%)	Permanent amenorrhea (mean age in years)
SPIES et al. (2001a)	200	21	90%	NA	91%	NA	38%a	58%a	0%	2% (NA)
WALKER and PELAGE (2002)	400	16.7	84%	79%	90%	86%	57%b	77%b	1%	7% (48.4)
PRON et al. (2003b)	538	8.2	83%	77%	NA	86%	35%c	42%c	NA	NA

NA, data not mentioned in the cited paper.

[a]Mean reduction at 12 months; [b]Median reduction at 9.7 months; [c]Median reduction at 3 months.

reported complete resolution of menorrhagia in 85% of patients with a mean follow-up of 30 months [10]. In a multicenter study reporting the use of tris-acryl microspheres larger than 500 µm, complete resolution of menorrhagia was observed in 84% of treated women at 24 months [23]. In a recent randomized study comparing tris-acryl microspheres and PVA particles for UFE, Spies demonstrated no significant difference between the two types of embolization particles in any of the outcome variables [24].

The recurrence rate after UFE has been reported to be lower than 10%, most cases beeing related to regrowth of fibroids not infarcted after the initial procedure [20]. The long-term rate of recurrence due to the growth of new fibroids in still to be determined [25].

10.4.4
Patient Satisfaction

Patient satisfaction with the clinical outcome of UFE has usually been measured with follow-up questionnaires and correlates well with symptomatic improvement [7, 26].

WORTHINGTON-KIRSCH et al. [26] surveyed their cohort of 53 patients for satisfaction with the procedure and reported that 79% of the patients interviewed would choose the procedure again. WALKER and PELAGE [7] reported that 97% of patients were pleased with the outcome and would recommend UFE to others. In their treatment of 200 consecutive patients, SPIES et al. [9] reported that patient satisfaction paralleled the symptom results and that these results remained stable during the course of follow-up.

10.4.5
Quality of Life After Embolization

A broader measure of outcome is the change in quality-of-life after UFE. Health-related quality-of-life questionnaires usually measure parameters such as energy, vitality, mood, pain, physical energy, social functioning, and sexual function [26, 27]. There has been relatively little written about the impact of UFE on quality-of-life, in part because until recently there have been few validated fibroid-specific quality-of-life questionnaires. Standardized quality-of-life questionnaires

such as the SF-36 and the SF-12 have been used to a limited extent in UFE [27]. SPIES et al. [27] found that there were significant improvements in health-related quality of life and fibroid-specific symptoms in 50 patients undergoing UFE. A disease-specific quality-of-life instrument for fibroids has been developed [28]. It has been used as one measure of outcome in a recent study comparing the outcome of UFE using PVA particles and tris-acryl microspheres [24]. SMITH et al. [29] confirmed significant improvement in health-related quality of life scores after UFE. High levels of satisfaction were observed even when subsequent therapies were necessary after UFE.

These published studies confirm the usefulness of measures of quality-of-life in assessing outcome and have particular utility when comparing relative outcome of UFE with other fibroid therapies.

10.4.6
Imaging Evaluation

10.4.6.1
Volume Reduction

Uterine volume reduction and fibroid shrinkage are evaluated after embolization as part of imaging outcome (Fig 10.4.1). Within 3–6 months after UFE, a 25%–60% reduction of uterine volume has been reported [4–7, 11, 19]. The reduction in volume of the dominant fibroid ranges between 33% to 68% at 3–12 months [5–7, 9, 11, 18, 19]. From the Canadian Trial with a cohort of 508 patients, published median uterine and dominant fibroid volume reduction were 35% and 42%, respectively [11]. In a cohort of 454 patients, RAVINA et al. [30] reported a marked 55% reduction in the size of the dominant fibroid at 6 months. WALKER and PELAGE [7] evaluated follow-up ultrasound imaging of fibroids in 400 patients who underwent UFE demonstrating 58% and 83% median reduction of uterine and dominant fibroid volumes, respectively, with a mean clinical follow-up of 16.7 months. Similar fibroid volume reductions have been reported with the use of gelatin sponge or tris-acryl microspheres [22, 31].

Fibroid location within the uterus may correlate with outcome. SPIES et al. [32] reported that smaller baseline leiomyoma size and submucosal location were more likely to result in a positive imaging outcome (Fig 10.4.2). JHA et al. [33] confirmed that

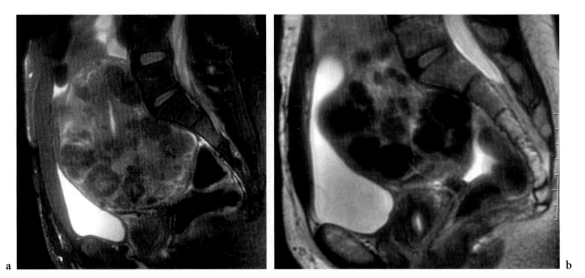

a   b

Fig. 10.4.1a,b. A 39-year-old woman with fibroid-related menorrhagia and pelvic pressure. **a** Pre-embolization sagittal T2-weighted MRI demonstrates a multifibroid uterus. **b** Post-embolization sagittal T2-weighted MRI obtained 6 months after embolization demonstrates a marked volume reduction of 55%. The patient's condition has also greatly improved

submucosal location was a strong positive predictor of fibroid volume reduction. MRI is also useful for quantitative assessment of signal intensity and morphological changes before and after UFE. BURN et al. [34] noted that the mean reduction in fibroid volume was 43% at 2 months and 59% at 6 months. In addition, pretreatment MRI findings may help predict the success of the procedure. They reported that high signal intensity on Tl-weighted images before UFE was predictive of a poor response and high signal intensity on T2-weighted images was predictive of a good response in terms of volume reduction [34]. DESOUZA and WILLIAMS [35] demonstrated that fibroid with high signal T2-weighted images before UFE showed significantly greater volume reduction than those low signal intensity.

Using three-dimensional color Doppler sonography, FLEISCHER et al. [36] found that hypervascular fibroids tend to decrease in size after UFE more than their isovascular or hypovascular fibroids. McLUCAS et al. [15] showed that the initial peak systolic velocity was positively correlated with the shrinkage of fibroids and uterine volume reduction.

In addition to volume reduction, the detection of new fibroids should be a priority since it is very common with other uterus-sparing therapies [20]. The remaining question is the duration between UFE and clinical recurrence due to new fibroids and whether this interval is different from that seen after myomectomy.

10.4.6.2
Residual Fibroid Perfusion

The MRI appearance of uterine fibroids after embolization has been well described [33]. The signal intensity increases on T1-weighted images indicating the presence of proteinaceous material related to hemorrhagic infarction [33]. In these fibroids, there is no enhancement after contrast injection (Fig. 10.4.2) [35]. In some cases however, some fibroids may not be completely infarcted after embolization and there may be some areas of residual perfusion [31, 37]. Arterial spasm leading to insufficient devascularization, unilateral embolization or additional fibroid supply from the ovarian artery have been shown to result in persistent fibroid perfusion (Fig. 10.4.3) [2, 37]. Because the technical goal of UFE is to cause complete infarction of all identified fibroids, it is important to assess after embolization the frequency with which the infarction occurs [37]. Complete devascularization of all the fibroids, is the necessary precursor of symptom improvement in the long term (Fig 10.4.2) [25, 37]. This has been demonstrated when viewing the long-term imaging outcome of embolization, because complete fibroid infarction does result in long-term improvement of symptoms, whereas incomplete infarction may predispose to regrowth and clinical recurrence (Fig. 10.4.3) [37].

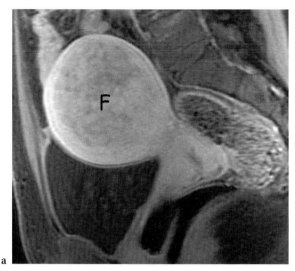
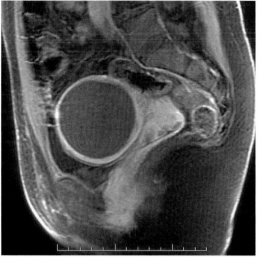

Fig. 10.4.2a,b. A 45-year-old woman with fibroid-related menorrhagia. **a** Pre-embolization sagittal contrast-enhanced MRI shows a single hypervascular intramural fibroid (*F*). **b** Post-embolization contrast-enhanced MRI obtained 3 months after embolization demonstrates a complete devascularization of the embolized fibroid with a normal myometrial perfusion The patient's condition has also greatly improved

In addition, the degree of gadolinium enhancement is not correlated with fibroid volume reduction [35, 37]. Therefore, these data suggest that ultrasound may not be useful for the imaging follow-up particularly in patients who have recurrent symptoms [37]. This observation may change if a more accurate means than color Doppler is developed to assess residual fibroid perfusion with ultrasound [38, 39].

10.4.7
Treatment Failures

Another measure of outcome is the effectiveness of UFE in avoiding other treatments for fibroids, as measured by subsequent medical therapies or additional surgery. For example, hysterectomy or additional hysteroscopic resection or myomectomy for clinical failure or recurrence after UFE is an important measure of safety and a key outcome measure of UFE [2]. SPIES et al. [9] reported nine (4.5%) hysterectomies out of 200 patients within 12 months of therapy. Seven of the patients underwent hysterectomy for clinical failure after UFE. The other two patients underwent incidental hysterectomy for treatment of a tubo-ovarian abscess and an adnexal mass. In a series of 400 women, WALKER and PELAGE [7] reported 23 (6%) clinical

failures or recurrence. Of these, nine (2%) required hysterectomy. In their ongoing clinical experience in 80 patients MARRET et al. [20] reported a 10% recurrence rate at a mean time of 27 months. In this study, hysteroscopic resection of submucosal fibroids was the most common intervention for recurrent fibroids and the number of hysterectomies was not mentioned [20]. Among the reported causes of failures, adenomyosis has been frequently involved [7, 40]. There are only four case series reporting the use of arterial embolization in patients with adenomyosis with or without uterine fibroids [41–44]. Uterine artery embolization is an effective procedure in the short-term but is associated with a high rate of clinical recurrence with up to 30% of embolized women ultimately requiring hysterectomy [43, 33]. Embolization may however be an option in young women with diffuse adenomyosis interested in future fertility since no uterus-sparing treatment is effective [44]. Even in the presence of two apparently normal uterine arteries, additional supply to the fibroids may come from other arterial sources, more commonly from the ovarian arteries [45–47]. The degree of ovarian supply varies but a potential predictor of clinical failure is the presence of ovarian artery supply not only to the uterus but also to portions of fibroids not supplied by the uterine arteries [2]. If the patient's condition does not improve after embolization and fibroids in the distribution of the ovarian supply do

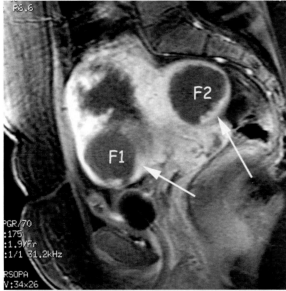

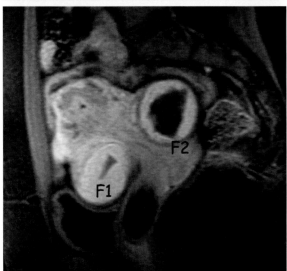

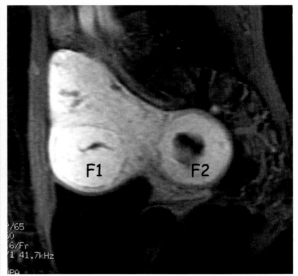

Fig. 10.4.3a-c. A 40-year-old woman with fibroid-related menorrhagia. **a** Immediate post-embolization sagittal contrast-enhanced MRI (obtained 24 h after embolization) shows two viable fibroids (*F1* and *F2*) with persistent enhancement of the peripheral portion (*arrows*). **b** At 6 months post-embolization contrast-enhanced MRI shows that F1 and F2 are still viable. The patient, however, reported marked improvement in symptoms. **c** At 12 months post-embolization contrast-enhanced MRI shows that F1 and F2 growing. The patient reported worsening symptoms and may consider another embolization procedure

not infarct, then additional ovarian artery embolization may be considered [2, 47].

10.4.8
Cost Analysis

Admittedly, measuring medical costs is very difficult. Nevertheless, in the current health care environment, in which cost considerations are important, careful study of the costs of UFE should be a priority. The cost information can be used to analyze the cost effectiveness of UFE compared to other

therapies for fibroids. The cost should include the overall hospital cost as well as the length of recovery after UFE. An initial analysis by SUBRAMANIAN and SPIES [48] evaluated the cost associated with UFE. They found that the facility cost of UEE compared favorably with that of hysterectomy. A subsequent comparative study conducted at the same institution concluded that procedure-related costs were lower with UFE than with abdominal myomectomy [49]. Using a decision model comparing the costs and effectiveness of UFE and hysterectomy, BEINFELD et al. [50] deduced that UFE was more effective and less expensive than hysterectomy. In Canada, AL-FOZAN et al. [51] reported that UFE was associated with a lower hospital cost and a shorter hospital stay compared with abdominal myomectomy, abdominal hysterectomy and vaginal hysterectomy. In France, it has been demonstrated that UFE was more cost-effective than vaginal hysterectomy [52].

10.4.9
Complications

Complications associated with UFE can be classified as minor or major based on their severity evaluated by the level of care required, the interventions necessary and the final outcome [53]. Two different systems (from the Society of CardioVascular and Interventional Radiology, SCVIR, and the American College of Obstetrics and Gynecology, ACOG) developed to allow standardized reporting of complication severity have been used to precisely assess complications following UFE [53]. From a cohort of 400 women, the peri-procedural morbidity was 8.5% according to the SCVIR classification system and 5% according to the ACOG system. Most complications were minor and occurred during the first 3 months after UFE. Five major complications (1.25%) were reported in this group of patients. There was only one hysterectomy (0.25%) for complication in this study [53]. From the Canadian trial, the overall complication rate after UFE was 8% [54]. In another study, the rate of readmission for complications from UFE was 17% [55]. All readmissions were due to infection, of which all but one were treated conservatively and median time to readmission was 3 weeks [55].

10.4.9.1
Peri-procedural Complications

10.4.9.1.1
Angiographic Complications

Complications that can occur at the common femoral artery puncture site include formation of a hematoma, pseudoaneurysm, or arteriovenous fistula, dissection or thrombosis of the common femoral artery, and infection [53, 56]. Vessel perforation is even more unusual than arterial dissection but may be problematic in that it could either cause occlusion of the uterine artery prior to embolization or can cause bleeding from the perforated vessel which may itself require embolization as treatment (Fig. 10.4.4) [56].

Arterial vasospasm is the most common complication associated with passage of the guidewire and catheter into the uterine artery. Because of its diameter and tortuosity, the uterine artery is prone to spasm. In theory, embolization of an artery in spasm may not result in a lasting occlusion since relaxation of the vessel can increase luminal diameter enough to allow flow around the embolization particles [2]. This may lead to a false angiographic end-point with secondary redistribution of the embolization particles [2, 10]. The systematic use of microcatheters and microguidewires has been shown to minimize the occurrence of spasm and medications such as nitroglycerin or papaverine may be effective to treat spasm [2].

10.4.9.1.2
Nontarget Embolization

The potential effects of non-target embolization warrant this type of monitoring and concern during uterine artery embolization procedures. An awareness of non-target embolization was established more than two decades ago in association with pelvic arterial embolization procedures performed for a variety of different indications [57]. This risk was highlighted by the report of a patient experiencing labial necrosis after uterine artery embolization [58]. The patient presented 5 days after embolization with vulvar pain and a tender, hypopigmented, necrotic appearing area on the labium. Ultimately, the labial lesion was self-limited, resolving completely within 4 weeks. This finding was attributed to non-target embolization into the internal pudendal artery, possibly due to retrograde reflux of embolic particles [58].

In 2000, Lai et al. [59] reported on a patient who experienced sexual dysfunction after uterine artery embolization. In this report, the patient experienced a loss of orgasm response to sexual stimulation after uterine artery embolization. These findings have been potentially attributed to embolization of the cervicovaginal branch of the uterine artery, again highlighting the potential risk of non-target embolization during UFE. The cervicovaginal branch can often be visualized angiographically arising from the distal descending segment or proximal transverse segment of the uterine artery [60]. It is believed that this vessel is responsible for supplying the uterovaginal plexus, which are the nerves surrounding and innervating the cervix and upper vagina [59]. This case has led many interventional-

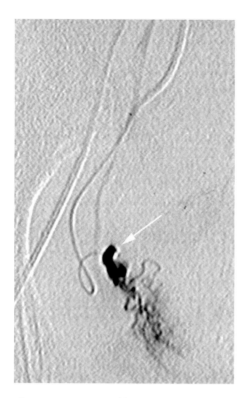

Fig. 10.4.4. A 48-year-old woman with fibroid-related menorrhagia. Selective catheterization of a thin right uterine artery was performed but vessel perforation occurred (*arrow*) without clinical consequence. However, superselective catheterization and embolization was successfully performed using a microcatheter

pulsed fluoroscopy, bilateral catheter technique with simultaneous embolization and focus on magnified fluoroscopy [7, 63].

10.4.9.2
Post-Procedural Complications

10.4.9.2.1
Post-Embolization Pain

After embolization, almost all patients experience a self-limited post-embolization pain lasting 6–24 h [5, 6, 12, 16, 64]. Some patients will even present with a post-embolization syndrome consisting of pelvic pain, nausea, vomiting, mild fever and general malaise [65]. Several strategies involving oral, intravenous, epidural and patient-controlled analgesia have been utilized to manage the pain associated with UFE [5, 6, 12, 16, 18, 26]. Most of the centers have been admitting their patients for 1–2 days to provide aggressive management of pain [5, 6, 12. WALKER and PELAGE [7] reported that post-embolization pain was stronger than period-type pain in 68% of women and worse than expected in 40% of cases. Recent approaches of the pain issue have included outpatient uterine artery embolization or less aggressive embolization of the uterine arteries [10, 65, 66]. When UFE is performed as an outpatient procedure, up to 10% of embolized women will ultimately require readmission for pain [66]. When a more limited embolization of the uterine arteries is performed, post-embolization pain seems to be less even if recent reports comparing aggressive and limited embolization have not demonstrated any difference in terms of pain [10, 67].

ists to adopt the practice of positioning their angiographic catheter or microcatheter beyond the origin of the cervicovaginal branch during uterine artery embolization procedures.

10.4.9.1.3
Radiation Exposure

Radiation doses during uterine artery embolization are higher than with common radiological procedures but within acceptable limits [34, 61, 62]. The mean estimated absorbed ovarian dose has been reported to be 22 cGy with a mean fluoroscopy time of 22 min and a mean number of 44 angiographic exposures [62]. These figures were compared to the published radiation dose for tubal recanalisation (3 cGy) and pelvic irradiation for Hodgkin's disease (up to 3,500 cGy). It is obvious that meticulous attention should be paid to cutting the screening times by coning and streamlining technique [63]. Radiation can also be limited by using low frequency

10.4.9.2.2
Ovarian Failure

The onset of amenorrhea and other symptoms of menopause is a well-documented complication following uterine artery embolization, with a reported incidence as high as 14% [68, 69]. Symptoms commonly associated with menopause including amenorrhea, vaginal dryness, hot flashes, mood swings, and night sweats have all been reported after uterine artery embolization [6, 7, 68, 70]. While the incidence of this complication can still be considered low (less than 4%), the impact of this complication can be quite significant, especially in patients wishing to preserve fertility options after embolization [53].

Several theories, however, have been proposed to serve as possible explanations for this complication. Small embolization particles administered within the uterine arteries can potentially make their way into the ovarian arterial circulation through patent uterine-to-ovarian anastomoses, increasing the risk of reduced ovarian perfusion and subsequent ischemia [6, 71]. This theory is supported by the demonstration of angiographically visible anastomoses between these two arterial beds in up to 10% of cases [71]. In addition, several reports described the presence of embolization particles in the ovarian arterial vasculature, within an oophorectomy specimen obtained after UFE [7, 72]. Microspheres smaller than 500 µm in diameter can pass within the ovarian arterial circulation after uterine artery embolization performed in sheep, which may offer some guidance as to particle size selection for this procedure [47].

Ovarian ischemia may also happen after aggressive embolization of both uterine arteries when to ovaries are supplied by the uterine arteries [47, 73]. Using ovarian Doppler flow measurements, RYU et al. [74] demonstrated that more than 50% of patients have decreased ovarian arterial flow after embolization of both uterine arteries to stasis. Nevertheless, the rate of amenorrhea mainly depends on the age of the patient at the time of treatment [68, 75]. CHRISMAN et al. [68] reported a 14% incidence of ovarian failure mainly in women over the age of 45. SPIES et al. [76] reported that patients older than 45 years of age are at an increased risk of experiencing significant increases in follicle-stimulating hormone (FSH) levels when compared to baseline. Based on this study, SPIES et al. [76] concluded that there is approximately a 15% chance of a significant change in FSH levels after uterine artery embolization in patients older than 45 years of age. Conversely, AHMAD et al. [77] reported no significant changes in menstruation or follicle-stimulating hormone (FSH) levels in patients younger than 45 years of age.

10.4.9.2.3
Uterine Necrosis and Infection

One of the potentially more serious complications of uterine artery embolization is the occurrence of an infection after embolization. Several studies have reported cases of pelvic sepsis after uterine artery embolization [6, 78, 79]. However, when several of the largest published series are considered in aggre-

gate, the overall rate of significant infection after embolization remains low and can be estimated at <1% [6, 7]. It has been suggested that submucosal fibroids, pedunculated subserosal fibroids or large uterine fibroids may be at increased risk for infection after embolization (Figs. 10.4.5 and 10.4.6) [61, 79]. The severity of this particular complication was made clear by the publication of the first death due to infection reported in a 51-year-old patient who underwent uterine artery embolization to treat abnormal bleeding attributed to submucosal fibroids [80]. After an immediate post-procedure period highlighted by a urinary tract infection the patient returned to the hospital 1 week later with abdominal pain, diarrhea, vomiting, and fever. Despite antibiotics, the infection required a total abdominal hysterectomy and bilateral salpingo-oophorectomy. Blood cultures ultimately were positive for *Escherichia coli*. Two weeks later, the patient died due to a multiorgan failure [80]. Most interventional radiologists consider that large pedunculated subserosal fibroids should not reasonably be embolized. Conversely, it has been reported that the rate of necrosis or infection of large uterine fibroids is not as high as generally considered [120].

It is often difficult to know exactly how to manage patients presenting with signs that might indicate the presence of a uterine infection after embolization [5, 82]. The diagnosis is made even more difficult by the fact that mild fever is often seen during the normal post-procedure recovery period [7]. Anyway, a patient presenting with increasing pelvic pain, high fever, vaginal discharge and leukocytosis a few weeks after uterine artery embolization should be immediately admitted for appropriate testing with imaging evaluation and treatment (Fig. 10.4.7) [5, 82, 83].

Bilateral occlusion of the uterine arteries during uterine artery embolization clearly increases the risk of global uterine ischemia and subsequent infarction in patients undergoing this procedure [10]. In fact, it is not unreasonable to assume that uterine ischemia occurs in all patients undergoing this procedure and that this ischemia likely contributes to the post-procedure pain that is commonly experienced by most patients after embolization. However, rarely this transient ischemia worsens to the point where the uterus becomes globally infarcted. There have been reports of diffuse uterine ischemia and necrosis after uterine artery embolization [84, 85]. The typical presentation of uterine ischemia consists of long-standing pelvic pain which persists for several weeks associated

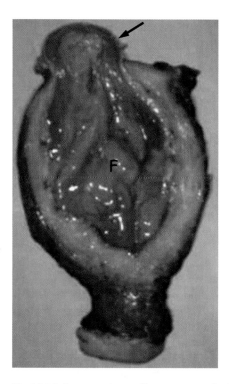

Fig. 10.4.5. Gross specimen of hysterectomy obtained 3 months after embolization in a 34-year-old woman with a large fundal fibroid (11 cm in diameter) associated with menorrhagia. Embolization was performed using small non-spherical PVA particles. A large infarcted fibroid (*F*) is seen in the uterine cavity and associated fundal perforation is seen (*arrow*)

with fever and elevated white blood cell count [7]. A contrast enhanced pelvic MRI may be useful in this setting to confirm the presence of uterine devascularization [121]. Ultimately, these patients may require a hysterectomy for pain relief [54]. In most cases however, imaging studies have been helpful in confirming myometrial perfusion and absence of myometrial ischemia in most patients after uterine artery embolization [81]. While the reported risk of uterine necrosis is far less than 1%, steps such as avoiding complete stasis during embolization or using large embolization particles may reduce this risk even more (PELAGE et al. 2003).

10.4.9.2.4
Vaginal Discharge and Expulsion of Uterine Fibroids

A reported complication after uterine artery embolization has been a persistent vaginal discharge [86]. This discharge, which is often characterized as brown or red-brown in color, can begin within days of the embolization procedure and can potentially last for several months [7]. Vaginal discharge may be more frequent in patients with submucosal fibroids or when embolization of the uterine arteries to stasis has been performed (Fig. 10.4.8) [7, 53].

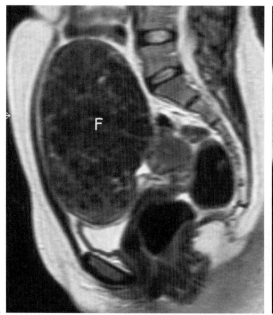
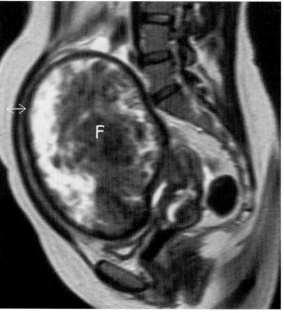

Fig. 10.4.6a,b. A 36-year-old woman with bulk-related symptoms. **a** Pre-embolization sagittal T2 weighted MRI shows a large pedunculated subserosal fibroid (*F*). **b** At 6 months post-embolization MRI shows a degenerative fibroid (*F*) with no volume reduction. The patient ultimately required myomectomy

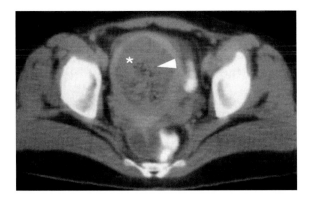

Fig. 10.4.7. A 47-year-old woman with high fever and pain after embolization. Computed tomography scan obtained 2 weeks after embolization because of pelvic pain and fever. A large infected fibroid (*asterisk*) containing air bubbles (*arrow*) is seen. The patient was treated by hysterectomy

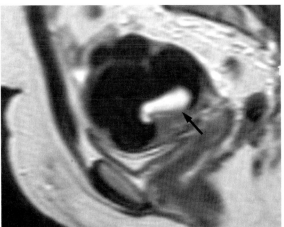

a

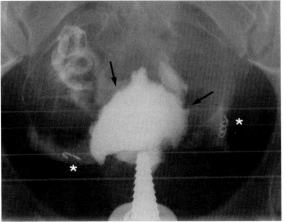

b

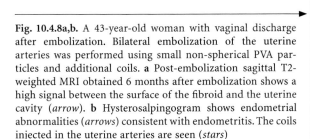

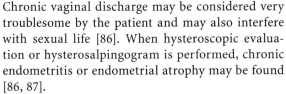

Fig. 10.4.8a,b. A 43-year-old woman with vaginal discharge after embolization. Bilateral embolization of the uterine arteries was performed using small non-spherical PVA particles and additional coils. **a** Post-embolization sagittal T2-weighted MRI obtained 6 months after embolization shows a high signal between the surface of the fibroid and the uterine cavity (*arrow*). **b** Hysterosalpingogram shows endometrial abnormalities (*arrows*) consistent with endometritis. The coils injected in the uterine arteries are seen (*stars*)

Chronic vaginal discharge may be considered very troublesome by the patient and may also interfere with sexual life [86]. When hysteroscopic evaluation or hysterosalpingogram is performed, chronic endometritis or endometrial atrophy may be found [86, 87].

The presence of a brown or red-brown vaginal discharge, however, is potentially a sign of impending transcervical passage of an embolized fibroid (Fig. 10.4.9) [7]. This event has been both well described and frequently reported [88–90]. This has been reported to occur both a few weeks after the embolization procedure and after a period of time as long as 4 years [88–91]. Typically, patients experiencing passage of a fibroid, report symptoms including vaginal discharge, hemorrhage and crampy pelvic pain [53]. Patients at an increased risk for expulsion include those with submucosal fibroids and those with intramural fibroids that have significant contact with the endometrial cavity [90]. Transcervical fibroid passage often occurs without incident (Fig. 10.4.10) [7]. In rare

cases, retention of fibroid fragments within the endometrial cavity can potentially increase the risk of infection after embolization. If retention of a fibroid fragment is confirmed by imaging evaluation, the fibroid can be resected hysteroscopically (Fig. 10.4.9) [7].

10.4.9.2.5
Pulmonary Embolism

As is the case with most invasive procedures, deep venous thrombosis and pulmonary embolus represent rare but potential complications of the uterine artery embolization procedure [53]. Patients taking oral contraception are known to be at increased risk for venous thromboembolic disease and there may be a transient hypercoagulability after embolization [92–94].

There have been at least two deaths reported in association with massive pulmonary embolism disease after uterine artery embolization [95]. While

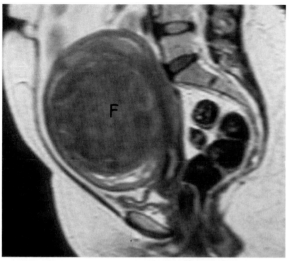 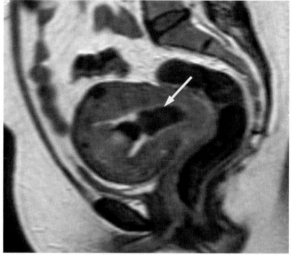

a   b

Fig. 10.4.9a,b. A 40-year-old woman with vaginal discharge and hemorrhage after embolization. **a** Preembolization sagittal T2-weighted MRI shows a large intracavitary fibroid (*F*). **b** A 2-months post-embolization MRI shows that most part of the fibroid has been expelled the residual part (*arrow*) is still attached and required hysteroscopic resection

the exact source of the thrombus was not determined in this case, it was likely from either deep venous thrombosis within the lower extremities or from pelvic vein thrombosis [96].

10.4.9.2.6
Uterine Sarcoma

It is inevitable that interventionalists will at some point perform the uterine artery embolization procedure on a patient with a leiomyosarcoma instead of the more common benign uterine fibroid [97]. Leiomyosarcomas of the uterus are very uncommon tumors, with an incidence of less than 0.2% of uterine fibroids [98–100]. The difficulty in distinguishing between a fibroid and a leiomyosarcoma is that there are no clinical or imaging features that clearly allow differentiation between these two entities [101, 102]. So far three patients with uterine sarcomas have been embolized [100, 103]. Common et al. [104] reported another case where uterine artery embolization was successfully performed, but continued growth of the fibroid prompted hysterectomy 6 months after embolization. These cases support the use of follow-up imaging, particularly contrast-enhanced MRI, after embolization because failure to respond to embolization would warrant consideration of a malignant diagnosis and a subsequent recommendation for hysterectomy [105].

10.4.9.2.7
Death

Four deaths have occurred following UFE, two from pulmonary emboli and two due to infection in approximately 50,000 cases [80, 85, 95]. A careful analysis of the two cases of infection suggests that early diagnosis and appropriate management would have probably avoided such a fatal consequence [106]. It should be remembered that the mortality rate for hysterectomy for benign disease excluding complications of pregnancy is 1:1,600 [107]. A recent review from Japan of 923 women having hysterectomy for fibroids found a 6% serious complication rate and one death due to pulmonary embolus [100].

10.4.10
Comparative Studies Between Uterine Fibroid Embolization and Surgery

10.4.10.1
Uterine Fibroid Embolization Versus Hysterectomy

Pinto et al. [108] reported the results of a randomized clinical trial in patients assigned to two groups: those given the option of UFE or hysterectomy and those not informed of alternative treatment. The overall clinical success of UFE was 86%. The hos-

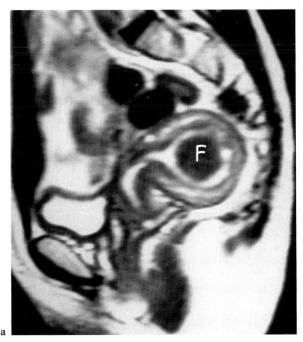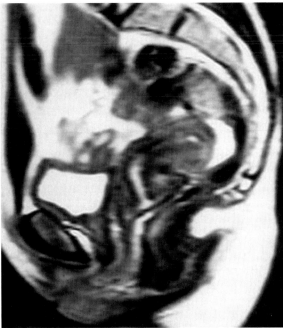

a   b

Fig. 10.4.10a,b. A 45-year-old woman with complete resolution of symptoms after embolization. **a** Pre-embolization sagittal T2-weighted MRI shows a small pedunculated submucosal fibroid (*F*). She underwent a failed attempt of hysteroscopic resection prior to embolization. **b** At 3-months post-embolization MRI shows that the whole fibroid has been spontaneously expelled. The uterus is virtually normal

pital stay for patients treated with UFE was 4.1 days shorter than for those who underwent hysterectomy (Table 10.4.2). Of women who underwent UFE, 25% had minor complications, in contrast to 20% of those who underwent hysterectomy having major complications [108].

A recent multicenter cohort study comparing UFE to hysterectomy has been completed by SPIES et al. [109]. For UFE patients, there were significant reductions in blood loss scores and menorrhagia questionnaire scores compared to baseline (Table 10.4.3). At 12 months, a larger proportion of hysterectomy patients had improved pelvic pain. There was no difference between the two groups in the proportion of patients with improvement in urinary symptoms or pelvic pressure. Similarly, no difference between both groups was found in terms of quality-of-life scores [109].

10.4.10.2
Uterine Fibroid Embolization Versus Myomectomy

At the time this chapter was written, only retrospective studies had been published [110–112]. In their retro-spective review of 16 myomectomies and 32 embolizations, McLUCAS and ADLER [17] found that myomectomy patients experienced longer hospital stays and more complications than UFE patients. In their retrospective review of subgroups of patients undergoing UFE and myomectomy, BRODER et al. [111] found that overall symptoms improved in 92% UFE patients and 90% myomectomy patients, respectively, and that 94% of UFE patients were satisfied with the choice of their procedure compared to 79% of myomectomy patients (Table 10.4.4). However, reintervention rates among myomectomy patients were lower than in UFE patients (3% vs. 29%, $p < 0.001$). In their analysis of 111 consecutive patients who underwent abdominal myomectomy or UFE, RAZAVI et al. [112] reported clinical success rates of 64% vs. 92% for menorrhagia ($p < 0.05$), 54% vs. 74% for pelvic pain (not significant) and 91% vs. 76% for bulk-related symptoms ($p < 0.05$) (Table 10.4.5). They found shorter hospitalization and recovery for patients treated with UFE, 0 vs. 2.9 days and 8 vs. 36 days respectively [112]. They concluded that efficacy appears to be greater with UFE in treatment of menorrhagia, and surgery may be a better choice for symptoms related to mass effect of fibroids. Several randomized studies are ongoing and should confirm these encouraging preliminary results.

Table 10.4.2. Results of a randomized trial comparing embolization to abdominal hysterectomy (PINTO et al. 2003)

	Embolization (n=40)	Hysterectomy (n=20)
Hospitalization (days)	1.71 ± 1.59	5.85 ± 2.52
Recovery (days)	9.50 ± 7.21	36.18 ± 20.47
Per-operative complications (%)	25	20
Minor post-operative complications (%)	50[a]	20[b]
Major post-operative complications (%)	2.5[c]	35[d]

[a] Hematoma at the puncture site, vaginal discharge.
[b] Parietal hematoma, urinary tract infection.
[c] Phlebitis of the lower limbs.
[d] Phlebitis of the lower limbs, parietal hematoma, bleeding requiring transfusion.

Table 10.4.3. Results of a prospective cohort study comparing embolization to hysterectomy (SPIES et al. 2004b)

	Embolization (n=102)	Hysterectomy (n=50)	Statistics
Improvement of pelvic pain (at 6 months)	83%	88%	NS
Improvement in urinary frequency (at 6 months)	75%	73%	NS
Post-operative complications (ACOG classification)	14.7%	34%	$p<0.01$
Post-operative complications (SCVIR classification)	3.9%	12%	NS

ACOG, American College of Obstetrics and Gynecology;
SCVIR, Society of CardioVascular and Interventional Radiology.

Table 10.4.4. Results of a study comparing embolization to abdominal myomectomy ([111])

	Embolization (n=51)	Myomectomy (n=30)	Statistics
Mean age (years)	44	38	p=0.001
Mean follow-up (months)	46	49	p=0.03
Clinical efficacy (%)	92	90	NS
Secondary treatment for failure or complication (%)	29	3	p=0.004
Secondary hysterectomy (%)	12	3	$p< 0.05$
Patient's satisfaction (%)	94	79	NS

Table 10.4.5. Results of a retrospective study comparing embolization to abdominal myomectomy ([112])

	Embolization (n=67)	Myomectomy (n=44)	Statistics
Mean age (years)	44.2	37.7	$p< 0.05$
Mean follow-up (months)	14.3	14.6	NS
Efficacy on menorrhagia (%)	92	64	$p< 0.05$
Efficacy on pelvic pain (%)	54	74	NS
Efficacy on pelvic pressure (%)	76	91	$p< 0.05$
Complication rate (%)	11[a]	25[b]	$p< 0.05$
Hospitalization (days)	0[c]	2.9	$p< 0.05$
Recovery (days)	8	36	$p< 0.05$

[a] Endometritis, prolonged post-embolization pain, amenorrhea.
[b] Abscess, transfusion, occlusion.
[c] Embolization performed as an outpatient procedure.

10.4.11
Fertility After Embolization

Fibroids can affect fertility and the incidence of miscarriage. The efficacy of UFE on pregnancy and fertility has yet to be fully established [113]. Patients who have had UFE have become pregnant and had successful deliveries [6, 7]. The ability of women treated with uterine artery embolization for different types of obstetrical or gynecological hemorrhage to conceive and deliver successfully is well-known and long-term follow-up is already available [114, 115]. However, in these cases the embolization agent has usually been resorbable gelatine sponge which does not produce as distal a block as non-resorbable particles and therefore may affect the uterus differently [13, 115]. Encouragingly, ultrasound and MRI observation of the uterus following embolization demonstrates rapid revascularization of the normal myometrium and an essentially normal appearance of the endometrium on 3- to 6-month MRI examinations [81]. The rapid revascularization may be due to the rich collateral supply in the pelvis which compensates for the complete occlusion of the uterine vessels produced by embolization [82]. The published evidence on fertility after embolization is still scanty whereas the literature on pregnancy following myomectomy is extensive. Until recently, most authors reserve UFE for women who no longer desire fertility [113]. Other groups like ours, have taken a more open approach and now offer embolization to patients who desire future fertility particularly if hysterectomy, repeat or multiple myomectomy is the only surgical alternative [10]. Even if at the moment, reports of pregnancy following uterine artery embolization remain anecdotal, questions of numerator (number of live births) and denominator (number of women attempting to conceive after embolization) will be determined soon by the results of large prospective registries. From available prospective studies, fecundity and delivery rates are encouraging and similar to those reported after myomectomy [30, 110, 116–119]. When pregnancy occurs, the rate of intrauterine growth retardation does not seem to be increased by potential alterations in uterine blood flow after embolization. Nevertheless, in interpreting fertility rates and pregnancy outcome following UFE, it should be taken into consideration that women undergoing UFE are not similar to the general obstetric population. Large prospective studies, including randomized trials comparing embolization and myomectomy in women interested in future pregnancy may answer the remaining questions.

It appears that after pluridisciplinary evaluation with gynecologists and interventional radiologists involved, UFE can be offered to women who plan future pregnancy if the only surgical options are repeated myomectomy or hysterectomy.

10.4.12
Conclusion

In conclusion, uterine artery embolization is both a safe and effective procedure to offer patients with symptomatic uterine fibroids. UFE has been described as a valuable alternative to hysterectomy and recurrent multiple myomectomy. Clinical success rates for control of heavy menstrual bleeding, pelvic pain and bulk-related symptoms have been reported to be 80%–95% of patients treated with a low rate of recurrence. The risk of major complications, including pulmonary embolism, uterine

infection and/or infarction and ovarian failure is low, with many of these complications potentially treatable without additional surgery. However, additional studies are needed to compare UFE to other uterine-sparing therapies such as single myomectomy and to provide pregnancy outcome after treatment. By gaining an understanding of results and complications described in this chapter, the practicing interventionalists can seek information from patients regarding their risk for certain complications and may be more comfortable when discussing indication for UFE with gynecologists.

References

1. Pron G, Bennett J, Common A et al. (2003a) Technical results and effects of operator experience on uterine artery embolization for fibroids: the Ontario Uterine Fibroid Embolization Trial. J Vasc Interv Radiol 14:545–554
2. Spies JB (2003) Uterine artery embolization for fibroids: understanding the technical causes of failure. J Vasc Interv Radiol 14:11–14
3. Nicholson T. Outcome in patients undergoing unilateral uterine artery embolization for symptomatic fibroids. Clin Radiol (2004) 59:186-191
4. Hutchins FL, Worthington-Kirsch R, Berkowitz RP (1999) Selective uterine artery embolization as primary treatment for symptomatic leiomyomata uteri. J Am Assoc Gynecol Laparosc 6:279–284
5. Goodwin SC, Vedantham S, McLucas B, Forno AE, Perrella R (1997) Preliminary experience with uterine artery embolization for uterine fibroids. J Vasc Interv Radiol 8:517–526
6. Pelage JP, Le Dref O, Soyer P et al. (2000) Fibroid-related menorrhagia: treatment with superselective embolization of the uterine arteries and midterm follow-up. Radiology 215:428–431
7. Walker WJ, Pelage JP (2002) Uterine artery embolization for symptomatic fibroids: clinical results in 400 women with imaging follow-up. Br J Obstet Gynaecol 109:1262–1272
8. Pelage JP. Polyvinyl alcohol particles versus tris-acryl gelatin microspheres for uterine artery embolization for leiomyomas (2004) J Vasc Interv Radiol 15:789-791
9. Spies JB, Ascher SA, Roth Arm, Kim J, Levy EB, Gomez-Jorge J (2001a) Uterine artery embolization for leiomyomata. Obstet Gynecol 98:29–34
10. Pelage JP, Le Dref OP, Beregi JP et al. (2003a) Limited uterine artery embolization with tris-acryl gelatin microspheres for uterine fibroids. J Vasc Interv Radiol 14:11–14
11. Pron G, Bennett J, Common A et al. (2003b) The Ontario uterine fibroid embolization trial: uterine fibroid reduction and symptom relief after uterine artery embolization for fibroids. Fertil Steril 79:120–127
12. Ravina JH, Herbreteau D, Ciraru-Vigneron N et al. (1995) Arterial embolisation to treat myomata. Lancet 346: 671–672

13. Siskin GP, Englander M, Stainken BF et al. (2000a) Embolic agent used for uterine fibroid embolization. Am J Roentgenol 175:767–773

14. Spies JB, Benenati JE, Worthington-Kirsch RL, Pelage JP (2001b) Initial experience with the use of trisacryl gelatin microspheres for uterine artery embolization for leiomyomata. J Vasc Interv Radiol 12:1059–1063

15. McLucas B, Adler L, Perrella R (2001a) Uterine fibroid embolization: nonsurgical treatment for symptomatic fibroids. J Am Coll Surg 192:95–105

16. Spies JB, Scialli AR, Jha RC et al. (1999a) Initial results from uterine fibroid embolization for symptomatic leiomyomata. J Vasc Interv Radiol 10:1149–1157

17. McLucas B, Adler L (2001) Uterine fibroid embolization compared with myomectomy. Int J Gynaecol Obstet 74:297–299

18. Andersen PE, Lund N, Justesen P, Munk T, Elle B, Floridon C (2001) Uterine artery embolization of symptomatic uterine fibroids. Acta Radiol 42:234–238

19. Brunereau L, Herbreteau D, Gallas S et al. (2000) Uterine artery embolization as the primary treatment of leiomyomas. Am J Roentgenol 175:1267–1272

20. Marret H, Alonso AM, Cottier JP, Tranquart F, Herbreteau D, Body G (2003) Leiomyoma recurrence after uterine artery embolization. J Vasc Interv Radiol 14:1395–1399

21. Khaund A, Moss JG, McMillan N, Lumsden MA (2004) Evaluation of the effect of uterine artery embolisation on menstrual blood loss and uterine volume. Br J Obstet Gynaecol 111:700–705

22. Katsumori T, Nakajima K, Mihara T, Tokuhiro M (2002) Uterine artery embolization using gelatin sponge particles alone for symptomatic uterine fibroids: midterm results. Am J Roentgenol 178:135–139

23. Joffre F, Tubiana JM, Pelage JP, FEMIC Group (2004) FEMIC (Fibromes Embolisés aux MICrosphères calibrées: uterine fibroid embolization using tris-acryl microspheres. A frendch multicenter study. CardioVasc Intervent Radiol 27:600–606

24. Spies JB, Allison SJ, Flick PA et al. (2004a) Polyvinyl alcohol particles and tris-acryl gelatin microspheres for uterine artery embolization for leiomyomas. J Vasc Interv Radiol 15:793–800

25. Pelage JP, Jacob D, Le Dref O, Laurent A (2004a) Leiomyoma recurrence after uterine artery embolization. J Vasc Interv Radiol 15:774–775

26. Worthington-Kirsch RL, Popky GL, Hutchins FL (1998) Uterine arterial embolization for the management of leiomyomas: quality of life assessment and clinical response. Radiology 208:625–629

27. Spies JB, Warren EH, Mathias SD, Walsh SM, Roth AR, Pentecost MJ (1999b) Uterine fibroid embolization: measurement of health-related quality of life before and after therapy. J Vasc Interv Radiol 10:1293–1303

28. Spies JB, Coyne K, Guaou-Guaou N, Boyle D, Skyrnarz-Murphy K, Gonzalves SM (2002a) The UFS-QOL, a new disease-specific symptom and health-related quality of life questionnaire for leiomyomata. Obstet Gynecol 99:290–300

29. Smith WJ, Upton E, Shuster EJ, Klein AJ, Schwartz ML (2004) Patient satisfaction and disease specific quality of life after uterine artery embolization. Am J Obstet Gynecol 190:1697–1706

30. Ravina JH, Ciraru-Vigneron N, Aymard A, Le Dref O, Merland JJ (2000) Pregnancy after embolization of uterine myoma: report of 12 cases. Fertil Steril 73:1241–1243

31. Banovac F, Ascher SM, Jones DA, Black MD, Smith JC, Spies JB (2002) Magnetic resonance imaging outcome after uterine artery embolization for leiomyomata with use of tris-acryl gelatin microspheres. J Vasc Interv Radiol 13:681–688

32. Spies J, Roth AR, Jha R et al. (2002b) Uterine artery embolization for leiomyomata: factors associated with successful symptomatic and imaging outcome. Radiology 222:45–52

33. Jha RC, Ascher SM, Imaoka I, Spies JB (2000) Symptomatic fibroleiomyomata: MR imaging of the uterus before and after uterine arterial embolization. Radiology 217:228–235

34. Burn P, McCall JM, Chinn R et al. (2000) Uterine fibroleiomyoma: MR imaging appearances before and after embolization of uterine arteries. Radiology 214:729–734

35. DeSouza NM, Williams AD (2002) Uterine arterial embolization for leiomyomas: perfusion and volume changes at MR imaging and relation to clinical outcome. Radiology 222:367–374

36. Fleischer AC, Donnelly EF, Campbell MG et al. (2000) Three-dimensional color Doppler sonography before and after fibroid embolization. J Ultrasound Med 19:701–705

37. Pelage JP, Guaou-Guaou N, Jha RC, Ascher SM, Spies JB (2004b) Uterine fibroid tumors: long-term MR imaging outcome after embolization. Radiology 230:803–809

38. Tranquart F, Brunereau L, Cottier JP et al. (2002) Prospective sonographic assessment of uterine artery embolization for the treatment of fibroids. Ultrasound Obstet Gynecol 19:81–87

39. Marret H, Tranquart F, Sauget S, Alonso AM, Cottier JP, Herbreteau D (2004a) Contrast-enhanced sonography during uterine artery embolization for the treatment of leiomyomas. Ultrasound Obstet Gynecol 23:77–79

40. Smith SJ, Sewall LE, Handelsman A (1999) A clinical failure of uterine fibroid embolization due to adenomyosis. J Vasc Interv Radiol 10:1171–1174

41. Siskin GP, Tublin ME, Stainken BF, Dowling K, Dolen EG (2001) Uterine artery embolization for the treatment of adenomyosis: clinical response and evaluation with MR imaging. Am J Roentgenol 177:297–302

42. Jha RC, Takahama J, Imaoka I et al. (2003) Adenomyosis: MRI of the uterus treated with uterine artery embolization. Am J Roentgenol 181:851–856

43. Kim MD, Won JW, Lee DY, Ahn CS (2004) Uterine artery embolization for adenomyosis without fibroids. Clin Radiol 59:520–526

44. Pelage JP, Jacob D, Fazel A, Namur J et al. (2005) Midterm results of uterine artery embolization for symptomatic adenomyosis: initial experience. Radiology 234:948–953

45. Nikolic B, Spies JB, Abbara S, Goodwin SC (1999) Ovarian artery supply of uterine fibroids as a cause of treatment failure after uterine artery embolization: a case report. J Vasc Interv Radiol 10:1167–70

46. Saraiya PV, Chang TC, Pelage JP, Spies JB (2002) Uterine artery replacement by the round ligament artery: an anatomic variant discovered during uterine artery embolization for leiomyomata. J Vasc Interv Radiol 13:939–941

47. Pelage JP, Walker WJ, Le Dref O, Rymer R (2003b) Ovar-

ian artery: angiographic appearance, embolization and relevance to uterine fibroid embolization. CardioVasc Intervent Radiol 26:227–233

48. Subramanian S, Spies JB (2001) Uterine artery embolization for leiomyomata: resource use and cost estimation. J Vasc Interv Radiol 12:571–574

49. Baker CM, Winkel CA, Subramanian S, Spies JB (2002) Estimated costs for uterine artery embolization and abdominal myomectomy for uterine leiomyomata: a comparative study at a single institution (2002) J Vasc Interv Radiol 12:1207–210

50. Beinfeld MT, Bosch JL, Isaacson KB et al. (2004) Cost analysis uterine artery embolization and hysterectomy for uterine fibroids. Radiology 230:1401–1404

51. Al-Fozan H, Dufort J, Kaplow M, Valenti D, Tulandi T (2002) Cost analysis of myomectomy, hysterectomy and uterine artery embolization. Am J Obstet Gynecol 187:1401–1404

52. Pourrat XJ, Fourquet F, Guerif F, Viratelle N, Herbreteau D, Marret H. Medico-economic approach to the management of uterine myomas: a 6- month cost-effectiveness study of pelvic embolization versus vaginal hysterectomy (2003) Eur J Obstet Gynecol Reprod Biol 111:59–64

53. Spies JB, Spector A, Roth AR, Baker CM, Mauro L, Murphy-Skrynarz K (2002c) Complications of uterine artery embolization for leiomyomata. Obstet Gynecol 100:873–880

54. Pron G, Mocarski E, Cohen M, Colgan T et al. (2003c) Hysterectomy for complications after uterine artery embolization for leiomyoma: results of a canadian multicenter clinical trial. J Am Assoc Gynecol Laparosc 10:99–106

55. Mehta H, Sandhu C, Matson M, Belli AM (2002) Review of readmissions due to complications from uterine fibroid embolization. Clin Radiol 57:1122–1124

56. Cragg AH, Nakagawa N, Smith TP et al. (1991) Hematoma formation after diagnostic arteriography: effect of catheter size. J Vasc Interv Radiol 2:231–233

57. Vedantham S, Goodwin SC, McLucas B, Mohr G (1997) Uterine artery embolization: an underused method of controlling pelvic hemorrhage. Am J Obstet Gynecol 176:938–948

58. Yeagley TJ, Goldberg J, Klein TA, Bonn J (2002) Labial necrosis after uterine artery embolization for leiomyomata. Obstet Gynecol 100:881–882

59. Lai AC, Goodwin SC, Bonilla SM et al. (2000) Sexual dysfunction after uterine artery embolization. J Vasc Interv Radiol 11:755–758

60. Pelage JP, Le Dref O, Soyer P et al. (1999) Arterial anatomy of the female genital tract: variations and relevance to transcatheter embolization of the uterus. Am J Roentgenol 172:989–994

61. Bradley EA, Reidy JF, Forman RG, Jarosz J, Braude PR (1998) Transcatheter uterine artery embolization to treat large uterine fibroids. Br J Obstet Gynaecol 105:235–240

62. Nikolic B, Spies JB, Lundsten MJ, Abbara S (2000) Patient radiation dose associated with uterine artery embolization. Radiology 214:121–125

63. Nikolic B, Spies JB, Campbell L et al. (2001) Uterine artery embolization: reduced radiation with refined technique. J Vasc Interv Radiol 12:39–44

64. Roth AR, Spies JB, Walsh SM, Wood BJ, Gomez-Jorge J, Levy EB (2000) Pain after uterine artery embolization for leiomyomata: can its severity be predicted and does severity predict outcome. J Vasc Interv Radiol 11:1047–1052

65. Siskin GP, Stainken BF, Dowling K et al. (2000b) Outpatient uterine artery embolization for symptomatic uterine fibroids: experience in 49 patients. J Vasc Interv Radiol 11:305–311

66. Klein A, Schwartz ML (2001) Uterine artery embolization for the treatment of uterine fibroids: an outpatient procedure. Am J Obstet Gynecol 184:1556–1563

67. Ryu RK, Omary RA, Sichlau MJ et al. (2003a) Comparison of pain after uterine artery embolization using tris-acryl gelatin microspheres versus polyvinyl alcohol particles. CardioVasc Intervent Radiol 26:375–378

68. Chrisman HB, Saker MB, Ryu RK et al. (2000) The impact of uterine fibroid embolization on resumption of menses and ovarian function. J Vasc Interv Radiol 11:699–703

69. Stringer NH, Grant T, Park J, Oldham L (2000) Ovarian failure aftere uterine artery embolization for treatment of myomas. J Am Assoc Gynecol Laparosc 7:395–400

70. Amato P, Roberts AC (2001) Transient ovarian failure: a complication of uterine artery embolization. Fertil Steril 75:438–439

71. Razavi MK, Wolanske KA, Hwang GL, Sze DY, Kee ST, Dake MD (2002) Angiographic classification of ovarian artery-to-uterine artery anastomoses: initial observations in uterine fibroid embolization. Radiology 224:707–712

72. Payne JF, Robboy SJ, Haney AF (2002) Embolic microspheres within ovarian arterial vasculature after uterine artery embolization. Obstet Gynecol 100:883–886

73. Ryu RK, Siddiqi A, Omary RA et al. (2003b) Sonography of delayed effects of uterine artery embolization on ovarian arterial perfusion and function. Am J Roentgenol 181:89–92

74. Ryu RK, Chrisman HB, Omary RA et al. (2001) The vascular impact of uterine artery embolization: prospective sonographic assessment of ovarian arterial circulation. J Vasc Interv Radiol 12:1071–1074

75. Beavis EL, Brown JB, Smith MA (1969) Ovarian function after hysterectomy with conservation of the ovaries in pre-menopausal women. J Obstet Gynaecol Br Commonw 76:969–978

76. Spies JB, Roth AR, Gonsalves SM et al. (2001c) Ovarian function after uterine artery embolization for leiomyomata: assessment with use of serum follicle stimulating hormone assay. J Vasc Interv Radiol 12:437–442

77. Ahmad A, Qadan L, Hassan N, Najarian K (2002) Uterine artery embolization treatment of uterine fibroids: effect on ovarian function in younger women. J Vasc Interv Radiol 13:1017–1020

78. Robson S, Wilson K, Munday D et al. (1999) Pelvic sepsis complicating embolization of a uterine fibroid. Aust N Z J Obstet Gynaecol 39:516–517

79. Rajan DK, Beecroft JR, Clark TWI et al. (2004) Risk of intrauterine infectious complications after uterine artery embolization. J Vasc Interv Radiol 15:1415–1421

80. Vashisht A, Stuff J, Carey A, Burn P (1999) Fatal septicaemia after fibroid embolization. Lancet 354:307–308

81. Katsumori T, Nakajima K, Tokuhiro M (2001) Gadolinium enhanced MR imaging in the evaluation of uterine

fibroids treated with uterine artery embolization. Am J Roentgenol 177:303–307

82. Walker WJ, Sutton C, Pelage JP (2002) Fibroid embolisation. Clin Radiol 57:325–331

83. Sabatini L, Atiomo W, Magos A (2003) Successful myomectomy following infected ischaemic necrosis of uterine fibroids after uterine artery embolisation. Br J Obstet Gynaecol 110:704–710

84. Godfrey CD, Zbella EA (2001) Uterine necrosis after uterine artery embolization for leiomyoma. Obstet Gynecol 98:950–952

85. De Blok S, de Vries C, Prinssen HM, Blaauwgeers HLG, Jorna-Meijer LB (2003) Fatal sepsis after uterine artery embolization with microspheres. J Vasc Interv Radiol 14:779–783

86. Walker WJ, Carpenter TT, Kent AS (2004) Persistent vaginal discharge after uterine artery embolization for fibroid tumor: cause of the condition, magnetic resonance imaging appearance and surgical treatment. Am J Obstet Gynecol 190:1230–1233

87. Tropeano G, Litwicka K, di Stasi C, Romano D, Mancuso S (2003) Permanent amenorrhea associated with endometrial atrophy after uterine artery embolization for symptomatic uterine fibroids. Fertil Steril 79:132–135

88. Berkowitz RP, Hutchins FL, Worthington-Kirsch RL (1999) Vaginal expulsion of submucosal fibroids after uterine artery embolization. A report of three cases. J Reprod Med 44:373–376

89. Abbara S, Spies JB, Scialli AR, Jha RC, Lage JM, Nikolic B (1999) Transcervical expulsion of a fibroid as a result of uterine artery embolization for leiomyomata. J Vasc Interv Radiol 10:409–411

90. Kroencke TJ, Gauruder-Burmester A, Enzweiler CN, Taupitz M, Hamm B (2003) Disintegration and stepwise expulsion of a large uterine leiomyoma with restoration of the uterine architecture after successful uterine fibroid embolization: case report. Hum Reprod 18:863–865

91. Marret H, Le Brun Keris Y, Acker O, Cottier JP, Herbreteau D (2004b) Late leiomyoma expulsion after uterine artery embolization. J Vasc Interv Radiol 15:1483–1485

92. Kim V, Spandorfer J (2001) Epidemiology of venous thromboembolic disease. Emerg Med Clin North Am 19:839–859

93. Nikolic B, Kessler C, Jacobs H et al. (2003) Changes in blood coagulation markers associated with uterine artery embolization for leiomyomata. J Vasc Interv Radiol 14:1147–1153

94. Vandenbroucke JP, Rosing J, Bloemenkamp KW et al. (2001) Oral contraceptives and the risk of venous thrombosis. N Engl J Med 344:1527–1535

95. Lanocita R, Frigerio LF, Patelli G, di Tolla G, Spreafico C (1999) A fatal complication of percutaneous transcatheter embolization for treatment of uterine fibroids. At: SMIT 1999; Boston, MA, USA

96. Tanaka H, Umekawa T, Kikukawa T, Nakamura M, Toyoda N (2002) Venous thromboembolic diseases associated with uterine myomas diagnosed before hysterectomy: a report of two cases. J Obstet Gynaecol Res 28:300–303

97. Seki K, Hoshihara T, Nagata I (1992) Leiomyosarcoma of the uterus: ultrasonography and serum lactate dehydrogenase level. Gynecol Obstet Invest 33:114–118

98. Leibsohn S, d'Ablaing G, Mishell DR, Schlaerth JB (1990) Leiomyosarcoma in a series of hysterectomies performed for presumed uterine leiomyomas. Am J Obstet Gynecol 162:968–997

99. Barbazza R, Chiarelli S, Quintarelli GF, Manconi R (1997) Role of fine needle aspiration cytology in the preoperative evaluation of smooth muscle tumors. Diagn Cytopathol 16:326–330

100. Takamizawa S, Minakami H, Usui R et al. (1999) Risk of complications and uterine malignancies in women undergoing hysterectomy for presumed benign leiomyomas. Gynecol Obstet Invest 48:193–196

101. Hata K, Hata A, Maruyama R, Hirai M (1997) Uterine sarcoma: can it be differentiated from uterine leiomyomas with Doppler ultrasonography? A preliminary report. Ultrasound Obstet Gynecol 9:101–104

102. Parker WH, Fu YS, Berek JS (1994) Uterine sarcoma in patients operated on for presumed leiomyoma and rapidly growing leiomyoma. Obstet Gynecol 83:414–418

103. Al-Badr A, Faught W (2001) Uterine artery embolization in an undiagnosed uterine sarcoma. Obstet Gynecol 97:836–837

104. Common AA, Mocarski EJM, Kolin A, Pron G, Soucie J (2001) Therapeutic failure of uterine fibroid embolization caused by underlying leiomyosarcoma. J Vasc Interv Radiol 12:1449–1452

105. Sterling KM, Vogelzang RL, Chrisman HB et al. (2002) Uterine fibroid embolization: management of complications. Techn Vasc Intervent Radiol 5:56–66

106. Pelage JP, Jacob D, Le Dref O, Lacombe P, Laurent A (2004c) fatal sepsis after uterine artery embolization with microspheres. J Vasc Interv Radiol 15:405–406

107. Wingo PA, Huezo CM, Rubin GL et al. (1986) The mortality risk associated with hysterectomy. Am J Obstet Gynecol 152:803–808

108. Pinto I, Chimeno P, Romo A et al. (2003) Uterine fibroids: uterine artery embolization versus abdominal hysterectomy for treatment: a prospective, randomized, and controlled clinical trial. Radiology 226:425–531

109. Spies JB, Cooper JM, Worthington-Kirsch R, Lipman JC, Mills BB, Benenati JF (2004b) Outcome of uterine embolization and hysterectomy for leiomyomas: results of a multicenter study. Am J Obstet Gynecol 191:22–31

110. McLucas B, Goodwin S, Adler L, Rappaport A, Reed R, Perrella R (2001b) Pregnancy following uterine fibroid embolization. Int J Gynaecol Obstet 74:1–7

111. Broder MS, Goodwin SC, Chen G et al. (2002) Comparison of long-term outcomes of myomectomy and uterine artery embolization. Obstet Gynecol 100:864–868

112. Razavi MK, Hwang G, Jahed A, Modanloo S, Chen B (2003) Abdominal myomectomy versus uterine fibroid embolization in the treatment of symptomatic uterine leiomyomas. Am J Roentgenol 180:1571–1575

113. Myers ER (2002) Uterine artery embolization: what more do we need to know? Obstet Gynecol 100:847–848

114. Stancato-Pasik A, Mitty H, Richard HM III, Eshkar NS (1997) Obstetric embolotherapy: effects on menses and pregancy. Radiology 204:791–793

115. Ornan D, White R, Pollak J, Tal M (2003) Pelvic embolization for intractable postpartum hemorrhage: long-term follow-up and implications for fertility. Obstet Gynecol 102:904–910

116. Goldberg J, Pereira L, Berghella V et al. (2004) Pregnancy

outcome after treatment for fibromyomata: uterine artery embolization versus laparoscopic myomectomy. Am J Obstet Gynecol 191:18–21

117. Goldberg J, Pereira L, Berghella V (2002) Pregnancy after uterine artery embolization. Obstet Gynecol 100:869–872

118. Pron G, Mocarski E, Bennett J, Vilos G, Common A, Vanderburgh L (2005) Pregnancy after uterine artery embolization for leiomyomata: the Ontario multicenter trial. Obstet Gynecol 105:67–76

119. Carpenter TT, Walker WJ (2005) Pregnancy following uterine artery embolisation for symptomatic fibroids: a series of 26 completed pregnancies. Br J Obstet Gynaecol 112:321–325

120. Katsumori T, Nakajima K, Mihara T (2003) Is a large fibroid a high-risk factor for uterine artery embolization? Am J Roentgenol 181:1309–1314

121. Gabriel H, Pinto CM, Kumar M et al. (2004) MRI detection of uterine necrosis after uterine artery embolization for fibroids. Am J Roentgenol 183:733–736

10.5 How to Minimize Failure after UFE

Jafar Golzarian and Jean Pierre Pelage

CONTENTS

10.5.1
Introduction

Ten years after Ravina et al. first introduced the concept of embolization as a definitive therapy for symptomatic fibroids, uterine fibroid embolization (UFE) is accepted as a safe alternative to surgical treatment of fibroid tumors. Technique and materials have been greatly refined. Much progress has been made in our understanding of fibroid vasculature, management of postoperative pain and complications, and causes of treatment failure. According to the literature, the failure rates vary between 6% and 14% [1, 2]; however, there is still some confusion as to how to define success, failure or recurrence. In this chapter, we discuss the causes of failure after UFE and the different options available to minimize them.

J. Golzarian, MD
Professor of Radiology, Director, Vascular and Interventional Radiology, University of Iowa, Department of Radiology, 200 Hawkins Drive, 3957 JPP, Iowa City, IA 52242, USA
J.-P. Pelage, MD, PhD
Department of Radiology Hôpital Ambroise Pare, 9, Avenue Charles De Gaulle, 92104 Boulogne Cedex, France

10.5.2
Definition

10.5.2.1
Clinical Success or Failure

Clinical success is measured by the resolution or the degree of improvement of symptoms [2]. The goal of UFE is to resolve or significantly improve symptoms. However, UFE is associated with no clinical benefit in some patients. This is one definition of failure. Another definition of failure is when a patient experiences clinical improvements in symptoms initially, but the improvements are not sustained long-term. This "recurrence" of symptoms may not necessarily be caused by new fibroid recurrence, however. The exact fibroid recurrence rate has not yet been established. One report indicated that the recurrence rate after UFE was lower than 10% in a patient population followed by ultrasound [3]. In early reports on uterine artery embolization (UAE), most imaging follow-ups were obtained by ultrasound, and the reduction of the volume was considered an important factor for success. The reduction of uterine and fibroid volumes, although important, are not determinant factors of success. Partial devascularization of fibroids is associated with partial necrosis of the tumors, resulting in volume reduction in most patients. With our better understanding of UFE, it is generally accepted that there is a high rate of regrowth of noninfarcted fibroids after the initial procedure. This is associated with a higher recurrence of symptoms. There is a shift to a new definition of success or failure based on the infarction of fibroids as demonstrated by imaging.

10.5.2.2
Imaging Success

Most authors agree that to obtain the best durable clinical outcome, complete devascularization of all fibroids is necessary [3, 4]. Although partial devascularization of fibroids can be associated with clinical improvement, failure to obtain complete devascularization may affect long-term clinical response and may lead to high recurrence rates [4]. Enhanced MRI best demonstrates fibroid perfusion after UFE. In cases of persistent perfusion of fibroid(s), patients need to be informed of the higher risk of recurrence of symptoms and require close follow-up. Thus, persistence of contrast enhancement of fibroid(s) after UFE should be considered no better than a partial success.

10.5.3
Failures Associated with UFE

Several causes of failure associated with UFE have been identified. These include the inability to cannulate uterine arteries, arterial spasm, flow restriction, variation of vascular anatomy, and/or misdiagnosis of fibroids as a cause of symptoms. Another important cause of failure is insufficient embolization, with recanalization of the fibroid vasculature occurring minutes to hours after the procedure's completion [5].

10.5.3.1
Catheterization Failure

To obtain technical success, both uterine arteries need to be embolized. Cannulation failure of one or both arteries can occur due to technical or anatomic conditions. Most technical failures of catheterization are related to anatomic variation. Vessel damage during the procedure is a rare cause of failure.

10.5.3.1.1
Vessel Damage

Perforation and dissection of the uterine artery are less common causes of failure [6]. These complications can occur with the use of hydrophilic guidewires associated to the arterial tortuosity (Fig. 10.5.1). Vasospasm occurring primarily in patients undergoing hormone therapy is an important cause of vessel damage. Careful catheterization, use of a microcatheter and experience of operator performing the procedure are all important factors in reducing this type of failure. In cases where

the perforation or dissection of the vessels prevent appropriate embolization, a second procedure is needed in order to obtain successful devascularization of all fibroids (Fig. 10.5.2).

10.5.3.1.2
Vascular Anatomy and Variants

There are some important anatomic variations associated with failure. These include tortuous artery, small uterine artery in one or both sides, absence of uterine arteries, ovarian artery supply of the fibroids and other less common variants such as a round ligament artery supply [7].

In the Ontario study, 5.8% of patients (32 patients) experienced failure of bilateral uterine artery embolization. In 18 out of 32 patients, uterine arteries were either too small or too tortuous to catheterize, or the vessel origin angles were too tortuous or steep for access [6]. In these situations, a second delayed procedure, usually with a contralateral approach, was successful most of the time [6].

Segmental arterial tortuosity may provoke flow limitation to the fibroids. Positioning the catheter past the tortuosity may increase the flow by correcting the curve of the artery; however, catheterization of the tortuous segment can increase the risk of spasm. The angulation of the origin of the uterine artery can be very acute, making distal catheterization more difficult, even with a microcatheter. If the microcatheter can be placed securely in the proximal uterine artery, embolization can be performed with a highly diluted embolic materials solution and a very slow injection.

10.5.3.1.3
Ovarian Artery

The role of ovarian arteries as a cause of failure is well known. Ovarian arteries may feed the fibroids through different pathways. The visualization of an ovarian artery is not systematically associated with failure. In one study, 25% of patients had large ovarian arteries before embolization [8]. Only arteries that directly participate in feeding the uterus cause failure. In cases of a small uterine artery or absence of one or both arteries, the ovarian artery supply should be suspected (Fig. 10.5.3). However, additional supply to the fibroids may come from the ovarian arteries, even if large sized bilateral uterine arteries are present [9, 10].

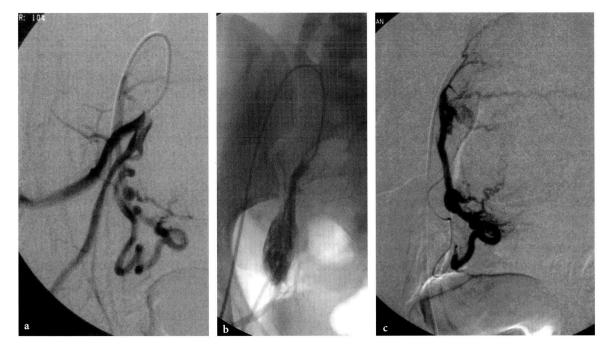

Fig. 10.5.1a–c. UFE in a patient with heavy bleeding. **a** Tortuous origin of the right uterine artery. **b** Perforation of the artery by the guidewire. **c** Distal uterine artery was successfully catheterized and embolization could be performed

There are few case reports on ovarian artery embolization with good clinical outcomes [11]. Embolization of ovarian arteries can be proximal with the use of Gelfoam torpedo, or they can be distal after selective catheterization of the ovarian artery distal to the tubo-ovarian artery using a microcatheter (Fig. 10.5.3). Although we always discuss the possibility of this variant pathway with patients, our policy is not to embolize the ovarian artery before discussing the problem with the patient in a second clinical visit.

10.5.3.2
Spasm

Embolization of uterine arteries for fibroids is based on preferential flow to the tumors, also called flow-directed embolization. The occurrence of spasm results in reduced flow to the perifibroid plexus, which is the target of embolization (Fig. 10.5.4). Thus, spasm may lead to insufficient delivery of embolic material to the fibroid tumors [5].

Spasm may be related to hormone therapy. For those patients undergoing hormone therapy (Lupron), the treatment should be discontinued prior to embolization. Embolization can only be performed once menstrual periods are resumed.

The most common cause for spasm is related to the catheterization. Careful catheterization is essential, although spasm can occur even in experienced hands. Use of a smaller catheter size (4 F) with hydrophilic coating and smaller hydrophilic guidewires (0.021" instead of 0.035") may reduce the occurrence of spasm. Systematic usage of the microcatheter is now recommended. The guiding catheter is placed at the origin of the uterine artery or even in the internal iliac artery. However, even with the systematic use of a microcatheter, spasm was present in 31% of cases in a recent study by Spies et al [1].

The use of the Roberts Uterine Catheter (Cook, Inc., Bloomington, IN) can be helpful to reduce the spasm. The benefit of this type of catheter is that the entire catheterization can be performed without a guidewire in the uterine artery, thus helping to prevent spasm (please see Chap. 10.3).

In our experience, use of vasodilators in the presence of spasm was not very helpful. When spasm occurs, the guiding catheter needs to be pulled out of uterine artery until the spasm is resolved. Sometimes the microcatheter should be pulled out of uterine artery as well. In cases of persistent spasm of the left uterine artery, one can remove the catheter and proceed to the embolization of the right uterine artery before re-catheterization of the left side. If a flow-limiting spasm persists, the use of smaller sized

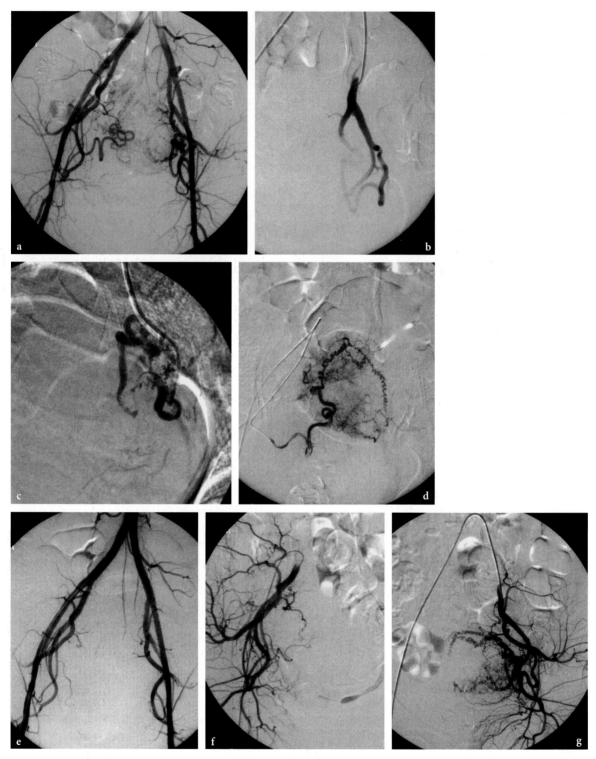

Fig. 10.5.2a–g. Heavy bleeding in a 42-year-old patient. **a** Pelvic angiogram demonstrates both uterine arteries. **b** Left hypogastric angiogram shows the left uterine artery with a proximal angulation. **c** Uterine artery angiogram demonstrates a dissection at the horizontal segment of the artery. **d** Patient underwent successful catheterization and embolization of the right uterine artery. **e** Pelvic angiogram at the end of the procedure shows no more fibroid blush and uterine artery. **f** Patient complained of symptoms recurrence after 6 months. A new procedure is performed. The right internal iliac angiogram demonstrates the persistence of uterine artery occlusion. **g** Left internal iliac angiogram shows the recanalization of the uterine artery with revascularization of the uterus. After successful embolization, patient is symptom free after 2 years

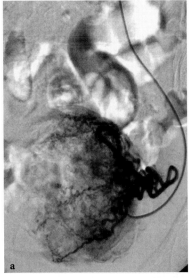
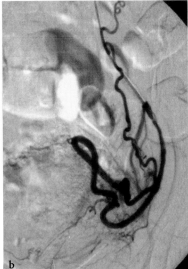
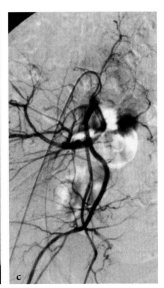
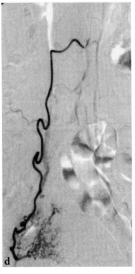
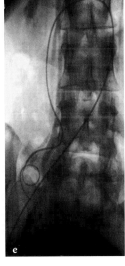

Fig. 10.5.3a–e. A 37-year-old patient with symptomatic fibroids. She was offered a hysterectomy as the only alternative. **a,b** Left uterine artery catheterization and embolization. The final angiogram at the termination of the embolization demonstrates the left ovarian artery (**b**). **c** Right internal iliac angiogram shows the absence of right uterine artery. **d** Catheterization of the right ovarian artery demonstrates the supply to the uterus by this artery. **e** Distal catheterization and embolization of the ovarian artery with successful clinical outcome

embolic materials associated with complete stasis of the uterine artery can reduce failure (Fig. 10.5.4).

10.5.3.3
Embolic Agents

The first embolic materials used for UFE were non-spherical polyvinyl alcohol (nPVA) particles, which were familiar to most interventional radiologists, readily available, inexpensive, and had a long history of being well tolerated. Variation in the size of the particles and the tendency for them to aggregate is thought to provoke a proximal vessel occlusion or unpredictable level of occlusion [12]. The aggregation of the particles may also cause microcatheter

occlusion. However, dilution and slow infusion of nPVA particles during the embolization procedure can reduce the tendency for particulate aggregation, which may subsequently lead to a more distal embolization [5, 13]. Diluted PVA solution is also associated with much less clumping and microcatheter occlusion [1, 14]. The accepted endpoint with nPVA has been complete stasis in the uterine artery as evidenced by a standing column of contrast.

Other newer agents have been introduced for use in UFE. Gelatin-coated trisacryl microspheres (Embospheres, Biosphere Medical Inc., Rockland, MA) were the first spherical agents and offered the theoretical advantage of a more uniform and targeted embolization of the perifibroid plexus [15]. Their compressibility also made microcatheter clog-

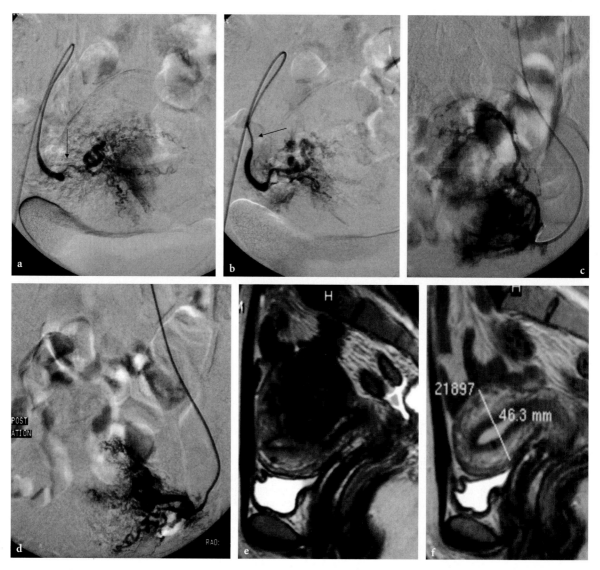

Fig. 10.5.4a–f. A 37-year-old patient with heavy bleeding related to a 7-cm intramural fibroid. **a,b** Right uterine artery angiogram demonstrates spasm (*arrow*) due to catheterization. **c** Left uterine artery angiogram shows the feeding artery to the fibroid (*arrow*). **d** Embolization of the main feeding artery and patency of the myometrial arteries. **e** MRI obtained prior to the embolization shows a large intramural mass. **f** MRI obtained 10 months after the embolization shows an almost normal uterus

ging less likely. A new endpoint was proposed with Embospheres, with a limited embolization of uterine arteries resulting in a "pruned-tree" appearance of the vasculature [15].

In a prospective, randomized study, Spies et al. [1] compared nPVA with Embospheres. There was a significantly higher rate of microcatheter clogging in the nPVA group, but no difference in success rates, either by imaging criteria (non-enhancement of all fibroids) or clinical outcome. Moreover, the intensity of pain and the complication rates were similar. In choosing between embolic agents with identical clinical outcomes, one needs to weigh the ease of handling, the total volume of particles required, the time for reaching the expected endpoint (with longer times being associated with higher radiation doses), and the cost of the agents.

In response to the rapid adoption of Embospheres for UFE, many companies have introduced the spherical PVA (sPVA) [16, 17]. Preliminary animal studies demonstrate that sPVA is safe, and the FDA has approved its clinical usage in UFE patients. An animal study has recently demonstrated a different penetration of sPVA particles compared to trisacryl microspheres. The authors have demonstrated that the sPVA particles have a more distal penetration than the trisacryl microspheres [18]. Interestingly, in clinical usage, the embolization endpoint is unpredictable and achieves much faster and with less embolic volume than with other embolic agents, witnessing a proximal occlusion. The number of vials needed to achieve the same endpoint with nPVA was at least twice as less. There are an increasing number of reports on failure after UFE with Contour SE (SPVA from Boston Scientific Corporation). At our institution, we have ceased using sPVA for UFE due to a high rate of imaging and clinical failure (Fig. 10.5.5). The reason for the higher failure rate associated with sPVA particles is not understood. One explanation for insufficient embolization could be a proximal occlusion of the uterine artery. LAURENT et al. have demonstrated that Contour SE particles are highly compressible (please see Chap. 10.6). This compressibility may be associated with the deformation of the spherical shape of the particles becoming more oval. The deformation of particles, as well as higher clamping, might explain the early proximal occlusion. However this proximal plug will move distally reopening the uterine artery. In fact, re-catheterization of the embolized

left uterine artery at the end of the procedure showed early reopening in some of our patients. PELAGE et al. suggested changing the embolization endpoint with the sPVA to a complete occlusion of the uterine artery [19]. With this new protocol, they have obtained a good fibroid infarction rate after UFE. Although this new technique might be effective, it has not yet been tested in a comparative study with any other accepted embolic agents. We believe that sPVA must be used with great caution, and patients should be carefully followed to ensure an acceptable outcome.

10.5.3.4
Patient Selection

10.5.3.4.1
Fibroid Location

Fibroid location within the uterus may influence the outcome of embolization. Submucosal fibroids were more likely to respond to UFE [20]. Submucosal location was a positive predictor of fibroid volume reduction after UFE [21]. The subserosal fibroids are also believed to be associated with less volume reduction after embolization (Fig. 10.5.6).

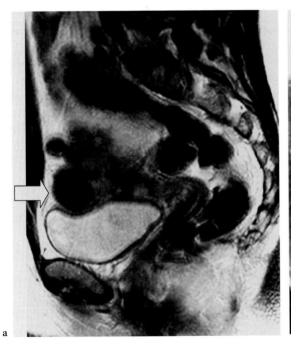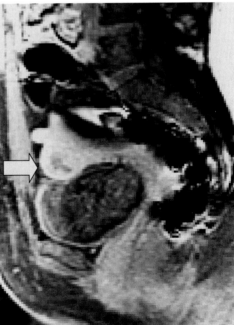

Fig. 10.5.5a,b. MRI obtained before and after embolization with sPVA. **a** *Arrow* demonstrates small fundal myomas before embolization. **b** Enhanced MR obtained 3 months post-embolization shows the persistent uptake in the partially necrosed fibroid (*arrow*)

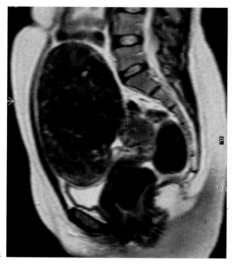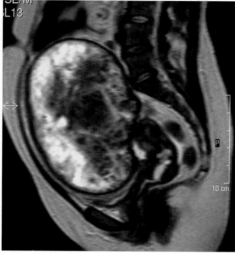

a   b

Fig. 10.5.6a,b. Patient with a 6-cm subserosal fibroid before and after embolization. **a** MRI before embolization shows a large sub-serosal fibroid. **b** Enhanced MRI obtained 6 months after embolization demonstrates no volume change with persistent uptake

Some authors suggest that in the presence of a large subserosal fibroid, the laparoscopic removal needs to be offered as the first option. In patients with multiple fibroids and a large subserosal fibroid, a combined laparoscopic resection of the subserosal fibroid and UFE is a good alternative to hysterectomy. Systematic use of MRI will help with appropriate patient selection, reducing the possibility of failure after UFE.

10.5.3.4.2
Adenomyosis

Early recurrence of symptoms can occur when uterine artery embolization is performed on patients with adenomyosis (please see Chap. 10.4). Uterine artery embolization for adenomyosis is reported to be effective to control the bleeding initially [22, 23]; however, this clinical success is short-term. There is a high rate of clinical recurrence after embolization of the uterine artery for adenomyosis. In a recent study by PELAGE et al., 44% of the patients required an additional treatment, including hysterectomies in 28% of the cases [24].

Undiagnosed adenomyosis [25, 26] can be a cause of failure after uterine artery embolization when MRI is not used as the imaging modality. Enhanced MRI is an excellent technique for diagnosing adenomyosis. To reduce the risk of failure related to improper patient selection, most centers use enhanced MRI as the screening technique of choice.

10.5.3.4.3
Undiagnosed Leiomyosarcomas

Unrecognized malignancy can be responsible for failure after UFE. This was a cause for treatment failure in two patients (2/538) in the Ontario trial [2]. However, the incidence of uterine leiomyosarcomas in UFE patients is less than 1% and would not be a common cause of failure [27]. Identifying a leiomyosarcoma is still difficult with imaging. The pre-embolization MRI aspect of sarcoma can be completely identical to a large leiomyoma with high cellularity. MRI findings of leiomyosarcoma include large heterogeneous masses and hemorrhage or cystic necrosis. However, even a histopathological diagnosis of uterine leiomyosarcoma is difficult to achieve.

Leiomyosarcoma should be considered in cases where uterine size increases and symptoms persist after a technically successful UFE. Close clinical and imaging follow-up is necessary to detect and treat potential malignancy after UFE.

10.5.4
Conclusion

Appropriate patient selection, careful catheterization and knowledge of different anatomic variants are important factors to minimize the failure after UFE. Systematic use of contrast-enhanced MRI is therefore essential, not only prior to the procedure, but also to monitor the perfusion of fibroids after embolization. The selection of embolic materials is also important. The newer materials need more clinical evaluations before being generally accepted.

References

1. Spies JB, Allison S, Flick P et al. (2004) Polyvinyl alcohol particles and tris-acryl gelatin microspheres for uterine artery embolization for leiomyomas: results of a randomized comparative study. J Vasc Interv Radiol 15:793–800
2. Pron G, Bennett J, Common A et al. (2003) The Ontario Uterine Fibroid Embolization Trial: uterine fibroid reduction and symptom relief after uterine artery embolization for fibroids. Fertil Steril 79:120–127
3. Marret H, Le Brun Keris Y, Acker O, Cottier JP, Herbreteau D (2004) Late leiomyoma expulsion after uterine artery embolization. J Vasc Interv Radiol 15:1483–1485
4. Pelage JP, Guaou-Guaou N, Jha RC, Ascher SM, Spies JB (2004) Uterine fibroid tumors: long-term MR imaging outcome after embolization. Radiology 230:803–809
5. Spies JB (2003) Uterine artery embolization for fibroids: understanding the technical causes of failure. J Vasc Interv Radiol 14:11–14
6. Pron G, Bennett J, Common A et al. (2003) Technical results and effects of operator experience on uterine artery embolization for fibroids: the Ontario Uterine Fibroid Embolization Trial. J Vasc Interv Radiol 14:545–554
7. Saraiya PV, Chang TC, Pelage JP, Spies JB (2002) Uterine artery replacement by the round ligament artery: an anatomic variant discovered during uterine artery embolization for leiomyomata. J Vasc Interv Radiol 13:939–941
8. Binkert CA, Andrews RT, Kaufman JA (2001) Utility of nonselective abdominal aortography in demonstrating ovarian artery collaterals in patients undergoing uterine artery embolization for fibroids. J Vasc Interv Radiol 12:841–845
9. Nikolic B, Spies JB, Abbara S, Goodwin SC (1999) Ovarian artery supply of uterine fibroids as a cause of treatment failure after uterine artery embolization: a case report. J Vasc Interv Radiol 10:1167–1170
10. Pelage JP, Walker WJ, Le Dref O, Rymer R (2003) Ovarian artery: angiographic appearance, embolization and relevance to uterine fibroid embolization. Cardiovasc Intervent Radiol 26:227–233
11. Barth MM and Spies BJ (2003) Ovarian artery embolization supplementing uterine embolization for leiomyomata. J Vasc Interv Radiol 14:1177–1182
12. Derdeyn C, Moran C, Cross D, Dietrich H, Dacey R (1995) Polyvinyl alcohol particle size and suspension characteristics. AJNR Am J Neuroradiol 16:1335–1343
13. Choe DH, Moon HH, Gyeong HK et al. (1997) An experimental study of embolic effect according to infusion rate and concentration of suspension in transarterial particulate embolization. Invest Radiol 32:260–267
14. Golzarian J, Torres C, Sun S, Valenti D (2004) Comparison of two different angiographic end-points for uterine fibroid embolization with PVA. A multicentre study (abstract). J Vasc Interv Radiol 15:S173
15. Pelage JP, LeDref O, Beregi JP et al. (2003) Limited uterine artery embolization with tris-acryl gelatin microspheres for uterine fibroids. J Vasc Interv Radiol 14:15–20
16. Redd D, Chaouk H, Shengelaia G et al. (2002) Comparative study of PVA particles, Embospheres and Gelspheres in a rabbit renal artery embolization model (abstract). J Vasc Interv Radiol 13:S57
17. Siskin GP, Dowling K, Virmani R, Jones R, Todd D (2003) Pathologic evaluation of a spherical polyvinyl alcohol embolic agent in porcine renal model. J Vasc Interv Radiol 14:89–98
18. Laurent A, Wassef M, Pelage JP et al. (2005) In vitro and in vivo deformation of TGMS and PVA microsphere in relation with their arterial location (abstract). J Vasc Interv Radiol 16:S77
19. Pelage JP (2005) Late breaking abstracts. 30th Annual Meeting of the Society of Interventional Radiology, New Orleans, LA, April 2
20. Spies J, Roth AR, Jha R et al. (2002) Uterine artery embolization for leiomyomata: factors associated with successful symptomatic and imaging outcome. Radiology 222:45–52
21. Jha RC, Ascher SM, Imaoka I, Spies JB (2003) Symptomatic fibroleiomyomata: MR imaging of the uterus before and after uterine arterial embolization. Radiology 217:228–235
22. Siskin GP, Tublin ME, Stainken BF, Dowling K, Dolen EG (2001) Uterine artery embolization for the treatment of adenomyosis: clinical response and evaluation with MR imaging. Am J Roentgenol 177:297–302
23. Pelage JP, Jacob D, Fazel A, Namur J et al. (2005) Midterm results of uterine artery embolization for symptomatic adenomyosis: initial experience. Radiology 234:948–953
24. Goodwin SC, McLucas B, Lee M et al. (1999) Uterine artery embolization for the treatment of uterine leiomyomata: mid-term results. J Vasc Interv Radiol 10:1159–1165
25. Smith SJ, Sewall LE, Handelsman A (1999) A clinical failure of uterine fibroid embolization due to adenomyosis. J Vasc Interv Radiol 10:171–1174
26. Common AA, Mocarski EM, Kolin A et al. (2001) Therapeutic failure of uterine fibroid embolization caused by underlying leiomyosarcoma. J Vasc Interv Radiol 12:1449–1452
27. Pattani SJ, Kier R, Deal R, Luchansky E (1995) MRI of uterine leiomyosarcoma. Magn Reson Imaging 13:331–333

10.6 Perspectives

ALEXANDRE LAURENT, JEAN-PIERRE PELAGE, and JAFAR GOLZARIAN

CONTENTS

10.6.1
Introduction

With several years of experience with uterine fibroid embolization, sufficient data are now available to allow some perspectives on the outcome of this procedure and discuss future directions for research. We have already learned that approximately 90% of patients will have symptomatic improvement while 10% will not improve [20, 30, 40]. As previously discussed in the chapter on how to minimize failure, there are different reasons for the procedure to fail.

A. LAURENT, MD, PhD
Associate Professor, Center for Research in Interventional Imaging (Cr2i APHP-INRA) Jouy en Josas, 78352 France
J.-P. PELAGE, MD PhD
Department of Radiology Hôpital Ambroise Pare, 9, Avenue Charles De Gaulle, 92104 Boulogne Cedex, France
J. GOLZARIAN, MD
Professor of Radiology, Director, Vascular and Interventional Radiology, University of Iowa, Department of Radiology, 200 Hawkins Drive, 3957 JPP, Iowa City, IA 52242, USA

Potential causes of failure are of technical origin (i.e. failed catheterization of the uterine artery, false angiographic end-point, uterine artery spasm or flow restriction), may be related to anatomical variations (ovarian artery supply to the fibroids in particular), or due to the presence of associated conditions (mainly adenomyosis) [42]. Beyond the short-term improvement in symptoms, the future acceptance of this procedure also depends on the durability of symptom control. Clinical failure or recurrence may be the outcome when some of the fibroids do not infarct following embolization [25, 26]. Optimization of the outcome from uterine fibroid embolization should be a priority for future clinical research. One of the primary clinical challenges in managing patients undergoing uterine fibroid embolization is the control of post-embolization pain [34, 47]. Post-procedural pain is the justification for performing uterine fibroid embolization as an inpatient procedure at most centers as opposed to an outpatient procedure which may be more easily accepted by both the patients and the referring gynecologists. As for liver chemoembolization, preclinical research is ongoing with drug eluting beads loaded with different types of medications. The same platforms may also be used to load hormones in order to achieve a greater degree of fibroid infarction or prevent the growth of new fibroids. The objectives of this chapter are to summarize the perspectives and future directions associated with uterine fibroid embolization.

10.6.2
How to Predict and Improve Long-Term Clinical Success

Given that short and mid-term outcomes indicate a safe procedure with a few major complications and symptomatic improvement in nearly all patients, one of the most important question is the durability of the procedure in the longer term. Three distinct types of treatment failure have already been reported after embolization.

- Early failure corresponds to temporary improvement or absence of clinical relief after embolization [42, 26]. Most of these failures are of technical or anatomical origin: unilateral uterine artery embolization, severe arterial spasm leading to a false angiographic end-point of embolization, additional arterial supply to the uterus from other sources such as the ovarian arteries [23, 42]. Prevention and identification of these causes of failures is mandatory in order to reduce the rate of early failures. As recently stated by SPIES [42] and our group [24], the systematic use of microcatheters may reduce the occurrence of spasm or flow-restriction and may allow better distribution of embolization particles and more targeted devascularization of all the fibroids. Ovarian artery supply to the fibroids should also be investigated and informed consent to perform additional embolization should be obtained from the patient [23]. Early failures are also related to associated conditions mimicking fibroid symptoms [16]. In our experience, long-term results observed in women with adenomyosis are not as good as in those with uterine fibroids (PELAGE et al. 2005). Finally, endometrial evaluation should always be performed in patients with irregular cycles, intermenstrual or continuous bleeding or periods lasting more than 14 days to exclude endometrial abnormalities accounting for bleeding symptoms [26].

- Clinical recurrence has been reported after an initial improvement and usually occurs within 2–3 years. This population of patients is of paramount importance for the future acceptance of embolization as a valuable alternative to myomectomy and other emerging uterus-sparing therapies. Most of these recurrences are related to progression of viable fibroids or regrowth of fibroids with partial devascularization after embolization [16]. As for the surgeons, small fibroids left in place during myomectomy or still perfused after embolization account for these secondary treatment failures [27]. We have already demonstrated that post-procedure imaging is crucial to predict such clinical recurrence. The use of contrast-enhanced MRI allows early detection of residual perfusion of the fibroids after embolization [27]. In our practice, we have found that a 24-h post-embolization contrast-enhanced MRI is strongly predictive of the 6- to 12-month post-embolization appearance [28]. In addition, there is a strong statistical correlation between residual fibroid perfusion and clinical recurrence, with virtually all patients with viable fibroids presenting with symptom recurrence at some time during the follow-up [28]. Future clinical studies comparing embolization to myomectomy should take the imaging appearance into consideration.

- Late recurrence is observed when new fibroids occur usually 5 years or later after embolization [26]. MRI may be useful to detect new fibroids actually even before the patient's symptoms worsen [27].

Recently, two minimally invasive therapies have been introduced to treat uterine fibroids. High frequency focused ultrasound and transvaginal paracervical clamping of the uterine arteries have been reported in the management of symptomatic uterine fibroids [10]. From our own experience with the use of uterine fibroid embolization, we know that unless complete devascularization of all identified fibroids is obtained after these therapies, the results in terms of recurrence will not be better than after myomectomy and may be higher than after embolization.

10.6.3
Technical Optimization for Uterine Fibroid Embolization

10.6.3.1
Reported Success Rates

The reported clinical success rates as high as 85%–90% in all studies may be considered disappointing to some skeptical observers. Similarly, the published reduction in uterine and dominant fibroid volumes is around 25%–60% and 33%–68% at 3–12 months [20, 30, 40, 47]. Even if it has been suggested that residual fibroid perfusion is more important than shrinkage after treatment, one may notice that these figures remain too low to compete with those of surgery where all the fibroids are actually resected. Thus, in one retrospective comparison between myomectomy and embolization, bulk-related symptoms were more quickly and more frequently resolved after surgery [32]. Is there a way to increase the percentage of fibroid and uterine volume reduction and can we get more consistent results from one patient to another? The technique of embolization has changed dramatically in recent years and the objectives were mainly to improve safety because efficacy was already well demonstrated in the first reports.

10.6.3.2
Calibrated Microspheres for Uterine Artery Embolization

Trisacryl-gelatin microspheres (TGMS) were developed to address some of the perceived shortcomings of non-spherical embolization particles of polyvinyl alcohol foam [14]. TGMS are compressible, which allows easy passage through a microcatheter with a luminal diameter smaller than that of the microspheres. The hydrophilic interaction of TGMS with fluids and a positive surface charge reduce the formation of aggregates. It has been demonstrated that calibrated TGMS are easy to deliver and unlikely to clump in vessels and lead to a rapid and reliable decrease in local blood flow [1, 6, 21, 24].

Theoretically, the calibration of microspheres should allow better control of the level of occlusion, which depends on the number of injected particles and the penetration of the embolic agent into the tissue [21]. Many interrogations were formulated about the advantages, risks, and effects of spherical agent by opposition to non-spherical PVA that were commonly used in uterine fibroid embolization [43]. The risk resulting from the use of small microspheres has been clearly understood and the rationale for choosing the proper size for uterine fibroid embolization is now defined [24, 25, 41]. New embolization techniques including the use of large microspheres and a more limited embolization of the uterine artery have been successfully used in several studies [11, 24, 25, 41]. The utility of calibrated microspheres is now accepted by a majority of operators. The introduction of the limited technique of uterine artery embolization with the use of large calibrated microspheres has opened a new era in the field of peripheral embolization [24. 25]. Widely used in neuroradiology, these more sophisticated techniques applied to uterine fibroid embolization have raised the issue of reduced efficacy compared to a more aggressive embolization [2].

Several spherical embolization materials are now available on the market. After the introduction of TGMS (Embosphere, Biosphere Medical), which was approved in Europe (CE approval) in 1997, in the USA (FDA approval) for general embolization in 2000 and specifically for uterine fibroid embolization in 2002, two PVA-based microspheres have been developed [33, 39]. Contour SE (Boston Scientific) and Bead Block (Biocompatibles) were approved recently in Europe and in the US. The three types of microspheres available have calibers within the same size ranges (100–300, 300–500, 500–700; 700–900; and 900–1200 μm).

Although calibrated and spherical in shape, the different types of microspheres are clearly different when considering their hydrophilic properties, superficial tension, ionic charge which therefore give different mechanical properties including rigidity and elasticity. For example, the rigidity at 70% compression is about 12 g for TGMS, a few grams for Bead Block and is quite absent for Contour SE (Fig. 10.6.1). In addition, Contour SE has a lower and incomplete elastic recovery than Bead Block and TGMS. PVA-based microspheres which are much less rigid and less elastic than TGMS may be deformed in microcatheters and arteries and may lead to a more distal occlusion [36].

In an experimental animal model, it has been found that after embolization of the kidney, the uterus, or the liver in the sheep with 500–700, 700–900 and 900–1200 μm microspheres that, for each caliber, the level of occlusion was more distal with Contour SE compared to TGMS of the same size [36]. These differences could be explained by a higher intravascular deformation of CSE compared to TGMS (Fig. 10.6.2). There were fewer differences in terms of location between TGMS and Bead Block (Fig. 10.6.2).

Clearly the differences between embolization microspheres available on the market have made the situation very complex for the users. Specific technical recommendations are necessary for each type of embolization materials and the use of such products

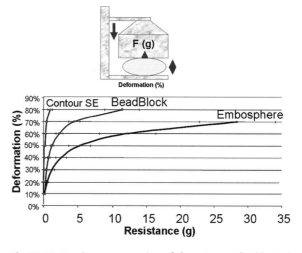

Fig. 10.6.1. In vitro compression of three types of calibrated microspheres available on the market

requires a learning curve for the operator. However, calibrated microspheres are so easy to handle and provide at least the same results as compared to non-calibrated particles, that the innovation will stay. Moreover, these microspheres also have the unique property of having the potential to be loaded with virtually any type of medication or drug. The clinical use of microspheres loaded with doxorubicin in patients with hepatocellular carcinoma has already started. It is too early to analyze the preliminary results but the revolution of embolotherapy is in motion. In order to enhance the effects of embolization to devascularization or shrink fibroids, the adjunct of hormones may be beneficial. In vitro and in vivo preclinical evaluation of such technologies have already started.

10.6.3.3
Microsphere Penetration in Vasculature and Vascular Topology

Vascularization of uterine fibroids comprises schematically dilated and tortuous peripheral vessels and smaller intra-tumoral vessels [37, 46, 50]. It has been recently demonstrated that a logical target for embolization is the peri-fibroid arterial plexus [24].

However, the sizes of these vessels have not been studied by means of plastic molding. One proposal could be to measure the microspheres and vessels sizes in histological specimens of patients operated after embolization, as was done for other tumors, and to confirm that there is a threshold for the pen-etration of calibrated microspheres inside the tumor [15].

It could be of great interest to verify that the size of these peripheral arteries ranges between 500 and 900 μm regardless of the size or location of the fibroid. Since drug-loaded microspheres will soon become available, for instance to prevent tumor recurrence, one could imagine that it could be of clinical interest to selectively occlude the intratumoral component.

10.6.3.4
Size, Number, and Dilution of Microspheres

Theoretically, small microspheres should distribute distally in small arterioles, and one could imagine completely filling a tumoral process with radioactive microspheres or drug-eluting beads. The pathological studies did not confirm this hypothesis: tissular distribution of beta-emitting microspheres smaller than 40 μm has been studied experimentally in rabbit liver and clinically [3, 29]. PILLAI [29] observed an inhomogeneous distribution of microspheres and a formation of clusters, while CAMPBELL [3] found that the median cluster size was ten times the size of the microsphere and the distance between the clusters.

In practical terms, this means that even small microspheres are not homogeneously distributed, contrary to what could be expected from their small size alone. Therefore, radiation or drug concentration could potentially be higher than expected in

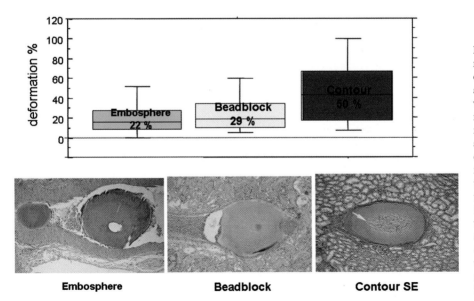

Fig. 10.6.2. In vivo deformation of three types of calibrated microspheres. The length and width of three types of microspheres has been measured on histological slides after embolization of sheep kidneys. The microsphere deformation was calculated by the formula: deformation (%) = 100 × (length–width)/width. The graph summarizes the results expressed in boxplots. A view of the deformation of each microsphere type is given below the graph

cluster areas, and low or null between the clusters. Several reasons may account for the formation of clusters of microspheres such as insufficient dilution, specific vascular topology or specific rheological conditions in small vessels.

The dilution is the unique factor which can be taken in consideration by the operator. Since the number of microspheres per millimeter of sediment is very high (about one million for small calibers), an adapted dilution has to be used. Without appropriate dilution, each 0.1 ml of sediment contains thousands of microspheres. The usual dilution recommended for clinical practice for microspheres is ×10, for instance 2 ml of microspheres in a 20-ml solution (contrast material and saline). One may suggest different optimal dilutions for larger sizes, i.e. over 600 µm and for smaller microspheres. Given the number of microspheres in a vial/syringe of 100 µm, higher dilutions (×100 or even ×1000) may be appropriate (Fig. 10.6.3). This has to be balanced with the acceptable amount of iodinated contrast medium injected.

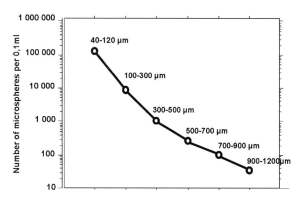

Fig. 10.6.3. Number of microspheres contained in 0.1 ml of microsphere sediment. This number is very high for small microsphere sizes (below 500 µm). A sufficient dilution (×10 or ×100) of these microspheres is mandatory to ensure a homogeneous distribution of the microspheres in the vascular network and to avoid the formation of clusters

10.6.4
New Generations of Spherical Embolization Particles

10.6.4.1
Detectability of Embolization Materials

The detectability of embolization particles has long been a matter of debate among interventional radiologists. Since calibrated microspheres have a high content in water, they are not detectable by fluoroscopy, CT, or MR scan, and operators cannot localize them during and after embolization.

Some favor radio-opaque particles in order to perform embolization without adding iodinated contrast material. Other potential advantages of being able to identify the location of microspheres include detection of non-target embolization, control of the homogeneity of distribution of the particles, evaluation of the intra- or extra-tumoral location of the microspheres, follow-up of the migration of the microspheres during time. The information regarding the distribution of the particles obtained at the time of embolization may have a significant impact on clinical practice with optimization of embolization protocols.

To obtain a radio-opaque microsphere, it is necessary to add a specific component that often radically changes the mechanical properties of the microspheres (compressibility and injectability) so that no product is available at the moment. We have chosen a completely different research approach. Since the goal of embolization is to produce targeted occlusion of the peri-fibroid arterial plexus and since the imaging tool used before and after embolization is MRI, it seemed logical to develop a microsphere detectable during MRI. Similarly to unenhanced computed tomographic studies obtained after arterial chemoembolization of the liver just by detecting the areas of trapped lipiodol, MRI detectable microspheres may be localized around the fibroids. Precise detection of the microspheres after embolization without using any contrast material could be helpful to optimize technique. Again, it could be of interest to confirm the diagnosis of non-target embolization in patients with unusual clinical manifestations after treatment [7, 18, 35, 49]. In vitro and in vivo preclinical results are encouraging since we have been able to successfully mark and detect with MRI the microspheres in different organs such as the kidneys, the uterus, and the liver (Figs. 10.6.4, 10.6.5).

10.6.4.2
Drug-Eluting Microspheres

Another potential application is to use the microspheres as a platform to load medications. Different manufacturing processes, which are coming from the drug industry for pharmaceutical purposes are

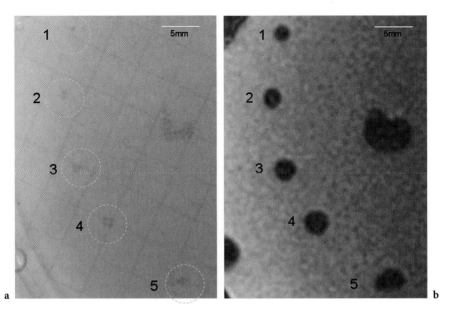

Fig. 10.6.4a,b. In vitro detectability of MR marked microspheres. Groups of *1, 2, 3, 4* and *5* microspheres are placed in a cup containing gelose (**a**) and then evaluated using MRI (**b**)

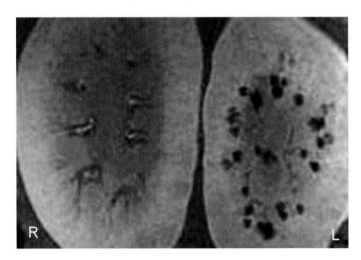

Fig. 10.6.5. In vivo detectability of 700–900 μm MR marked microspheres after renal artery embolization in the sheep. The left kidney has been embolized with trisacryl-gelatin microspheres containing an MR marker (L), and the right kidney with control trisacryl-gelatin microspheres (*R*). MRI study of the explanted kidneys was performed 24 h after embolization (3D SPGR T1, slice thickness). MR marked microspheres are detectable in the cortical area. No control microsphere is detected in the opposite side

being transposed to drug delivery embolic devices. The first products already available in the field of interventional radiology have been developed to treat liver disease. Two types of microspheres are available: those which behave like sponges able to absorb large amounts of drug in solution or those produced from specific polymers able to adsorb a given drug which reaches high concentration inside the biomaterial (GESCHWIND JF, unpublished data). In the first case the release system can be considered as a ready-to-load platform for water-soluble drugs, but a release can occur in the medium before and during injection. In the second, the product is more susceptible to release on long term.

Similarly, drug-loaded microspheres for fibroid embolization can be developed in different directions. Vasoactive drugs, prothrombotic agents, and antiangiogenic factors can enhance or prolong the duration of arterial occlusion. Hormones, growth factor inhibitors, and antimitotics may prevent local tumor regrowth. Antalgic or anti-inflammatory drugs may reduce post-embolization pain after fibroid embolization. Post-embolization pain is the reason for keeping patients in hospital after embolization at most centers. Following initial experience with the use of embolization, there have been several attempts to reduce pain at the time of embolization by, for example, mixing lidocaine with the particles. Post-embolization pain is usually considered as a local effect of embolization on the fibroids and on the myometrium [34]. Reduction in the intensity of ischemia or inflammation observed in the uterus may help to reduce post-embolization pain [47]. Different research projects are ongoing to evaluate the feasibility and the effects of loading of analgesics or anti-inflammatory drugs in calibrated microspheres (Fig. 10.6.6).

The theoretical advantages of drug-loaded implants are numerous: a higher local concentration and a lower total dose of drug compared to a systemic administration and finally the possibility of using drugs that are potentially toxic via the systemic route (Fig. 10.6.6). Preliminary tests should be conducted in order to evaluate the diffusion of the drug. The diffusion area is composed of the vessel wall and the perivascular space, which comprises veins, lymphatic ducts and interstitial tissue. Within the few hours following embolization, a foreign body reaction develops around the microsphere. This inflammatory response may modify the drug release in two ways: either by creating a barrier which reduces the diffusion of the drug, or by eliminating the drug in the process.

For these reasons the drug release is a very promising strategy but its efficiency needs to be demonstrated experimentally first in animals and then in patients. In animals it has to be proven that: first, the systemic level of the drug is null or much lower than after a systemic administration, second that the microsphere can release the loaded drug in significant amounts, third that there are evident signs of the biological action of the drug, fourth that no adverse local or general event or side effect occurs, and finally that the primary effect of the micro-

spheres is not changed by the loaded drug. Therefore, it remains to be proven in patients that drug-loaded microspheres are safe and effective in terms of symptoms or tumor recurrence.

10.6.4.3
Resorbable Embolization Materials for Uterine Fibroid Embolization

It may be hypothesized that, compared to materials which are slowly degradable, resorbable embolics would be more able to restore uterine artery integrity. A gelatin sponge is mainly used to perform hemostatic embolization [19]. This biodegradable intravascular embolization agent has also been successfully used for fibroid embolization. Mid-term results seem to be comparable to those obtained with non-spherical PVA particles or calibrated microspheres [12].

However, the main advantage of resorbable embolics for uterine fibroid embolization is still not proven. The gelatin sponge can be supplied in three forms: as a powder containing small fragments, as a sheet from which different sized sections can be cut or as thicker blocks or cubes making it possible to obtain large pledgets [12, 19, 38]. The major limitations associated with its use for uterine fibroid embolization are the absence of calibration and the great variability in the resorption speed, which is influenced by many factors such as nature, homogeneity, size, enzymatic potential, and local inflammatory response [39]. Recanalization after arterial embolization using gelatin sponge ranges from 3 weeks to 4 months and even long-term occlusion has been reported [39].

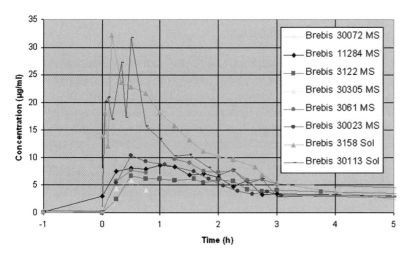

Fig. 10.6.6. Comparison of plasmatic levels of ibuprofen after injection in the uterine arteries (two sheep labeled sol) or after embolization of the uterine arteries with microspheres loaded with the same amount of ibuprofen (sheep MS). The peak is obtained immediately after intra-arterial injection whereas a more progressive plasmatic distribution is observed with the loaded microspheres

Resorbable calibrated microspheres with controlled resorption time could be advantageously proposed for uterine fibroid embolization. Theoretically, such a product could better guarantee that uterine artery and branches recover a complete functionality after embolization than non-resorbable particles.

10.6.5
How Can We Improve Uterine Functionality after Embolization?

Fertility is still a controversial issue among interventional radiologists and gynecologists.

Once hemorrhage is stopped or necrosis of the tumor is obtained, occlusion of uterine arteries and vessels is no longer necessary. A long-lasting arterial occlusion may alter the uterine artery functionality. The stakes include the preservation of the uterine artery to maintain the functionality of the uterus (fertility, sexuality) but also possibilities of re-embolization in case of recurrence.

Since embolization may become a first-line treatment in women still wishing to conceive, it becomes of paramount importance that embolization not only preserve the uterus but also its functionality. Surprisingly, uterine artery functionality after embolization is unknown and no angiographic, MRI, or Doppler study has ever addressed this issue.

Embolization may lead to a reduced uterine blood flow during gestation and it is well known that uterine blood flow is crucial for fetal growth and survival [8, 48]. A bilateral uterine artery embolization blocks the main arterial supply to the embryo and it has been demonstrated that the reduction in uteroplacental blood flow using ligation [5], clamp [4], occlusion [13] or embolization [45] significantly affects fetal and placental weight.

An experimental study has demonstrated that PVA and TGMS had a varying impact on fertility in the sheep [22]. When PVA particles used for uterine artery embolization were compared to TGMS, a significant decrease in subsequent fertility and lower birth weight of the newborns were observed suggesting intra-uterine growth retardation [22]. These functional results strongly suggest that embolization with these two embolic agents lead to vascular occlusions at different sites and with different long-term consequences. The histopathological analysis of resected sheep uteri confirmed this hypothesis. PVA particles tend to form large-sized aggregates,

which obstruct the trunk and first branches of the uterine artery [25]. In contrast, because of its blockade of more distal vessels, TGMS may exert a weaker impact on resistance of uterine and/or fetal umbilical arteries.

Even if the rate of recanalization for PVA and TGMS was not significantly different in our long-term implantation study, the transvascular migration was very different between the two products (Fig. 10.6.7) [25]. Transvascular migration of embolization particles was first described by TOMASHEFSKI et al. [44]. PVA aggregates were found almost exclusively in the intima, and no PVA particle was observed outside of the vessel (Figs. 10.6.7, 10.6.8) (PELAGE et al. 2003c). Conversely, TGMS were found in intima (about 50%) in media adventitia (25%) and outside the vessel (25%) (Figs. 10.6.7, 10.6.8). Thus, a more proximal location associated with the absence of transvascular migration of PVA aggregates could create a permanent blockade of the uterine artery accounting for the intra-uterine growth retardation. Cases of intra-uterine growth retardation have already been reported after uterine artery embolization in human [17]. In his retrospective analysis of 50 published cases of pregnancy after uterine artery embolization, GOLDBERG et al. [9] found that women who become pregnant after UAE are at risk of conceiving newborns with smallness for gestational age. However, in agreement with our experimental results, hypotrophy of newborns after UAE is not systematically related to a premature delivery. Thus, among the four cases of newborns (22% of live births) small for gestational age (≤ 5th percentile) reported recently by PRON et al. [31] three were delivered at term.

10.6.6
Conclusion

It is our goal to perfect our technique in order to get more consistent results, reduce complications, and establish uterine fibroid embolization for a durable time period. Large calibrated microspheres are equally effective to smaller non-calibrated particles to target the peri-fibroid arterial plexus. Calibrated microspheres are so easy to deliver through microcatheters that one may predict the progressive replacement of non-spherical particles in the near future. MRI has become the reference imaging tool before and after embolization. The use of contrast-enhanced studies allows early detection

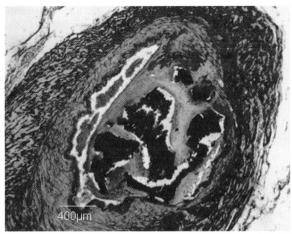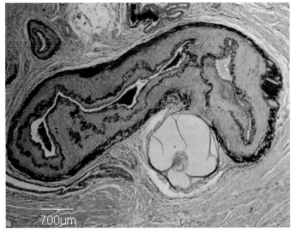

a

b

Fig. 10.6.7a,b. Transvascular migration of non-spherical PVA particles and tris-acryl microspheres: bilateral uterine artery embolization in the sheep was performed 30 months earlier (orcein staining). **a** An aggregate of PVA particles (in *black*) is located in the media. No PVA particle is seen in the media or outside of the vessel. The internal elastic limitans is ruptured. A recanalization of the embolized artery is visible. **b** One tris-acryl microsphere (in *white*) is visible outside the vessel. Both internal and external elastic limitans are ruptured and indicate the trajectory of the microsphere exclusion. A recanalization of the embolized artery is also visible

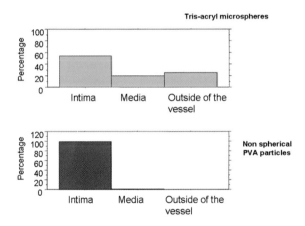

Fig. 10.6.8. Distribution of non-spherical PVA particles and tris-acryl microspheres: bilateral uterine artery embolization in the sheep was performed 30 months earlier

of viable portions of fibroids which are associated with clinical recurrence in the long-term in a more sensitive way than Doppler ultrasound. Given the experience of liver chemoembolization where the effects of embolization particles and drugs are combined, the future of uterine fibroid embolization will probably consist in the use of X-rays or MRI detectable microspheres loaded with hormones, analgesics or anti-inflammatory drugs. As stated recently, "in ten years from now, who will remember that the revolution of embolotherapy started with uterine fibroids…".

References

1. Andrews TA, Binkert CA (2003) Relative rates of blood flow reduction during transcatheter arterial embolization with tris-acryl gelatin microspheres or polyvinyl alcohol: quantitative comparison in a swine model. J Vasc Interv Radiol 14:1311–131

2. Bendszus M, Klein R, Burger R, Warmuth-Metz M, Hofmann E, Solymosi L (2000) Efficacy of trisacryl gelatin microspheres and polyvinyl alcohol particles in the preoperative embolization of meningiomas. Am J Neuroradiol 21:255–261

3. Campbell AM, Bailey IH, Burton MA (2000) Analysis of the distribution of intra-arterial microspheres in human liver following hepatic yttrium-90 microsphere therapy. Phys Med Biol. 45:1023–1033

4. Clark KE, Durnwald M, Austin JE (1982) A model for studying chronic reduction in uterine blood flow in pregnant sheep. Am J Physiol 242:H297–H301

5. Creasy, RK, Barrett C T, de Swiet M, Kahanpaa K V, Rudolph AM (1972) Experimental intrauterine growth retardation in the sheep. Am J Obstet Gynecol 112:566–573

6. Derdeyn CP, Graves VB, Salamat MS, Rappe A (1997) Collagen-coated acrylic microspheres for embolotherapy: in vivo and in vitro characteristics. Am J Neuroradiol 18:647–653

7. Gabriel H, Pinto CM, Kumar M, et al. (2004) MRI detection of uterine necrosis after uterine artery embolization for fibroids. Am J Roentgenol 183:733–736

8. Gilbert M, Leturque A (1982) fetal weight and its relationship to placental blood flow and placental weight in experimental intrauterine growth retardation in the rat. J Dev Physiol 4: 237–246

9. Goldberg J, Pereira L, Berghella V (2002) Pregnancy after uterine artery embolization: Obstet Gynecol 100:869–872

10. Hindley J, Gedroyc WM, Regan L, et al. (2004) MRI guidance of focused ultrasound therapy of uterine fibroids: early results. Am J Roentgenol 183:1713–1719

11. Joffre F, Tubiana JM, Pelage JP and the FEMIC group (2004) FEMIC Fibromes Embolisés aux Microsphères calibrées. uterine fibroid embolization using tris-acryl microspheres: a french multicentric study. CardioVasc Intervent Radiol 27: 600–606

12. Katsumori T, Nakajima K, Mihara T, Tokuhiro M (2002) Uterine artery embolization using gelatin sponge particles alone for symptomatic uterine fibroids: midterm results. Am J Roentgenol 178:135–139

13. Lang U, Baker RS, Khoury J, Clark KE (2000) Effects of chronic reduction in uterine blood flow on fetal and placental growth in the sheep. Am J Physiol Regul Integr Comp Physiol 279:R53–R59

14. Laurent A, Beaujeux R, Wassef M, et al. (1996) Trisacryl gelatin microspheres for therapeutic embolization, I: development and in vitro evaluation. Am J Neuroradiol 17: 533–540

15. Laurent A, Wassef M, Chapot R, Wang Y, Houdart E, Feng L, Tran Ba Huy P, Merland JJ. Partition of calibrated tris-acryl gelatin microspheres in the arterialvasculature of embolized nasopharyngeal angiofibromas and paragangliomas.J Vasc Interv Radiol. 2005 Apr;16(4):507–513

16. Marret H, Alonso AM, Cottier JP, Tranquart F, Herbreteau D, Body G (2003) Leiomyoma recurrence after uterine artery embolization. J Vasc Interv Radiol 14:1395–1399

17. Nizard J, Barrinque L, Frydman R, Fernandez H (2003) Fertility and pregnancy outcomes following hypogastric artery ligation for severe post-partum haemorrhage. Hum Reprod 18:844–848

18. Payne JF, Robboy SJ, Haney AF (2002) Embolic microspheres within ovarian arterial vasculature after uterine artery embolization. Obstet Gynecol 100:883–886

19. Pelage JP, Le Dref O, Mateo J, et al. (1998) Life-threatening primary postpartum hemorrhage. Treatment with emergency selective arterial embolization. Radiology 208:359–362

20. Pelage JP, Le Dref O, Soyer P, et al. (2000) Fibroid-related menorrhagia: treatment with superselective embolization of the uterine arteries and midterm follow-up. Radiology 215: 428–431

21. Pelage JP, Laurent A, Wassef M, et al. (2002a) Acute effects of uterine artery embolization in the sheep: comparison between polyvinyl alcohol particles and calibrated microspheres. Radiology 224: 436–445

22. Pelage JP, Martal J, Huynh L, Rymer R, Merland JJ, Laurent A (2002b) Bilateral uterine artery embolization in the sheep: Impact on fertility. Radiology 225 (P): 306

23. Pelage JP, Walker WJ, Le Dref O, Rymer R (2003a) Ovarian artery: angiographic appearance, embolization and relevance to uterine fibroid embolization. CardioVasc Intervent Radiol 26:227–233

24. Pelage JP, Le Dref OP, Beregi JP, et al. (2003b) Limited uterine artery embolization with tris-acryl gelatin microspheres for uterine fibroids. J Vasc Interv Radiol 14:11–14

25. Pelage JP, Wassef M, Namur J, Bonneau M, Martal J, Laurent A (2003c) Pathological findings two years after uterine artery embolization in the sheep: comparison of tris-acryl-gelatin microspheres and non-spherical PVA particles. Cardiovasc Intervent Radiol 2003: 17

26. Pelage JP, Jacob D, Le Dref O, Laurent A (2004a) Leiomyoma recurrence after uterine artery embolization. J Vasc Interv Radiol 15:774–775

27. Pelage JP, Guaou-Guaou N, Jha RC, Ascher SM, Spies JB (2004b) Uterine fibroid tumors: long-term MR imaging outcome after embolization. Radiology 230:803–809

28. Pelage JP, Brouard R, Jacob D, Boudiaf M, Abitbol M, Le Dref O (2004) Perfusion of uterine fibroids evaluated using contrast-ehanced magentic resonance imaging performed 24 hours after embolization as a predictor of clinical outcome [abstract]. Radiology (P): 613

29. Pillai KM, McKeever PE, Knutsen CA, Terrio PA, Prieskorn DM, Ensminger WD (1991) Microscopic analysis of arterial microsphere distribution in rabbit liver and hepatic VX2 tumor. Sel Cancer Ther 7:39–48

30. Pron G, Bennett J, Common A, et al. (2003b) The Ontario uterine fibroid embolization trial: Uterine fibroid reduction and symptom relief after uterine artery embolization for fibroids. Fertil Steril 79: 120–127

31. Pron G, Mocarski E, Bennett J, Vilos G, Common A, Vanderburgh L (2005) Pregnancy after uterine artery embolization for leiomyomata: the ontario multicenter trial. Obstet Gynecol 105:67–76

32. Razavi MK, Hwang G, Jahed A, Modanloo S, Chen B (2003) Abdominal myomectomy versus uterine fibroid embolization in the treatment of symptomatic uterine leiomyomas. Am J Roentgenol 180:1571–1575

33. Redd D, Chaouk H, Shengelaia G, et al. (2002) Comparative study of PVA particles, Embospheres and Gelspheres in a rabbit renal artery embolization model [abstract]. J Vasc Interv Radiol 13:S57

34. Roth AR, Spies JB, Walsh SM, Wood BJ, Gomez-Jorge J, Levy EB (2000) Pain after uterine artery embolization for leiomyomata: can its severity be predicted and does severity predict outcome. J Vasc Interv Radiol 11:1047–1052

35. Ryu RK, Chrisman HB, Omary RA, et al. (2001) The vascular impact of uterine artery embolization: prospective sonographic assessment of ovarian arterial circulation. J Vasc Interv Radiol 12:1071–1074

36. Saint-Maurice JP, Wassef M, Namur J, Merland JJ, Laurent A (2003) Vascular distribution of two types of microspheres (Embosphere and Contour SE): a comparative study [abstract]. Presented at the annual meeting of the Cardiovascular and Interventional Radiological Society of Europe, Antalya, Turkey, September 20–24

37. Sampson J. The blood supply of uterine myomata (1912) Surg Gynecol Obstet 14:215–234

38. Siskin GP, Englander M, Stainken BF, et al. (2000) Embolic agent used for uterine fibroid embolization. Am J Roentgenol 175:767–773

39. Siskin GP, Dowling K, Virmani R, Jones R, Todd D (2003) Pathologic evaluation of a spherical polyvinyl alcohol embolic agent in porcine renal model. J Vasc Interv Radiol 14:89–98

40. Spies JB, Ascher SA, Roth Arm, Kim J, Levy EB, Gomez-Jorge J (2001a) Uterine artery embolization for leiomyomata. Obstet Gynecol 98:29–34

41. Spies JB, Benenati JE, Worthington-Kirsch RL, Pelage JP (2001b) Initial experience with the use of trisacryl gelatin microspheres for uterine artery embolization for leiomyomata. J Vasc Interv Radiol 12:1059–1063

42. Spies JB (2003) Uterine artery embolization for fibroids:

understanding the technical causes of failure. J Vasc Interv Radiol 14:11–14

43. Spies JB, Allison SJ, Flick PA, et al. (2004) Polyvinyl alcohol particles and tris-acryl gelatin microspheres for uterine artery embolization for leiomyomas. J Vasc Interv Radiol 15:793–800

44. Tomashefski JF, Jr., Cohen AM, Doershuk CF (1988) Long-term histopathologic follow-up of bronchial arteries after therapeutic embolization with polyvinyl alcohol (Ivalon) in patients with cystic fibrosis. Hum Pathol 19:555–561

45. Trudinger BJ, Stevens D, Connelly A, et al. (1987) Umbilical artery flow velocity waveforms and placental resistance: the effects of embolization of the umbilical circulation. Am J Obstet Gynecol 157:1443–1448

46. Walocha JA, Miodonski AJ, Szczepanski W, Skrzat J, Stachura J. Two types of vascularisation of intramural uterine leiomyomata revealed by corrosion casting and immunohistochemical study (2004) Folia Morphol 63:37–41

47. Walker WJ, Pelage JP (2002) Uterine artery embolization for symptomatic fibroids: clinical results in 400 women with imaging follow-up. Br J Obstet Gynaecol 109:1262–1272

48. Wigglesworth J (1974) Fetal growth retardation. animal model: uterine vessel ligation in the pregnant rat. Am J Pathol 72: 347–350.

49. Yeagley TJ, Goldberg J, Klein TA, Bonn J (2002) Labial necrosis after uterine artery embolization for leiomyomata. Obstet Gynecol 100:881–882

50. Farrer-Brown G, Beilby JO, Rowles PM. Microvasculature of the uterus. An injection method of study. Obstet Gynecol. 1970 Jan;35(1):21–30

11 Pelvic Congestion Syndrome

Lindsay Machan

CONTENTS

11.1
Introduction

The association between varicose veins in the pelvis and pelvic pain in women has been known since the description of tubo-ovarian varicocele by RICHET in 1857 [1]. However, it was not until 1976 that the phrase "pelvic congestion syndrome" was coined by HOBBS [2] to describe a syndrome of chronic pelvic pain and heaviness due to pelvic varicosities. The pelvic varicosities are almost always secondary to reversed flow in the ovarian vein, in essence a female

L. MACHAN, MD
Department of Radiology, UBC Hospital, 2211 Wesbrook Mall, Vancouver BC, V6T 2B5, Canada

varicocele; however, the clinical syndrome of pelvic pain in women resulting from gonadal vein reflux is less appreciated than the corresponding entity of symptomatic varicocele in men. In addition it is being increasingly recognized that visible varicose veins of the buttocks, labia, or lower extremities may be secondary to ovarian vein reflux.

11.2
Pathophysiology

Pelvic congestion is a complex subject. When considering the pathophysiology, two components must be considered (Fig. 11.1); gonadal vein reflux, which is the commonest cause of pelvic varicosities, and the pelvic varicosities themselves, which are felt to be the principle cause of pain in pelvic congestion syndrome. Each may be seen without the other, and both can be present in asymptomatic patients.

11.2.1
Gonadal Vein Reflux

Reversed flow in the ovarian veins can occur because of absent or incompetent valves, or because of structural or functional obstruction. Anatomical studies show that 13%–15% of women lack valves in the left ovarian vein and approximately 6% on the right and that when valves are present, 43% on the left and 35%–41% on the right are incompetent [3, 4]. When the valves are incompetent, mean ovarian venous diameter increases from the normal of 3.8 mm to 7.5 mm [5].

Some authors suggest that renal vein obstruction is a common etiology of ovarian vein reflux. This does not reflect the author's experience. A Belgian study of 48 patients with pelvic congestion syndrome found that 83% had extrinsic compression of the left renal vein between the aorta and the superior mesenteric artery resulting in the "nutcracker phenom-

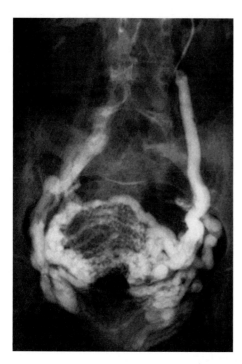

Fig. 11.1. Pelvic congestion syndrome. Selective injection of the left ovarian vein reveals retrograde flow in a dilated left ovarian vein and results in opacification of an extensive network of pelvic varicosities

enon" [6] (Fig. 11.2). The ovarian and internal iliac veins can serve as important collateral pathways when there is obstruction of the iliocaval venous system. The significant interconnections and relative paucity of valves can result in ovarian venous blood flow in either direction [7].

11.2.2
Pelvic Varicosities

The evidence that pelvic varicose veins cause pain is indirect. Pelvic varicosities are more frequently seen in women with pelvic pain than in asymptomatic patients. In one study of transuterine venography, 91% of patients with chronic pelvic pain had evidence of pelvic varicosities compared with 11% of control patients [8]. When intravenous dihydroergotamine (a vasoconstrictor), is administered to women during an acute attack of pelvic pain there is both a decrease of pelvic venous diameter and a significant reduction in pain [9].

Ovarian varicosities are more frequent after pregnancy [10] due to hemodynamic and physiologic factors which result in pelvic venous hypertension during pregnancy. The capacity of the ovarian veins

may increase 60 times over the non-pregnant state contributing to both venous dilatation and valvular incompetence. As the veins dilate during pregnancy, the valve cusps separate and become incompetent [11].

Pelvic veins are uniquely predisposed to become dilated, even without pregnancy. Many pelvic veins are devoid of valves and have weak attachments between the adventitia and supporting connective tissue [12]. Although this is different from veins elsewhere in the body the histology of pelvic varicosities is similar to that of varicose veins elsewhere, including fibrosis of the tunica intima and media, muscular hypertrophy and proliferation of capillary endothelium.

There are many possible reasons to explain why some patients with ovarian vein reflux have no pain while others are in agony. Most importantly, there are marked individual differences in how pain of any kind is perceived and significant variations between women in the density of nerves in the ovarian vein [13]. There may also be physical changes in the pelvic organs of women with pelvic congestion. Compared with normal women of similar age and parity, women with chronic pain due to pelvic congestion have a larger uterus and thicker endometrium and as many as 56% have cystic changes in their ovaries [14]. In addition menstrual disorders such as menorrhagia and polymenorrhea are more frequent in women with pelvic congestion syndrome [15].

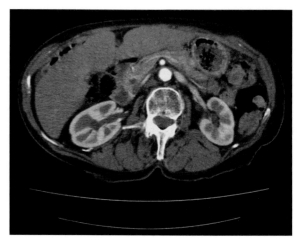

Fig. 11.2. "Nutcracker phenomenon". Axial CT image demonstrates contrast in the distal left renal vein does not extend through narrowed central vein compressed between aorta and SMA. Contrast drained preferentially through retrograde flow in left ovarian vein

11.3
Clinical Considerations

The symptom complex of pelvic congestion syndrome includes pelvic heaviness or pain of varying severity typically exacerbated by long periods of standing, with exercise, or at the end of the day. These symptoms may be worst in the premenstrual period. Associated dyspareunia is frequent, manifesting as pain at the time of sexual intercourse or intense pelvic cramping immediately after. Some women note that intercourse is painful at the end of the day but not in the morning, presumably because venous engorgement of the pelvic tissues which had occurred after a day of standing is relieved by hours spent supine.

In addition to paraovarian varicosities many patients have labial varicosities and varicose veins in their legs secondary to, or exacerbated by, ovarian vein reflux. Clues to the presence of ovarian vein reflux include varicosities on the buttocks and posterior aspect of the thigh, or varicose veins of the leg which recur immediately after surgical repair. Treatment of these visible varicosities can occur as a part of the therapy in women presenting with pelvic congestion syndrome who are also troubled by cosmetically or physically symptomatic superficial veins. With the resurgent interest in the treatment of lower extremity varicosities, patients are more frequently presenting solely for treatment of vulvar or lower extremity varicose veins. When questioned, these patients often report minor levels of pelvic discomfort. In a recent study of 160 women presenting primarily for treatment of lower limb varicose veins, 26 (16%) were found to incidentally have symptoms of pelvic congestion syndrome [16]. Twenty four of the 26 women underwent ovarian venography, and ovarian vein reflux was demonstrated and treated by embolization in 24 (92%).

The diagnostic criteria for pelvic congestion syndrome are not universally agreed upon [17]. Some physicians make the diagnosis on clinical grounds without the aid of imaging. Others use transuterine venography and base the diagnosis on the diameter of the ovarian veins, distribution of vessels, and delay in clearance of contrast medium, viewing the presence or absence of ovarian vein reflux as irrelevant. However, the majority of modern literature bases the diagnosis on the presence of pelvic varicose veins filled by ovarian vein reflux, this is the model preferred by the author. In our experience, true pelvic varicosities without ovarian vein reflux are rare.

Pelvic congestion syndrome is controversial and is not accepted as an entity by many practitioners. Like retrograde flow in the gonadal vein in men, critical analysis of both the disorder and its treatment are difficult because of the lack of standardized diagnostic criteria, the fact that pelvic varicosities are seen in many asymptomatic women, and because there are numerous causes of chronic pelvic pain. Experienced gynecologists will frequently comment that they see dilated pelvic veins at laparoscopy in parous women who do not have symptoms of pelvic congestion. As described earlier, physiologic venous ectasia can be a normal consequence of pregnancy but flow should be antegrade in dilated but otherwise normal veins whereas in pelvic congestion syndrome the patients have retrograde flow in tortuous varicosities.

Chronic pelvic pain is defined as pelvic pain present for at least 6 months. It is common, affecting approximately one in seven women [18] and accounting for 10% of all referrals to gynecologists [19]. Potential causes of chronic pelvic pain are listed in Table 11.1. In laparoscopic studies of women with chronic pelvic pain, approximately one third of patients will have endometriosis, one third other visible pathology such as PID, pelvic adhesions or ovarian cysts, and one third will have no obvious findings [20]. Whether utilizing the resources of a multidisciplinary pain clinic or applying surgical interventions, at least 20% of women with chronic pelvic pain can not be effectively treated [21, 22]. Due at least in part to the difficulties in accurate diagnosis and lack of effective therapy, there is often significant psychological overlay [23]. Any physician investigating or treating a patient with chronic pelvic pain may be faced with a frustrated complex patient whose symptoms are difficult to elucidate, diagnosis is elusive, and in chronic pain that has been refractory even to aggressive therapy.

11.3.1
Pre-procedure Workup

All patients with chronic pelvic pain should have the benefit of clinical evaluation and shared care by a physician with expertise in chronic pelvic pain. A laparoscopy and pelvic ultrasound should be performed prior to radiologic interventions. Their role is to exclude other diagnoses, not to make the diagnosis of pelvic congestion. If the clinical presentation is recurrent lower extremity varicose veins or

Table 11.1. Common causes of chronic pelvic pain

Physiologic

   Ovulation
   Menstruation

Pelvic inflammatory disease

Genitourinary

   Ovarian/paraovarian cysts
   Endometriosis
   Fibroids
   Malignancy
   Prolapse
   Cystitis
   Calculi

Gastrointestinal

   Ulcerative colitis
   Crohn's disease
   Diverticulitis
   Irritable bowel syndrome
   Malignancy

Musculoskeletal

   Lumbar disc
   Sacral canal stenosis
   Spondylolisthesis
   Perineum syndrome

labial varicosities, these investigations are not necessary prior to venography in most cases.

Laparoscopy. Laparoscopy is the most effective means of diagnosing other causes of chronic pelvic pain and virtually all women with chronic pelvic pain should undergo this procedure. In particular, minimal lesion endometriosis, the most common cause of chronic pelvic pain, will not be detected by ultrasound and may only be detected by an expert laparoscopist. Dilated veins, however, often cannot be seen because of their retroperitoneal position and the increased intra-abdominal pressure and increased venous drainage with Trendelenburg positioning that are part of laparoscopic examination. It should be noted that a negative laparoscopy in a woman with chronic pelvic does not exclude pelvic congestion.

11.3.1.1
Cross-Sectional Imaging

Although imaging can demonstrate pelvic varicose veins [24], direct visualization of tortuous and dilated ovarian veins with venography is still felt to be the gold standard for accurate diagnosis of pelvic congestion. The author reserves cross-sectional imaging as a means to exclude other causes of pelvic pain, and does not view a normal noninvasive imaging study as a contraindication to ovarian venography when there are symptoms which might be due to pelvic congestion.

Ultrasound. Ovarian and pelvic varices are seen as multiple dilated tubular structures with venous Doppler signal around the uterus and ovary on both transabdominal or transvaginal US with color Doppler. Sonographic diagnostic criteria for pelvic congestion have been published. These include: (a) a tortuous pelvic vein with a diameter greater than 4 mm, (b) slow blood flow (about 3 cm/s), and (c) a dilated arcuate vein in the myometrium that communicates between bilateral pelvic varicose veins [25]. The author prefers to rely on abnormal accentuation of blood flow with Valsalva maneuver (Fig. 11.3) rather than utilizing strict size criteria. Venous diameter can vary considerably with body position, nervousness or hydration, or there may be physiologic ectasia from prior pregnancies, but without valvular incompetetence.

Ovarian cysts may be seen in women with pelvic congestion syndrome ranging from a few cysts to polycystic ovary syndrome produced by estrogen overstimulation.

CT and MRI. On CT and MRI pelvic varices are seen as dilated tortuous paraovarian or parauterine tubular structures, frequently extending to the broad ligament and pelvic sidewall or paravaginal venous plexus [26, 27] (Fig. 11.4a,b).

Dilated ovarian veins are frequently seen on CT scans in asymptomatic women, highlighting the importance of correlating the imaging and clinical findings. ROZENBLIT et al. (2001) reported seeing dilated ovarian veins in 63% of parous women without symptoms of pelvic congestion and in 10% of nonparous women [28].

On T1-weighted MR images, pelvic varices have no signal intensity because of flow-void artifact; on gradient-echo MR images the varices have high signal intensity. After the intravenous administration of gadolinium, T1 gradient-echo sequences demonstrate blood flow in pelvic varices with high signal intensity. On T2-weighted MR images they usually appear as an area of low signal intensity; however, possibly because of the relatively slow flow through the vessels, hyper intensity or mixed signal intensity may also be noted (Fig. 11.4c).

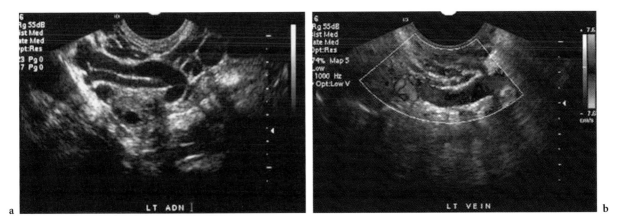

Fig. 11.3a,b. Ultrasound imaging of pelvic varicosities. **a** Transvaginal grey scale ultrasound demonstrating multiple left adnexal varicosities. **b** With Valsalva maneuver there is strong accentuation of flow within the varicosities. This can be a useful sign to differentiate physiologic venous ectasia from ovarian vein reflux

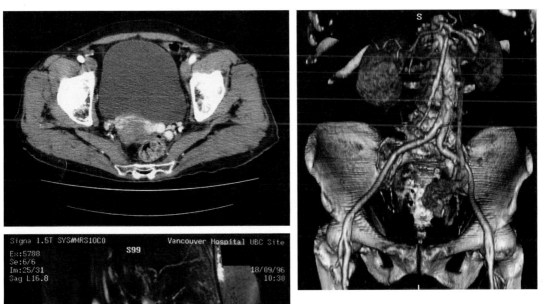

Fig. 11.4a–c. Cross sectional imaging of pelvic congestion syndrome. **a** Transverse CT image demonstrating contrast filled tortuous varicosities posterior to the bladder. **b** 3D reconstructed image from a CT angiogram showing a dilated left ovarian vein and a cluster of varicosities in the left side of the pelvis. **c** Sagittal T_2 weighted fat suppressed MR image demonstrating dilated pelvic veins posterior to the bladder

11.4
Alternative Therapies

Therapeutic modalities which have been applied to pelvic congestion syndrome include psychotherapy, physiotherapy, analgesia alone, pharmacologic ovarian suppression, surgery, and embolization. Critical comparison of treatment outcomes between different therapies is difficult, if not impossible. Not only are a wide variety of therapeutic endpoints described, but diagnostic criteria are different (or not described at all) in virtually every study.

Multiple surgical treatments have been performed for pelvic congestion syndrome. Bilateral oophorectomy and hysterectomy with subsequent hormone replacement has been reported with symptom improvement in 66% of women [29]. Surgical ligation of the left ovarian vein has been described resulting in improvement in 73% of women [30], and left nephrectomy (at time of renal donation) with an 77.9% symptom improvement [31]. In the latter study of 273 female renal donors, 27 had evidence of left ovarian venous reflux, of whom 22 completed a questionnaire about symptoms. Of these, 13 reported pelvic pain and ten had reduced or absent symptoms after left nephrectomy.

Isolated cases of laparoscopic ovarian vein ligation have been reported [32]; however, there are no large series published to date. Non-embolic interventional treatments such as venous stenting and surgical bypass have been reported in small numbers of patients when the varicosities are secondary to venous obstruction [33].

11.5
Anatomy

The entire venous network of the female pelvis is interconnected by an extensive anastomotic network that is virtually devoid of valves. The ovarian plexus drains superiorly via the ovarian veins: the left ovarian vein almost always drains into the left renal vein and the right usually directly into the vena cava , although in 8.8% there is drainage into the right renal vein [4]. The visceral system is composed of venous plexuses that surround the rectum, bladder, vagina, uterus and ovaries. The large uterine and vaginal plexuses drain mainly through two or three veins at the uterine pedicle. Although the latter two systems drain predominantly into the internal iliac veins there are extensive communications with the ovarian venous plexus (Fig. 11.5a).

11.6
Technique of Ovarian Venography and Embolization

Ovarian venography is performed in the same manner as venography of the spermatic veins. The author favors performing ovarian venography on a tilting table with the patient at least 45° upright, however the majority of interventionists perform the procedure with the patient flat. There is no data ascribing an advantage to either method. It cannot be overstressed that the diagnosis of pelvic congestion syndrome cannot be made on venographic criteria alone, correlation with the clinical presentation is mandatory!

11.6.1
Transjugular Route

Under ultrasound guidance a sheath is introduced into the left internal jugular vein. The sheath is used for patient comfort during the procedure. A catheter, usually multipurpose shape, is positioned into the peripheral portion of the left renal vein. A left renal venogram is performed with the patient performing a Valsalva maneuver. In the authors' opinion, only retrograde flow within the ovarian vein with the visualization of paraovarian varicosities constitutes a positive study (Fig. 11.1). Reflux of contrast down to the ovary without opacification of varicosities constitutes a negative venogram regardless of the diameter of the ovarian vein (Fig. 11.5a,b).

If there is ovarian vein reflux and varicosities, the catheter is then advanced into the distal left ovarian vein and forceful injection is performed to identify all collateral channels. The catheter is then directed into each of the major branches and embolization of the main ovarian vein and all visible collateral channels with glue, tetradecyl sulfate, or Gianturco coils is performed, extending cranially to within 2 cm of the ovarian vein origin (Fig. 11.6). The author's preferred method is place the catheter selectively into the origin of each of the two or three caudal branches of the main ovarian vein and inject tetradecyl sulphate 3% (2 cc mixed with 0.5 cc of contrast) with the patient performing a Valsalva maneuver as the liquid is being injected (have the patient do this

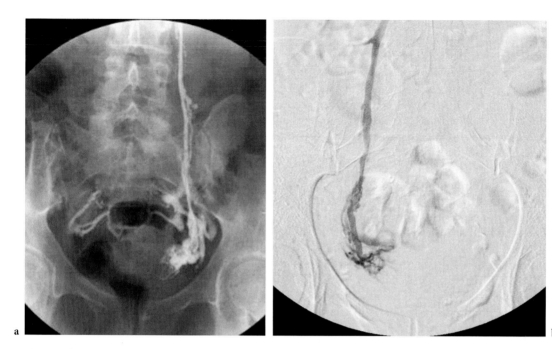

a   b

Fig. 11.5a,b. Normal ovarian venography. **a** Selective left ovarian venogram demonstrating reflux of contrast into the paraovarian plexus and normal collaterals communicating with the left internal iliac vein. No varicosities are seen. **b** Selective right ovarian subtraction venogram. The paraovarian plexus is opacified but no dilated irregular venous structures typical of pelvic varicosities

only during injection or they will faint!). I continue this until static sclerosant is seen at the catheter tip. Depending on the anatomy, I will occasionally "cap off" these the distal ovarian vein branches with a Gianturco coil (Cook, Inc, Bloomington, IN). These most distal coils (usually 38-5-5) are extruded holding the catheter firmly in place, while advancing the guidewire, resulting in a tightly coiled, compact configuration. Once all major branches of the ovarian vein have been injected with sclerosant (this may take up to 15 cc, but typically is less) there will typically be hazy, static opacification of the pelvic varicosities. I will then withdraw the catheter leaving a trail of the same contrast opacified tetradecyl sulphate 3% mixture by injecting as the catheter is withdrawn to immediately above the iliac crest. After the sclerosant is injected, it is critical not to flush the catheter vigorously, or the sclerosant will at best be diluted, and at worst distributed elsewhere. A coil is laid immediately above this (usually 30-8-10) in an elongated configuration to within 2 cm of the ovarian vein origin. This is achieved by holding the guidewire in place and withdrawing the catheter as the coil is deployed. The elongated configuration is favored to decrease the likelihood of recanalization. A gentle venogram is then performed to confirm occlusion, appropriate position of the upper

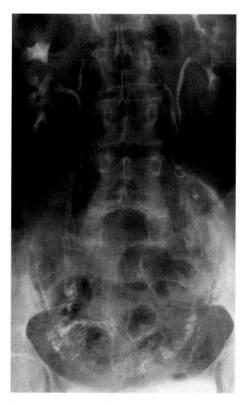

Fig. 11.6. Post-embolization image of patient in Fig. 11.1 demonstrates opacified sclerosant in the pelvic veins and coils occluding the proximal ovarian veins bilaterally

coils, and that there is not a parallel channel which occasionally will opacify only after the main ovarian vein is occluded. If there is still rapid retrograde flow in the ovarian vein after elongated coil deployment, we overlap a second elongated coil with the first in the configuration of a double helix. At the proximal end of the ovarian vein it is critical that the coil does not protrude into the renal vein or inferior vena cava. If the coil does project it should be removed with a nitinol snare and replaced.

The same multipurpose shape catheter is then directed into the right ovarian vein. A right ovarian venogram and, if needed, embolization are performed in the same fashion as described for the left. If the ovarian venograms are negative, then bilateral internal iliac venograms are performed as rarely isolated pudendal vein reflux will cause symptomatic pelvic varicosities (Figs. 11.7a,b). We do not routinely study the internal iliac veins if ovarian vein reflux is found; however, other interventionists do this routinely [34].

11.6.2
Transfemoral Route

A catheter, usually a Cobra catheter is introduced into the right femoral vein and directed into the peripheral left renal vein. Selective ovarian venog-

raphy and embolization are performed using the same diagnostic criteria and methods as described for the transjugular route (Fig. 11.8). The catheter is then exchanged for a Simmons II catheter or equivalent and right ovarian venogram performed. This approach has the disadvantage that a 180° bend is required for selective catheterization. This can be particularly troubling for cannulation of the right ovarian vein as pushing the catheter may result in advancement of the entire catheter up the IVC rather than advancement of the catheter tip.

11.6.3
Post-procedural Care

Patients are kept in bed for 1 h post procedure. Unless sedation was used, no special recording of vital signs is necessary. Mild pelvic cramping is common for which over the counter anti-inflammatory agents are taken as needed and instructions are given to avoid any activity involving Valsalva maneuver such as lifting, vigorous, or "hitting type" sports (including golf) for 3 full days beginning the day after the procedure. The patient should be advised that if she has persistent discomfort at the end of 3 days she should continue these instructions until resolution. There are no restrictions on resumption of sexual activity. For reasons not clear to the author, the first

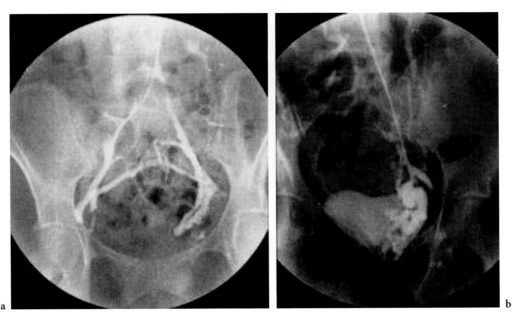

a   b

Fig. 11.7a,b. Internal iliac venography. **a** Normal study. Selective injection of contrast in right internal iliac vein demonstrates prominent pelvic anastomotic connections, but no varicosities are seen. **b** Pelvic varicosity in internal iliac venous system. There is bulbous dilation of the left pudendal vein. On delayed images sluggish drainage of contrast was seen

period after embolization is often unusually heavy and patients should be warned of this and the fact that this is almost invariably transient.

11.6.4
Follow-up

The patient should be seen approximately 3 months post-procedure for clinical examination and ultrasound. Post-treatment ultrasound will normally reveal persistent dilated veins in the pelvis, but normal or no accentuation of flow with Valsalva maneuver on duplex exam (Fig. 11.9).

11.6.5
Sclerosis of Labial or Buttock Varicosities

The varices are directly cannulated using a 25 gauge butterfly needle (or standard needle with extension tube) under direct vision or (rarely) ultrasound guidance (Figs. 11.10a,b). I prefer to have the patient on a tilt table at approximately 45 degrees upright to allow distension of the veins as they often collapse with the patient supine. Contrast is then gently injected, not to evaluate drainage, but to allow estimation of the amount of sclerosant needed. I prefer 1% tetradecyl sulfate, although some practitioners use other agents such as polydoconal or sclerosant foam. The same amount of sclerosant is injected as contrast was needed to opacify the veins. The patient is instructed to wear tight underwear for the rest of the day, otherwise there are no specific instructions.

The most important aspect of treating labial, buttock or lower limb varicosities that might be related to ovarian vein reflux is to treat the highest point of reflux first. This implies doing ovarian venography and embolization and then waiting at least 3 months before treating more distal veins. The author's experience is that approximately 25% of veins will subside adequately just with ovarian vein embolization although this has not been confirmed by data.

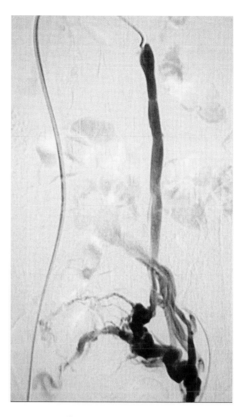

Fig. 11.8. Left ovarian venogram via femoral route demonstrating dilated ovarian vein and paraovarian varicosities which drain into the left internal iliac venous system

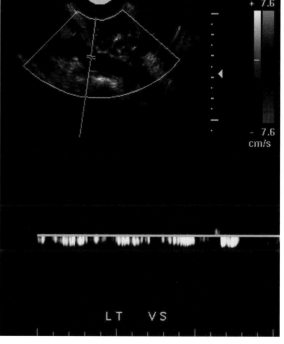

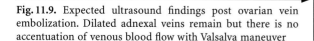

Fig. 11.9. Expected ultrasound findings post ovarian vein embolization. Dilated adnexal veins remain but there is no accentuation of venous blood flow with Valsalva maneuver

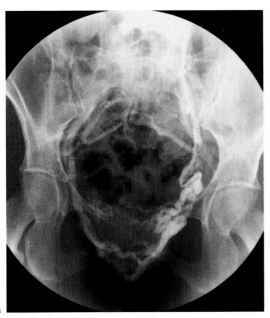
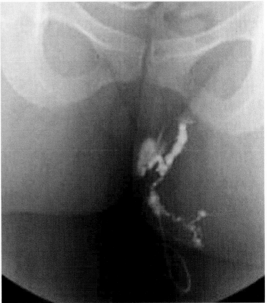

a

b

Fig. 11.10a,b. Labial varicosities. **a** Left ovarian vein injection. There are multiple pelvic sidewall varicosities and faint opacification of labial varices. Very delayed images are often required. **b** Left labial venogram using butterfly needle

Cookbook: (Materials)

First choice:
- 7-F 11-cm long sheath (Cordis or Terumo)
- 7-F Multipurpose catheter (Cordis) (we use 7-F instead of 5-F because puncture hole size is not important in venous procedures as it is in arterial studies. The stiffness of the 7-F catheter is a considerable advantage when catheterizing the right ovarian vein)
- 0.035 TSCF guidewire (Cook)
- 0.035 Angle-tipped Glidewire (Terumo)
- Gianturco coils (Cook)
- 3% Tetradecyl sulphate (Omega, Montreal)

In case of severe spasm or aberrant anatomy:
- 3-F Microcatheter (Boston Scientific)
- Microcoils (Cook)
- Cyanoacrylate
- For femoral approach: 5-F Cobra catheter for left ovarian vein
- 5-F Sos or Simmons type II catheter for right ovarian vein

11.7
Other Techniques

There are other methods for directly opacifying dilated pelvic veins besides selective catheterization of ovarian veins. These include transuterine injection of contrast material and direct injection of contrast material into vulval varices [8]. Except as a precursor to sclerosis of vulvar varicosities, these techniques are rarely used now because most radiologists are less comfortable both with the techniques and interpretation of the findings, and they do not allow direct progression to therapy. Noninvasive imaging modalities have nearly replaced these forms of venography for purely diagnostic investigation of pelvic varicose veins.

11.8
Tips and Tricks

11.8.1
Technical Difficulties in Right Ovarian Vein Cannulation

Inability to locate or cannulate the right ovarian vein is the most common reason for technical failure. The right ovarian vein origin is more variable in location than the left. It is usually located immediately anterior and inferior to the right renal vein orifice. The author's approach is to perform a right renal venogram to insure that the ovarian vein does not arise from the renal vein, and assess for accessory renal veins. I then withdraw the catheter to the renal vein orifice, rotate 2° anteriorly and advance the catheter 1–2 cm, rotating anteriorly another 2° with each pass if unsuccessful. If the ovarian vein orifice is not found, gentle probing along the IVC wall in an up and down motion extending from the right renal vein orifice to the iliac confluence is performed, beginning laterally, and rotating anteriorly slightly between each sweep. It may arise to the left of the midline. The right ovarian vein arises from the inferior vena cava at an acute angle, which can make catheterisation from the femoral route especially difficult. Use of a multipurpose shaped catheter from the jugular route greatly facilitates this.

11.8.2
Venous Spasm

If spasm of the ovarian vein occurs during selective catheterization then forceful injection of 5 cc of normal saline followed by a wait of 4–5 min is usually sufficient to allow resolution. The use of injectable vasodilators such as nitroglycerin has not been successful in the author's hands. If resolution of spasm is not possible, the procedure can be attempted on another occasion and at that instance the patient provided with sublingual nifedipine and intravenous sedation prior to the procedure.

11.9
Results

EDWARDS et al. (1993) reported the first published case of ovarian vein embolization for pelvic congestion syndrome [35]. Since then, the treatment of pelvic congestion syndrome by embolization has been reported using coils alone [36], glue alone [37], or by coils with glue [38], gelatin sponge [39], alcohol [40], sodium morulate [34], or tetradecyl sulfate [41]. Most authors embolize one or both of the ovarian veins, although others routinely occlude the internal iliac veins in addition [34, 36]. As previously noted when discussing alternative therapies, critical comparison between embolic techniques is difficult due to lack of common diagnostic and therapeutic criteria. The variability of the literature is illustrated by the sampling of reported series that follows. It is also apparent, however, that regardless of the technique or embolic agent used there is a striking similarity in patient outcomes.

After embolization of 40 patients with enbucrylate and lipidized oil and 1 with enbucrylate and coils, MALEUX et al. (2000) found that 58.5% of their patients had complete symptom relief and 9.7% partial symptom resolution at 19.9 months [36]. Technical success rate was 98%. The authors found no difference in rate of symptomatic response whether ovarian venous reflux was bilateral (nine patients) or unilateral (32 patients).

Using enbucrylate and coils CARPASSO et al. (1997) reported the results of embolization in 19 women with pelvic congestion syndrome [36]. A total of 13 patients required unilateral embolization and six bilateral. Five patients developed recurrence treated successfully by embolization. Initial technical success rate was 96.7%, and there were no complications. At mean follow-up of 15.4 months, 73.7% of patients reported improved symptoms with pain relief rated as complete in 57.9%. The authors noted that the eight patients who had only partial or no relief suffered from dyspareunia and felt this was a negative prognostic factor. (By comparison, most studies report that dyspareunia is a symptom that does respond to treatment).

CORDTS et al. (1998) described ovarian vein embolization in nine women with symptoms of pelvic congestion syndrome using coils and absorbable gelatin sponge [37]. Embolization of both ovarian veins was performed in four women, of the left ovarian vein alone in four patients, and of a left obturator vein that communicated with vulvar varices in one patient. The authors reported that eight of the nine women (88.9%) had more than 80% immediate relief but that two women had a mild to moderate return of the symptoms at 6 and 22 months. Improvement in symptom relief varied from 40% to 100% at a mean time of 13.4 months.

Clinical outcomes appear similar when the internal iliac veins are routinely occluded. VENBRUX et al. (1999) followed 56 women for a mean of 22.1 months after embolization with coils and sodium morulate [36]. The internal iliac veins were also occluded in 43 of 56 patients at a separate procedure 3 to 10 weeks after ovarian vein embolization. The technical success rate was 100%. Three patients developed recurrent varices, two of whom were treated with repeat embolization. Using visual analogue scales to measure pain, a mean 65% decrease in VAS score was recorded. Two patients (4%) reported no change in their symptoms, no patients had worsening of their pain after embolization.

In the aforementioned studies embolization was performed in patients with ovarian vein reflux due to absent or incompetent valves. In a Belgian study in which 83% of 48 patients had pelvic congestion syndrome due to extrinsic compression of the left renal vein between the aorta and the superior mesenteric artery (nutcracker syndrome), the technical success rate of ovarian vein embolization was 96% [6]. The initial clinical success rate was 86% with long-term pain reduction in 75% of the patients. No difference in outcome was described between patients who had renal vein compression and those who did not.

In one of the most intriguing studies of the treatment of pelvic congestion syndrome to date, CHUNG and HUH (2003) reported on 106 women with pelvic congestion syndrome confirmed by laparoscopy and venography who did not respond to medication after 4–6 months treatment [42]. The patients were prospectively randomized into three groups: embolization with Gianturco coils; hysterectomy with bilateral oophorectomy and hormone replacement therapy; and hysterectomy with unilateral oophorectomy. At 12-month evaluation by visual analog scale pain scores was carried out: embolotherapy was significantly more effective at reducing pelvic pain, compared to the two surgical therapies.

11.10
Complications

Ovarian vein embolization is generally remarkably benign; most authors report no complications of the procedure and no worsening of symptoms. In our first review of our own patients, 9% developed a transient worsening of their pelvic pain immediately after embolization, felt most likely to be related to post-embolization ovarian phlebitis [39]. Both patients returned to their baseline symptoms within weeks, with only anti- inflammatory and analgesic therapy. An analogous condition is seen in men after varicocele embolization. VENBRUX et al. (1999) [35] and CHUNG and HUH (2003) [42] each reported two patients in whom coils embolized to the pulmonary circulation; the coils were snared without clinical sequelae in all four cases.

11.11
How to Prevent or Troubleshoot Complications

From a physicians' perspective, the principle "complication" is dealing with patients in whom the procedure has not successfully relieved the symptoms. The two most important aspects to minimize the impact of this are excluding other causes of chronic pelvic pain before embolization, and managing patient expectations. The first is accomplished by working with clinicians with expertise in pelvic pain or pelvic congestion syndrome, the second by communication with the patient and the referring clinicians. Most series report symptom improvement in 70%–80% of patients. This implies that it will not be effective in 20%–30% of women undergoing the procedure. The reasons for this include the following: the pain may not have been related to pelvic congestion (and the pelvic varicosities were an incidental finding), inadequate embolization or recanalization of the pelvic vessels (uncommon), or adequate time may not have passed since the procedure. It may take up to 6 months for a chronic pain syndrome of any type to respond to therapy, even after removal of the stimulus, and in pelvic congestion this is certainly true. It is critical to tell the patient, the referring doctor, and the patient's primary care physician this fact before and at the time of the procedure or the radiologist will be the recipient of innumerable communications .

11.12
Conclusion

There are two distinct patient groups to whom ovarian embolization can be applied. The more frequent and traditional indication is chronic pelvic pain. Pelvic congestion syndrome remains a poorly understood entity whose existence, let alone appropriate criteria for diagnosis and methods of investigation and treatment are still under question. The similarity of outcomes between a wide variety of surgical procedures and varied methods of radiologic embolization do suggest that it is a real entity but we are lacking a robust method of identifying those patients in whom intervention is likely to result in symptom relief. Until the unlikely arrival of such a tool, it bears repeating that there are few areas of interventional radiology where the correlation of clinical presentation and radiologic findings is of more importance than pelvic congestion. It is essential that any radiologist treating women with chronic pelvic pain work closely with a gynecologist or pain specialist.

A second patient group presents with varicose veins of the perineum or legs. This indication has become more important as endovascular treatments for lower limb varicosities have increased. Although these patients require less complicated clinical management, specific knowledge or shared clinical care with an expert in lower extremity venous disease is essential to good clinical results.

References

1. Richer NA (1857) Traite practique d'anatomie medico-chururgiale. E Chamerot, Librairie Editeur, Paris
2. Hobbs JT (1976) The pelvic congestion syndrome. Practitioner 216:529–540
3. Ahlberg NE, Bartley O, et al. (1965) Circumference of the left gonadal vein. An anatomical and statistical study. Acta Radiol 3:503–512
4. Ahlberg NE, Bartley O, et al. (1966) Right and left gonadal veins. An anatomical and statistical study. Acta Radiol 4:593–601
5. Kennedy A, Hemingway A (1990) Radiology of ovarian varices. Br J Hosp Med 44:38–43
6. d'Archambeau O, Maes M, et al. (2004) The pelvic congestion syndrome: role of the «nutcracker phenomenon» and results of endovascular treatment. JBR-BTR 87:1–8
7. LePage PA, Villavicencio JL, et al. (1991) The valvular anatomy of the iliac venous system and its clinical implications. J Vasc Surg 14:678–683
8. Beard RW, Highman JH, et al. (1984) Diagnosis of pelvic varicosities in women with chronic pelvic pain. Lancet 2:946–949
9. Reginald PW, Kooner JS, et al. (1987) Intravenous dehydro ergotamine to relieve pelvic congestion with pain in young women. The Lancet 8:351–353
10. Hodgkinson CP (1953) Physiology of the ovarian veins during pregnancy. Obstet Gynecol 1: 26–37
11. Chidekel N (1968) Female pelvic veins demonstrated by selective renal phlebography with particular reference to pelvic varicosities. Acta Radiol 193:1–20
12. Viala JL, Flandre O, et al. (1991) Histology of the pelvic vein. Initial approach. Phlebologie 44:369–372
13. Stones RW (2000) Chronic pelvic pain in women: new perspectives on pathophysiology and management. Reprod Med Rev. 8:229–240
14. Adams J, Reginald PW, et al. (1990) Uterine size and endometrial thickness and the significance of cystic ovaries in women with pelvic pain due to congestion. Br J Obstet Gynecol 97:583–587
15. Beard RW, Reginald PW, et al. (1988) Clinical features of women with chronic lower abdominal pain and pelvic congestion. Br J Obstet Gynecol 95:153–161
16. Black CM, Collins J, et al. (2005) Pelvic venous congestion syndrome and lower extremity superficial reflux disease. Presented at Society of Interventional Radiology Annual Meeting, April
17. Stones RW (2003) Pelvic vascular congestion – half a century later. Clinical Obst Gyn 46:831–856
18. Mathias SD, Kuppermann M, et al. (1996) Chronic pelvic pain: prevalence, health-related quality of life, and economic correlates. Obstet Gynecol 87:321–327
19. Reiter RC (1990) A profile of women with chronic pelvic pain. Clin Obstet Gynecol 33:130–136
20. Robinson JC (1993) Chronic pelvic pain. Curr Opin Obstet Gynecol 5:740–743
21. Kames LD, Rapkin AJ, et al. (1990) Effectiveness of an interdisciplinary pain management program for the treatment of chronic pelvic pain. Pain 41:41–46
22. Carter JE (1998) Surgical treatment for chronic pelvic pain. J Soc Laparoendosc Surg 2:129–139
23. Fry RP, Beard RW, et al. (1997) Sociopsychological factors in women with chronic pelvic pain with and without pelvic venous congestion. J Psychosom Res 42:71–85
24. Kuligowska E, Deeds L et al. (2005) Pelvic pain: overlooked and underdiagnosed gynecologic conditions. Radiographics 25:3–20
25. Beard RW, Highman JH, et al. (1984) Diagnosis of pelvic varicosities in women with chronic pelvic pain. Lancet 2:946–949
26. Coakley FV, Varghese SL, et al. (1999) CT and MRI of pelvic varices in women. J Comput Assist Tomogr 23:429–434
27. Desimpelaere JH, Seynaeve PC, et al. (1999) Pelvic congestion syndrome: demonstration and diagnosis by helical CT. Abdom Imaging 24:100–102
28. Rozenblit AM, Ricci ZJ, et al. (2001) Incompetent and dilated ovarian veins: a common CT finding in asymptomatic parous women. AJR 176:119–122
29. Beard RW, Kennedy RG, et al. (1991) Bilateral oophorectomy and hysterectomy in the treatment of intractable pelvic pain associated with pelvic congestion. Brit J Obstet & Gynaecol 98:988–992
30. Rundqvist F, Sandhold IE, et al. (1984) Treatment of pelvic varicosities causing lower abdominal pain with extraperitoneal resection of the left ovarian vein. Ann Chir Gynaecol 2:946–951
31. Belenky A, Bartal G, et al. (2002) Ovarian varices in healthy female kidney donors: incidence, morbidity, and clinical outcome. Am J Roentgenol 179:625–627
32. Gargiulo T, Mais V, et al. (2003) Bilateral laparoscopic transperitoneal ligation of ovarian veins for treatment of pelvic congestion syndrome. J Am Assoc Gynecol Laparosc 10:501–504
33. Scultetus AH, Villavicencio JL, et al. (2001) The nutcracker syndrome: its role in the pelvic venous disorders. J Vasc Surg. 34:812–819
34. Venbrux AC, Chang AH, et al. (2002) Pelvic congestion syndrome (pelvic venous incompetence): impact of ovarian and internal iliac vein embolotherapy on menstrual cycle and chronic pelvic pain. J Vasc Interv Radiol 13:171–178
35. Edwards RD, Robertson IR, et al. (1993) Case report: pelvic pain syndrome – successful treatment of a case by ovarian vein embolisation. Clin Rad 47:429–430
36. Venbrux AC, Lambert DL (1999) Embolization of the ovarian veins as a treatment for patients with chronic pelvic pain caused by pelvic venous incompetence. Curr Opin Obstet Gynecol 11:395–399
37. Maleux G, Stockx L, et al. (2000) Ovarian vein embolization for the treatment of pelvic congestion syndrome: long-term technical and clinical results. JVIR 11:859–864
38. Carpasso P, Simons C, et al. (1997) Treatment of symptomatic pelvic varices by ovarian vein embolization. Cardiovasc Intervent Radiol 20:107–111

39. Cordts PR, Eclavea A, et al. (1998) Pelvic congestion syndrome: early clinical results after transcatheter ovarian vein embolization. J Vasc Surg 28:862–868

40. Tarazov PG, Prozorovski, KV et al. (1997) Pelvic pain syndrome caused by ovarian varices. Treatment by transcatheter embolization. Acta Radiol 38:1023–1025

41. Machan LS and Martin ML (2000) Ovarian vein embolization for pelvic congestion syndrome. Semin Intervent Radiol 17:277–284

42. Chung MH, Huh CY (2003) Comparison of treatments for pelvic congestion syndrome. Tohoku J Exp Med 201:131–138

Genitourinary

12 Varicocele Embolization

David Hunter and Galia T. Rosen

12.1
Introduction

Varicocele is defined as an abnormal distention of veins in the pampiniform plexus.

The association between testicular atrophy and dilated scrotal veins was noticed as early as in the first century AD [1]. Ivanissevich in a 1960 article [2] remarked that the clinical association of varicocele with pain symptoms had been noted as early as 1541 by Ambrois Pare who described the varicocele as "a compact pack of vessels filled with melancholic blood". In the same article Ivanissevich described one of the earliest extensive experiences with suprainguinal ligation of the internal spermatic vein as a curative measure [2]. In the late nineteenth century it was first shown that correction of varicocele could

D. Hunter, MD; G. T. Rosen, MD
Department of Radiology, J2-447 Fairview-University Medical Center, University of Minnesota, 500 Harvard Street S.E., Minneapolis, MN 55455, USA

result in restoration of fertility [3]. Widespread acceptance of the relationship between varicocele and male factor infertility, however, came only in the 1950s based on work by Tuloch [4].

Surgical correction has always been the main therapeutic option for correction of varicocele. In 1980 Iaccarino [5] was the first to describe a percutaneous method for treatment of varicocele. The steady advancement in embolization techniques and materials has led to the development of the modern percutaneous procedure that is considered to be a safe, simple and effective alternative to surgery.

12.2
Anatomy

The veins of the spermatic cord form a loose, tortuous plexus after emerging from the mediastinum of the testis. These vessels are named the pampiniform plexus. The veins in the anterior portion of the plexus coalesce to form the internal spermatic vein (ISV). The ISV passes through the inguinal canal and then ascends through the retroperitoneum alongside the spermatic artery, until it drains into either the left renal vein on the left side, or the infrarenal IVC on the right side. Additional venous drainage of the testis, which becomes important following occlusion of the ISV, includes the external pudendal, vasal and cremasteric veins (Fig. 12.1). Alternative drainage pathways of the ISV include the peri-renal, retroperitoneal and lumbar veins.

Other anastomoses can exist between the ISV and other venous outflow channels in the retroperitoneum and pelvis. These anastomoses can permit reflux and varicocele formation even in the presence of a competent valve in the proximal ISV. The resulting condition is termed an aberrantly supplied varicocele. The reported rate of this phenomenon is 17%–19% of patients examined with spermatic venography. Percutaneous treatment of this type of varicocele is possible, but requires occlusion of the

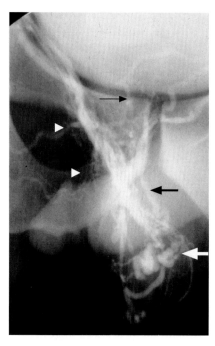

Fig. 12.1. Accessory veins. Perivesical (*thin arrow*), External pudendal (*arrowheads*), Cremasteric (*white arrow*), Vasal (*thick arrow*)

ISV at the very least above and below the segment of the vessel at the level of the venous collateral communication. Treatment of a varicocele with this type of complex anatomy has a success rate that is somewhat lower than one with classical anatomy [6].

12.3
Pathophysiology

There is still debate about how, when, and to what extent varicocele affects fertility. A total of 10% of all men have a varicocele. Most are both asymptomatic and not associated with infertility. However, among infertile couples the incidence of a varicocele increases to 30% [7]. Why should the dilatation of the veins of the pampiniform plexus impair spermatogenesis? A related question in patients with a unilateral varicocele, is how unilateral venous abnormality produces bilateral testicular dysfunction? Several theories have been postulated to explain the pathophysiology of varicocele. The most popular among the theories involves the adverse effect of elevated testicular temperature on spermatogenesis [8]. Another theory is that reflux of adrenal or renal metabolites that could inhibit spermatogenesis reach the left testicle by back flow from

the renal vein, particularly in cases with renal vein outflow obstruction due the compression of the vein between the aorta and superior mesenteric artery, the so-called nutcracker effect. Proponents of either theory further postulate that a bilateral effect could occur by venous crossover to the right testis [8].

There are conflicting opinions about the laterality of varicocele. Some authors feel that the condition is predominantly left-sided, with at most 30% of patients having a bilateral problem [9]. In other studies [10, 11], including one in which venograms were performed bilaterally regardless of the physical exam findings [11], bilateral ISV incompetence to an enlarged pampiniform plexus was found in 70%–80% of patients.

12.4
Diagnosis

The clinical assessment of varicocele must start with a careful physical examination. The patient should be examined in a warm room in the standing position, and preferably after standing for 5 min. The examination should include palpation and Doppler of the scrotum during a Valsalva maneuver. The grading system as developed by DUBIN and AMELAR [12] is the most commonly used to classify varicoceles, and includes the following categories:
- Grade 1, varicocele palpable only during a Valsalva maneuver.
- Grade 2, varicocele palpable in the standing position.
- Grade 3, varicocele detectable by visual scrutiny alone.

However, the limitations of physical examination are well documented [13], and the standard of care involves employment of additional diagnostic methods. These include thermography, color flow Doppler sonography, and venography [14–16]. Although each of these tests has reported standards that are used to make the diagnosis of varicocele, the standards are not universally accepted and the accuracy of each test has frequently been called into doubt. A varicocele that is present on an imaging study but not on physical examination is termed a subclinical varicocele. Embolization or surgical treatment of subclinical varicocele is a frequent practice in subfertile males with no other explanation for infertility.

Those who advocate treating subclinical varicocele claim that even though the angiographically demonstrated degree of reflux is indeed lower in subclinical cases, the improvement in semen analysis and fertility rates that is seen after embolization, appears to be about equal for the clinical and subclinical varicocele patients [17].

12.5
Clinical Considerations

Varicocele can result in pain and infertility, and either or both may be present in any patient. One important additional group of patients that has been studied in several prospective studies in Europe is adolescent boys. In most cases of adolescent varicocele, the diagnosis is made incidentally on routine physical examination. Pain and dysfunctional spermatogenesis with or without testicular atrophy is an unfortunately frequent outcome for these patients and many advocate preemptive treatment for them as well [18].

The most common semen abnormality in patients with varicocele and infertility is poor sperm motility, followed by abnormal morphology, and then depression of sperm count. The isolated finding of abnormal sperm motility has been referred to as a stress pattern. The normal World Health Organization (WHO) values [13] for the commonly evaluated parameters studied during semen analysis include the following:

- Volume: 1.5–5.0 ml
- Sperm count or density: greater than 20 million sperm/ml
- Motility: greater than 60% normal motility
- Morphology: greater than 60% normal forms
- Forward Progression (scale 1–4): 2+
- Viscosity: no hyperviscosity
- White blood cells: 0–5 per high power field

12.6
Alternative Therapy

Until the development of the percutaneous approach, surgical ligation of the ISV was the only available therapy. Several surgical procedures can be used, which differ primarily based on the level of ligation of the spermatic vein. The common sites for surgical ligation are retroperitoneal, inguinal or subinguinal. Laparoscopic methods of performing the ligation, and microsurgical operations that treat the

varicocele directly are becoming more common [19]. The techniques for surgical ligation have improved adequately so that percutaneous options are often not discussed with patients unless the patient has read about it, usually on the Internet, and requests the information directly. This approach clearly limits the number of percutaneous procedures performed.

12.7
Percutaneous Embolization

The percutaneous treatment of varicocele is aimed at decreasing the engorgement of the pampiniform plexus by occluding the incompetent ISV and its collaterals.

The use of percutaneous sclerotherapy as a treatment for varicocele was first described in 1980 [5]. The most commonly used embolization method in the USA, which is the use of metal coils (Fig. 12.2), was described in 1978 [20]. Ever since, additional materials and methods have been reported including modified coils such as the new Amplatz vascular plug, boiling contrast, detachable balloons,

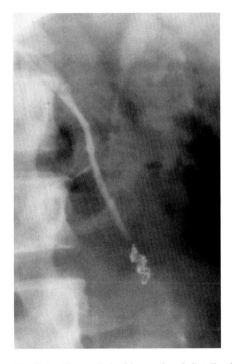

Fig. 12.2. After coils had been placed distally, these two coils were placed above the only large collateral. Notice how they are nested tightly inside each other. It was not considered necessary to place coils closer to the ISV origin

tissue adhesives, and sclerosing agents such as concentrated dextrose, sodium morrhuate, Sotradecol (sodium tetradecyl sulfate) [21], Varicocid [18], ethanolomine [10], and alcohol [22].

12.8
Catheterization Technique

Most studies have reported using a femoral vein approach. The left spermatic vein requires a double curve catheter to reach the ISV origin, and the right ISV is best entered with a sidewinder type catheter. Because of the double curve required to get into either spermatic vein, the femoral technique frequently requires coaxial catheters or a catheter exchange to reach an appropriate level in the ISV.

In our experience, a right trans-jugular approach to both the right and the left spermatic veins is preferable as it facilitates deep catheterization and therefore accurate delivery of the sclerosing agent or occlusion device, obviates a femoral vein puncture and the small but important risk of femoral DVT, and allows a more rapid discharge post-procedure with essentially no bleeding risk [11]. There is a small chance that manipulation through the right atrium may induce a dysrhythmia but such rhythm disturbances are almost always short-lived and resolve spontaneously. A heat re-shaped 5- or 6-F Headhunter catheter with two to six sideholes in the distal 2–3 cm (Fig. 12.3) can be used to select the left renal vein. The lordotic tertiary curve should be re-shaped into a kyphotic curve. While the catheter is being heated with a heat gun, a guidewire is kept in the lumen of the catheter to maintain catheter patency. The distal-most 3–4 mm of the tip of the catheter must be further modified to "point downstream" for selection of the right spermatic vein. Alternative catheters such as angled tip catheters (JB 1 or Vert shape), Cobra shape catheters, and variations of these shapes have all been tried but with less success.

Coming from the jugular or femoral approach, the most common first maneuver is to catheterize the left renal vein. The "C" shape of the reformed headhunter catheter makes this extremely easy from the jugular approach. Entry into the left renal vein from the IJ approach occasionally requires advancing the wire far into the renal vein and then applying a counterclockwise twist or torque, thus pointing the catheter tip posteriorly. If the catheter tip passes either inferiorly or seems to be "caught" in the cen-

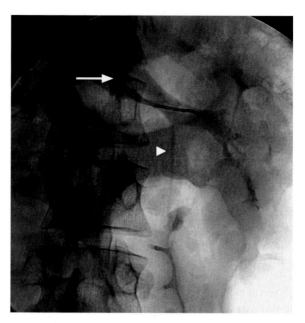

Fig. 12.3. The lordotic tertiary curve has been reformed into a kyphotic "C" shape (*arrow*). There is slight reflux into the left ISV (*arrowhead*)

tral left renal vein territory, a gentle hand injection of contrast can be done to check position. If the hand injection reveals that the catheter is in a lumber vein, the catheter should be pulled back and rotated slightly clockwise or anteriorly, as the lumbar vein orifice is always posterior to the left renal vein orifice. Once the catheter tip is in the mid-portion of the left renal vein, a left renal venogram is done during a forceful Valsalva maneuver to document L ISV incompetence (Fig. 12.4) and also to establish landmarks for selective L ISV catheterization. The left spermatic vein itself is also accessed using a counterclockwise rotation as the tip is pulled back, which rotates the tip of the catheter first posterior and then inferior since the curve is braced against the left renal vein origin. If the catheter tip enters the collateral from the proximal left renal vein to the adjacent paralumbar, hemiazygous system, the tip is rotated gently clockwise to point it slightly to the left and anterior where the origin of the adjacent L ISV is always located. Once the L ISV origin has been engaged, and assuming that incompetence has already been documented by the renal venogram, the catheter is advanced only 2–3 cm into the vein and the first selective diagnostic venogram is done. A forceful hand injection is performed into the L ISV using 10 cc of diluted contrast media, with the catheter tip just past the origin of the vessel. The patient is instructed once again to perform a Val-

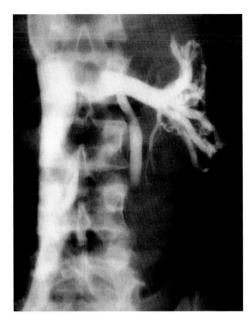

Fig. 12.4. During the left renal venogram with the catheter tip nicely positioned in the mid-left renal vein, a forceful Valsalva maneuver refluxes contrast not only down the incompetent L ISV but also down the IVC

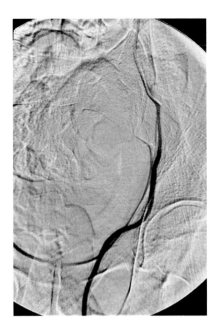

Fig. 12.5. Injection into the mid L ISV demonstrates a very atypical finding of a single dominant channel of the L ISV passing down through the inguinal canal

salva maneuver, while the operator looks carefully to both confirm reflux into the incompetent spermatic vein and also to define the upper L ISV anatomy. If free reflux is seen, confirming incompetence of the valve, the wire is advanced to the level of the mid to upper third of the SI joint and the catheter rotated down over the wire to the same position in approximately the mid L ISV. The catheter should be rotated and not "pushed" since that can cause buckling in the IVC or right atrium. Injections are done at approximately the mid-SI joint level to clearly define the remainder of the L ISV anatomy, confirm abnormal retrograde flow into a distended pampiniform plexus (Figs. 12.5, 12.6), and delineate any connections to other veins that could act as sources for aberrant varicocele filling or as collaterals if the L ISV is eliminated. Only after all of the diagnostic studies have been completed, can a meaningful and accurate embolization or sclerotherapy be carried out.

If no reflux is seen into the L ISV on either the left renal venogram or selective L ISV origin injection, but there is clear sonographic or physical examination evidence of a varicocele, we routinely assume that the patient has retroperitoneal or pelvic bypassing collaterals and believe that embolization of the ISV is still indicated. If, however, the only abnormality is the semen analysis, and there is no physical exam or imaging evidence of reflux or varicocele,

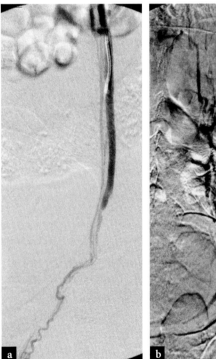
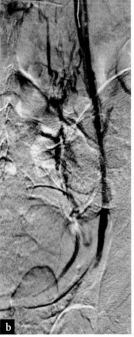

Fig. 12.6a,b. Two patients who had recurrence of pain following surgical ligation of the L ISV. With the catheter tip in the mid L ISV just below the mid-portion of the L SI joint, injection in patient (**a**) demonstrates one small channel through the inguinal canal, whereas patient (**b**) has no patent vessels that would suggest a recurrence. Patient (**a**) was treated, (**b**) was not

and a competent valve is clearly seen on the L ISV origin injection, the procedure on that side can be terminated.

The procedure on the right side is similar although there is no way to do a preliminary venogram to confirm incompetence. This fact alone may have led to a substantial underestimation of right-sided incompetence reflected in much of the varicocele literature. Coming from the femoral approach, the origin of the right ISV is easy to enter using a standard sidewinder catheter. From the IJ approach, the headhunter that was used for the L ISV needs to be modified so that the tip points more inferiorly (Fig. 12.7). The R ISV origin is usually located just anterior and inferior to the right renal vein. In order to find it, the catheter is placed into the right renal vein then pulled out, rotated slightly counterclockwise, pushed down below the renal vein level and manipulated up and down on the vein wall until it "catches" on the R ISV orifice. Once the tip of the catheter just barely enters the origin, the first injection is done with a gentle Valsalva to avoid dislodgement of the catheter. If the catheter tip is allowed to go too deep into the vein, the valve at the origin, which is frequently the only valve, can be bypassed, and an incorrect diagnosis of incompetence made. Once incompetence has been documented, the catheter is advanced over a floppy wire to the mid to upper third of the R ISV (Fig. 12.8), the anatomy of the remainder of the vein is clarified, and embolization or sclerotherapy performed.

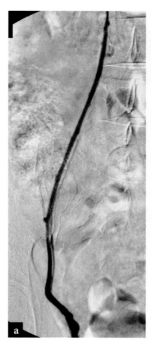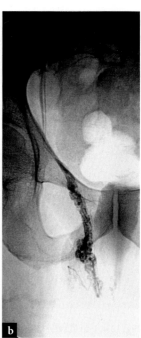

Fig. 12.8a,b. Injection above (**a**) and at (**b**) the mid R ISV, demonstrates the typical parallel collaterals and multiple channels at the level of the inguinal ligament that make complete treatment with coil placement or surgical ligation challenging

12.9
Hot (Boiling) Contrast Sclerotherapy

The use of heat to occlude veins is a well-documented and tested technique. Various heat sources have been used including boiling liquids, lasers, and radiofrequency electrodes. One distinct advantage of heat is that it induces spasm and wall damage leading to occlusion with relatively minimal thrombosis. Embolization and non-heated liquid sclerotherapy techniques result in a large amount of thrombus, which, along with any mechanical blockade causes secondary venous obliteration. The same contrast that is used during the diagnostic part of the procedure can be heated in a metal container over a heating plate for the sclerotherapy. This makes boiling contrast quick, inexpensive, universally available, non-toxic, and easily visible and therefore controllable. The advantage of a boiling liquid over other heat sources and over all embolization techniques, is that it can flow into and obliterate any potential collaterals. While the patient is receiving extra sedation and the contrast is coming to a boil, the multisideholes catheter is allowed to drain so that the ISV is as empty as possible. When boiling temperature is reached, which is signified by the liquid dem-

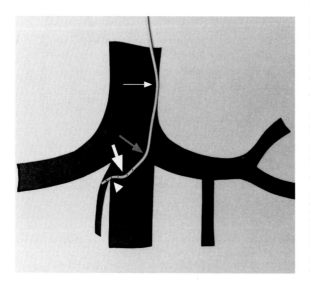

Fig. 12.7. Tertiary (*thin arrow*), Secondary (*grey arrow*), Primary (*thick arrow*) curves are all still kyphotic, but the distal tip is bent to point downward (*arrowhead*)

onstrating the bubbling action of a "rolling boil", the operator fills, as best as possible, a 10 cc plastic syringe with the boiling contrast, eliminates extra air, and injects the remaining 6–9 cc directly into the catheter under careful fluoroscopic control. No stopcocks or connectors are used to minimize any heat loss. A senior member of the team concurrently compresses the ISV where it crosses over the superior pubic ramus (Fig. 12.9) to prevent any flow of boiling material into the pampiniform plexus. Any sclerosant or boiling liquid that is allowed to enter the veins of the pampiniform plexus will cause a very painful scrotal swelling and potentially testicular atrophy. Injections are done without moving the catheter since the spread of the boiling contrast in volumes of 6–9 cc is usually adequate to cover the entire extent of the ISV as well as any collaterals. In most cases, three sequential injections of 6–9 cc of boiling contrast are sufficient to ensure a complete obliteration of the injected vein unless it is exceptionally large.

Overall, the angiographic or imaging success rate of the boiling contrast and other liquid sclerosing agents is considered very high with a reported recurrence rate of 2%–19% [23].

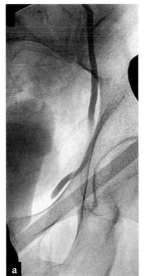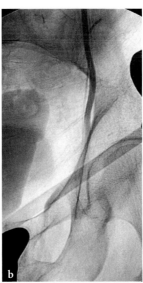

Fig. 12.9a,b. Compression on the ramus (**a**) occludes retrograde flow whereas compression slightly off the ramus (**b**) or tilted does not

12.10
Coil Embolization

The most common percutaneous technique in current use is that of coil embolization. Its primary and significant advantage over sclerotherapy techniques especially boiling contrast is that it is relatively painless requiring far less sedation. Gianturco coils (Cook), ranging in size from 5 mm to 8 mm are the most common sizes used [24], although some authors report using smaller or larger coils as needed based on the size of the vein.

Coil sizing, stacking, and placement are clearly of paramount importance for technical success and avoiding complications particularly coil embolization to the heart and lungs. The size of the coil should be 10%–20% larger than the diameter of the ISV at the level of deployment. Sizing the coil too small can result in pulmonary embolization, which is aesthetically and emotionally unpleasant, but due to the size of the coils is usually without any clinical consequences. Coil removal from the pulmonary artery can usually be done with minimal problems using a snare or grasper [25]. Usually more than one coil is deployed at any given site since a single coil

has a higher recanalization and failure rate than two or more "stacked" or "nested" coils. With the development of special tapered shape coils that are tapered in one or two directions, the need for multiple coils is no longer clear although it has not been rigorously tested. The Amplatz Vascular Plug (AGA Medical, Minneapolis, MN) is a coil type device that is longer and more completely occlusive than standard coils, is recapturable until a good "final position" has been confirmed, and will likely find an important role in the treatment of varicocele. Coils must be deployed proximal and distal to any major collaterals. If there are parallel veins, often both must be separately occluded. The minimal distance of the coils from the orifice of the ISV is somewhat debatable. Most European literature cites a distance of 6 cm from the origin as safe and effective, while others claim that embolization up to the level of the origin is preferable to avoid "dead space" in which clot could accumulate and potentially embolize.

Some authors [26] favor the combination of coils and sodium tetradecyl sulfate (Thromboject 3%; Omega, Montreal, QC, Canada). The coils are delivered relatively distally, at the level of the inguinal canal, not only to occlude the vein at that level but also to prevent reflux into the pampiniform plexus. The sclerosant is delivered proximal to the coils to occlude all the side branches that could become collaterals. If necessary, coils can also be deposited in the proximal portion of the ISV to prevent pulmonary emboli. One coil that was never used in the

USA deserves special mention. This coil was made from tungsten, which obviously would markedly improve visibility. Unfortunately, one feature of the tungsten coil is that it was biodegradable leading to increased tungsten levels in the blood [27–29]. Though no adverse effects of tungsten in humans were ever described, the observation was concerning enough that their usage for this application has been discontinued.

12.11
Tissue Adhesives

The most commonly used liquid tissue adhesives are cyanoacrylates. Their low viscosity makes their delivery easy through small coaxial microcatheters. However, their rapid polymerization when in contact with blood, can make precise and safe occlusion challenging. Usually they are mixed with an oil-based contrast media, such as Ethiodol (Savage Laboratories, Melville, NY). The contrast serves to both opacify the cyanoacrylate and slows the polymerization time [30].

Another tissue adhesive that has been reported is enbucrylate (Histoacryl; B. Braun, Tuttlingen, Germany). It can be used when multiple collaterals are seen that are too small to be selectively catheterized [26].

12.12
Detachable Balloons

The use of detachable balloons to occlude the ISV was first described in 1981 [31]. Due to a lack of FDA approval for some of the devices and manufacturer related issues, the balloons have not always been readily available in the USA. From a technical standpoint, balloons were similar to coils in that they needed to be deployed above and below collateral connections. However, since the balloon occluded the vein completely, much like the Amplatz Vascular Plug, only one was necessary at any given site. As with coils, it was common for users of balloons to perform some type of sclerotherapy on the vein segments between balloons to decrease the development of collaterals. Balloons suffered from two major drawbacks that severely limited their more widespread acceptance. The first was cost. The other was that the size of the catheter required to deliver

a large balloon of 7–10 mm diameter was 7 or 8 F. In addition, the introducer catheter had to be placed to the level of the desired occlusion, a feat that was often technically very challenging especially from the femoral approach.

12.13
Complications

A unique, and fortunately rare, but significant risk of the hot contrast or other liquid sclerotherapy, is distal reflux of the sclerosing agent. Inadvertent injection of a sclerosing agent into the pampiniform plexus can result in painful scrotal swelling, phlebitis, and testicular damage with depression of spermatogenesis and even irreversible testicular atrophy [11].

To prevent that a preliminary run with contrast is carried out to verify that the occlusion of the inflow into the pampiniform plexus is indeed complete and efficient. A specially designed device, which is essentially a gently curved piece of plastic with padding on the edge that will press against the skin, was developed specifically to address this and was shown to be highly effective [32]. The device must be held exactly at a 90' angle to the bone. Fluoroscopy is used to verify its end-on position and to ensure that all contrast stays above the compressor during the injection.

A different kind of complication is proximal reflux of the sclerosing agent, which can result in renal vein thrombosis.

Other complications are extravasation and dissection. The ISV is a very thin-walled structure that can easily be torn by overly aggressive catheter manipulations or the use of glidewires. Gentle maneuvers and the use of a carefully controlled floppy wire will almost always prevent ISV damage. On occasion, however, a small vein may go into spasm around the wire and catheter resulting in vein avulsion or disruption during attempts to extract it. Hot contrast or sclerosants should definitely be prevented from reaching the retroperitoneum since they can cause ureteral or muscle injury and severe pain. Contrast extravasation at the time of catheter placement should prompt a change of the embolization method to one using coils or other mechanical devices.

Another consideration with the use of sclerosing agents is the pain that is associated with their injection. However it is usually of very short duration, most commonly 10–15 s, although rare instances lasting up to several minutes in poorly sedated patients have been seen. The pain can be both alleviated and "forgotten" with the use of agents such as Fentanyl and Versed.

12.14
Efficacy of Treatment and Comparison to Surgery

Success of the embolization or sclerotherapy treatment can be defined as a technical success, which is the immediate angiographic closure of the ISV. It can also be defined as a long-term technical success based on the finding of persistent closure on the delayed or follow-up angiographic or other imaging study. Of particular note, the thermal damage caused by boiling contrast may result in some immediate spasm and stasis of contrast, but the vein generally remains patent acutely. Success can also be defined as clinical success, that is, partial or complete resolution of the clinical signs and symptoms associated with varicocele. In particular, the most meaningful definition of success in couples with an infertility issue is the successful achievement of a pregnancy.

The two parameters that are usually evaluated in the assessment of the clinical efficacy of the treatment are semen analysis changes and the pregnancy rate.

There is great controversy in the literature about the effectiveness of varicocele embolization. According to one recent Cochrane analysis, the existing prospective randomized trials that satisfied their criteria for inclusion showed improvement in semen parameters and symptoms, but no difference in pregnancy rate compared to no treatment [33]. However, some of the individual studies in that analysis did show a very significant improvement in pregnancy rate of the treated group [34]. When retrospective data or non-randomized control groups are included in the analysis, most authors do find a significant difference in pregnancy rates between treatment and no treatment for varicocele. The historical rates that seem to have the most widespread acceptance suggest that the pregnancy rate for couples in whom there is documented male infertility as the sole cause of infertility is approximately 30% if the male receives either surgical or percutaneous treatment of the varicocele. This compares to a pregnancy rate of 16% for couples with the same history who undergo no therapy [35]. Thus, many clinicians and infertile couples are still interested in treatment for varicocele.

When the percutaneous procedure is compared to surgical ligation, varicocele embolization has been shown to be an equally effective means of treatment and is associated with less post procedure discomfort and more rapid return to normal activities [24, 36–38].

The overall reported technical success rate as cited by the JVIR quality improvement guidelines are 83%–96% with a clinical or imaging detected recurrence rate at 6 weeks of 7%–16% [23]. All of the analyses of procedural and clinical efficacy are obviously influenced and potentially severely confounded by several poorly controlled variables. One problem is that the need for treatment of both sides has never been clarified and it is clear that different authors have had markedly different opinions and angiographic findings on the subject. Another problem is that imaging follow-up is infrequent and impossible to quantify in a meaningful fashion. Therefore, the impact of aggressive and extensive treatment such as with coils plus sclerosants, boiling contrast or sclerosants is difficult to compare with simple coil or ligation therapy. In addition, the inclusion criteria, particularly with respect to semen analysis variables are poorly controlled. As an example, patients who present with a very low sperm count, below 2 million/ml, seem to have a lower response rate to treatment and yet are usually lumped with more favorable patients in most analyses.

One place where embolization or sclerotherapy appears to have established a definite niche is in the treatment of recurrence or failure following surgical ligation. In these cases, repeat surgery can be done with a different technique, but fearing another failure, most surgeons will refer the patient for percutaneous diagnosis and treatment. A total of 31 patients out of 40 with recurrence after surgery in one study [16], and 33 out of 39 patients in another [39] had successful diagnoses and treatment. The ISV venogram allows a precise anatomical definition of the cause and location of the veins responsible for the recurrent varicocele and the use of steel-coil embolization in both studies provided an effective means of treatment with improvement in semen quality and pregnancy rates [16, 39].

12.15
Conclusion

Even though some controversy exists about the justification for any type of treatment of varicocele with wide variation in results between different studies, we feel that current recommendations should advocate percutaneous embolization of varicocele as a safe, effective and potentially first-line treatment. Its overall efficacy is comparable to that of surgical ligation with a shorter recovery period and less pain, permitting it to be conducted as an outpatient procedure.

Our preferred embolization method is using boiling contrast. Other embolization techniques, such as coils, vascular plugs, other sclerosing agents, and detachable balloons are acceptable, and clearly less painful although more complex alternatives. The primary and important risk of any sclerosant type procedure is reflux into the pampiniform plexus, which might lead to orchitis and even testicular atrophy. The best way to avoid this complication is to use a compression device, rather than relying on manual compression.

Cookbook:

Catheter:
- IJ approach #1:
  Heat reformed Headhunter 1 with extra sideholes
- IJ approach #2:
  Heat reformed JB 1 with extra sideholes
    Femoral approach, renal double curve guider left and Sidewinder 1 right

Microcatheter:
None needed from the IJ approach
    Renegade from the femoral approach

Embolic agent:
Boiling contrast
    Amplatz vascular occluder, or coils, preferably with a tornado or other complex shape, and always at least two at each point of embolization

References

1. Page H (1989) Estimation of the prevalence and incidence of infertility in a population: a pilot study. Fertil Steril 51:571–577
2. Ivanissevich O (1960) Left varicocele due to reflux; experience with 4,470 operative cases in forty-two years. J int coll surg 34:742–755
3. Barwell R (1885) One hundred cases of varicocele treated by subcutaneous wire loop. Lancet 1:978
4. Tulloch WS (1952) A consideration of sterility factors in the light of subsequent pregnancies. IISubfertility in male. Trans Edinb Obst Soc 59:29–34
5. Iaccarino V (1980) A nonsurgical treatment of varicocele: trans-catheter sclerotherapy of gonadal veins. Ann Radiol 23:369–370
6. Marsman JW (1995) The aberrantly fed varicocele: frequency, venographic appearance, and results of transcatheter embolization. AJR 164: 649–657
7. Schlessinger MH, Wilets IF, Nagler HM (1994) Treatment outcome after varicocelectomy. Urol Clin North Am 21: 517–529
8. Goldstein M, Eid JF (1989) Elevation of intratesticular and scrotal skin surface temperature in men with varicocele. J Urol. 142: 743–745
9. Bigot JM, Le Blanche AF, Carette MF, Gagey N, Bazot M, Boudghene FP (1997) Anastomoses between the spermatic and visceral veins: a retrospective study of 500 consecutive patients. Abdom Imaging. 22:226–232
10. Gat Y, Bachar GN, Zukerman Z, Belenky A, Gornish M (2004) Varicocele: a bilateral disease. Fertil Steril. 81:424–429
11. Hunter DW, King NJ 3rd, Aeppli DM, Yedlicka JW Jr, Castaneda-Zuniga WR, Hulbert JC, Kaye K, Amplatz K (1991) Spermatic vein occlusion with hot contrast material: angiographic results. J Vasc Interv Radiol 2:507–515
12. Dubin L, Amelar RD (1970) Varicocele size and results of varicolectomy in selected subfertile men with varicocele. Fertil Steril 21:606–609
13. World Health Organization (1985) Comparison among different methods for the diagnosis of varicocele. Fertil Steril 43:575–582
14. Chiou RK, Anderson JC, Wobig RK, Rosinsky DE, Matamoros A Jr, Chen WS, Taylor RJ (1997) Color Doppler ultrasound criteria to diagnose varicoceles: correlation of a new scoring system with physical examination. Urology 50:953–956
15. Hamm B, Fobbe F, Sorensen R, Felsenberg D (1986) Varicoceles: combined sonography and thermography in diagnosis and posttherapeutic evaluation. Radiology 160:419–424
16. Morag B, Rubinstein ZJ, Madgar I, Lunnenfeld B (1985) The role of spermatic venography after surgical high ligation of the left spermatic veins: diagnosis and percutaneous occlusion. Urol Radiol 7:32–34
17. Marsman JW (1985) Clinical versus subclinical varicocele: venographic findings and improvement of fertility after embolization. Radiology 155:635–638
18. Braedel HU, Steffens J, Ziegler M, Polsky MS (1990) Outpatient sclerotherapy of idiopathic left-sided varicocele in children and adults. Br J Urol 65: 536–540
19. Donovan JF, Winfield HN (1992) Laparoscopic varix ligation. J Urol 147:77–81
20. Lima SS, Castro MP, Costa OF (1978) A new method for the treatment of varicocele. Andrologia 10:103–106
21. Trombetta C, Salisci E, Deriu M, Paoni A, Sanna M, Ganau A, Belgrano E (1993) Echo-flowmetric control 6 years after percutaneous treatment of varicocele. Arch Ital Urol Androl 65:363–367
22. Usuki N, Nakamura K, Takashima S, Takada K, Kaminoh T, Tsubakimoto M, Matsuoka T, Nakatsuka H, Oda J,

Minakuchi K, et al. (1994) Embolization of varicocele with ethanol. Nippon Igaku Hoshasen Gakkai Zasshi 54:870–875 (Japanese)

23. Drooz AT, Lewis CA, Allen TE, Citron SJ, Cole PE, Freeman NJ, Husted JW, Malloy PC, Martin LG, Van Moore A, Neithamer CD, Roberts AC, Sacks D, Sanchez O, Venbrux AC, Bakal CW (2003) Society of Interventional Radiology Standards of Practice Committee. Quality improvement guidelines for percutaneous transcatheter embolization. J Vasc Interv Radiol 14(9 Pt 2): S237–242

24. Shlansky-Goldberg RD, VanArsdalen KN, Rutter CM, Soulen MC, Haskal ZJ, Baum RA, Redd DC, Cope C, Pentecost MJ (1997) Percutaneous varicocele embolization versus surgical ligation for the treatment of infertility: changes in seminal parameters and pregnancy outcomes. J Vasc Interv Radiol 8:759–767

25. Chomyn JJ, Craven WM, Groves BM, Durham JD (1991) Percutaneous removal of a Gianturco coil from the pulmonary artery with use of flexible intravascular forceps. J Vasc Interv Radiol 2: 105–106

26. Tay KH, Martin ML, Lisl Mayer A, Machan LS (2002) Selective spermatic venography and varicocele embolization in men with circumaortic left renal veins. J Vasc Interv Radiol 13:739–742

27. Barrett J, Wells I, Riordan R, Roobottom C (2000) Endovascular embolization of varicoceles: resorption of tungsten coils in the spermatic vein. Cardiovasc Intervent Radiol 23:457–459.

28. Kampmann C, Brzezinska R, Abidini M et al. (2002) Biodegradation of tungsten embolisation coils used in children. Pediatr Radiol 32:839–843

29. Wells IP (2003) Biodegradation of tungsten embolisation coils used in children. Pediatr Radiol 33:288

30. Pollak JS, White RI (2001) The use of cyanoacrylate adhesives in peripheral embolization. J Vasc Interv Radiol 12:907–913

31. White RI Jr, Kaufman SL, Barth KH, Kadir S, Smyth JW, Walsh PC (1981) Occlusion of varicoceles with detachable balloons. Radiology 139:327–334

32. Hunter DW, Bildsoe MC, Amplatz K (1989) Aid for safer sclerotherapy of the internal spermatic vein. Radiology 173:282

33. Evers J, Collins J (2004) Surgery or embolisation for varicocele in subfertile men. Cochrane Database Syst Rev 3: CD000479

34. Madgar I, Weissenberg R, Lunenfeld B, Karasik A, Goldwasser B (1995) Controlled trial of high spermatic vein ligation for varicocele in infertile men. Fertil Steril 63:120–124

35. Skoog SJ, Roberts KP, Goldstein M, Pryor JL (1997) The adolescent varicocele: what's new with an old problem in young patients? Pediatrics 100:112–122

36. Dewire DM, Thomas AJ, Falk RM, Geisinger MA, Lammert GK (1994) Clinical outcome and cost comparison of percutaneous embolization and surgical ligation of varicocele. J Androl 15[suppl]:38–42

37. Nieschlag E, Behre HM, Schlingheider A, Nashan D, Pohl J, Fischedick AR (1993) Surgical ligation vs. angiographic embolization of the vena spermatica: a prospective randomized study for the treatment of varicocele related infertility. Andrologia 25:233–237

38. Parsch EM, Schill WB, Erlinger C, Tauber R, Pfeifer KJ (1990) Semen parameters and conception rates after surgical treatment and sclerotherapy of varicocele. Andrologia 22:275–278

39. Punekar SV, Prem AR, Ridhorkar VR, Deshmukh HL, Kelkar AR (1996) Post-surgical recurrent varicocele: efficacy of internal spermatic venography and steel-coil embolization. Br J Urol 77:124–128

13 Embolization Therapy for High-Flow Priapism

JIM A. REEKERS

CONTENTS

13.1
Introduction

Priapism is named after the Greek god, Priapus, son of Aphrodite and Dionysus.

Priapism is a persistent erection of the corpora cavernosa of the penis, originating from disturbances to the mechanisms that control penile detumescence. This affects only the corpora cavernosa. The corpora spongiosum of the glans penis and surrounding the urethra are not part of the process.

The overall incidence of priapism is 1.5 per 100000 person-year [1]. Priapism is broadly classified as high-flow and low-flow. Arterial high-flow priapism (HFP) is usually secondary to the laceration of a cavernous artery with unregulated flow into the lacunar spaces. This type of priapism is most of the times not painful because there is no ischemia. HFP is rare and only 200 cases have been reported in the literature. Nonetheless, because it is painless, it is possible that HFP is under reported. The other type is veno-occlusive priapism which is usually caused by corporeal veno-occlusion, and can be very painful due to ischemia.

J. A. REEKERS, MD, PhD
Department of Radiology, G1-207, Academic Medical Center, University of Amsterdam, Meibergdreef 9, AZ 1105 Amsterdam, The Netherlands

The clinical presentation of these two types of priapism is different. HFP is often seen after an acute injury, and the onset can be delayed. This delayed onset may be due to initial vessel spasm, hemostasis with clot formation or a compressing hematoma. Reabsorption of this clot or hematoma is the mechanism for the late onset. The HFP is often less tumescent when compared with venous priapism. Priapism secondary to arterial causes may be, as mentioned before, significantly less painful than venous priapism and is not considered as an emergency. The major etiology of HFP is trauma, especially in children or young adults; in older men, HFP is a rare event mainly caused by malignancy [2]. High-flow priapism in acute lymphatic leukaemia has also been reported [3].

Veno-occlusive priapism presents with a painful erection, which can already have been there for days. Prolonged veno-occlusive priapism results in fibrosis of the penis and a loss of the ability to achieve an erection. Significant changes at the cellular level are noted within 24 h in veno-occlusive priapism, whereas arterial priapism is not associated with fibrotic change. Veno-occlusive priapism most commonly is idiopathic, although there is a long list of other causes which include leukemia and multiple myeloma, sickle cell disease, thalassemia, spinal cord injury, spinal anesthesia and drugs.

13.2
Diagnosis

Careful patient history and clinical signs and symptoms are of paramount importance. As stated previously, history of trauma with a painless priapism favors HFP. Cavernous blood coloration and gas measurement are very useful and easily available to distinguish between HFP and venous priapism. A bright red appearance of the cavernous blood is more in favor of HFP, which in turn is associated with a high po2 and low pco2. General diagnostic tests include complete blood count, platelets, differential white blood cell count and reticulocyte count and urine analysis for drugs.

13.3
Imaging

Penile ultrasound and Doppler testing may be necessary to differentiate high-flow from low-flow priapism. In HFP, ultrasound reveals an hypoechoic, well-circumscribed region in the corpus cavernosum. The Doppler will show an increased flow in the penile artery, uni-or bilateral, and an arterio-cavernosal fistula (Fig. 13.1). In patients with high-flow priapism, selective penile angiography may be required in order to identify the site of the fistula. Angiography should however not be done as a diagnostic procedure, but always in combination with a planned therapeutic embolization.

13.4
Therapy

The goal of all treatment is to treat the priapism while preserving future erectile function. This paper will only discuss the treatment options in HFP.

There are some alternative treatment options for high-flow priapism, like ice packs where ice is applied to the penis and perineum to reduce swelling, corporal aspiration, massage, and pressure dressings. Pharmacological interventions are also used. This includes the use of alpha-agonists (e.g., metaraminol bitartrate) or methylene blue. Alpha-agonist agents counteract smooth muscle relaxation. However, they may cause significant systemic hypertension. Methylene blue inhibits guanylate cyclase and has a second messenger inhibitory effect; thus, it inhibits smooth muscle relaxation. The effect of methylene blue is relatively short-lived, and priapism may recur. Any of these treatment options are often of little use in high-flow priapism, as a rupture of the artery does not subside spontaneously. Surgical ligation of the fistula is an operation which is redundant now that embolization is widely used; however it is still performed. One of the main potential complications of this procedure includes long-term impotence. For HFP caused by inherited diseases, and malignancy conservative therapy is mandatory.

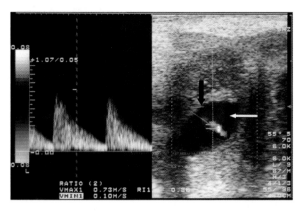

Fig. 13.1. Ultrasound with Doppler in a patient after a bicycle trauma. Doppler shows high systolic velocity of 73 cm/s. Color Doppler demonstrates a fistula (*black arrow*) within a well-circumscribed hypoechoic hematoma or laceration in the corpus cavernosum.

13.5
Embolization Therapy

The blood supply of the penis derives from the internal pudendal artery (IPA). The common penile artery is a distal branch of the IPA and gives rise to the bulbourethral artery at the base of the penis, subsequently dividing into the dorsal penile and cavernosal arteries. The anatomy of the internal pudendal artery has many variations, but usually comes from the anterior division. The most common presentation is shown in Fig. 13.2. One has to take in consideration that the inferior rectal artery derives from the IPA, which off course prevents selective embolization from the origin of the IPA with a flow guided embolic agent like particles as they will end also in the rectal mucosa. However, when a selective position cannot be achieved, proximal coil embolization in the IPA might be performed (Fig. 13.3). In high-flow priapism one can see arteriovenous fistulas or pseudoaneurysms, resulting in abnormal arterial inflow, which exceeds venous outflow capacity, resulting in tumescence. Fistulas can be uni-lateral or bilateral, and to achieve optimal results, all fistulas should be occluded (Fig. 13.4) [4, 5].

13.6
Technique of Embolization

In our experience contra lateral access, over the aortic bifurcation, gives the best stability and freedom of movement for selective catherization. If the

Fig. 13.2. a The most common anatomy of the internal pudendal artery origin. **b** Selective catheterization of the internal pudendal artery with distal division into the deep and dorsal branch

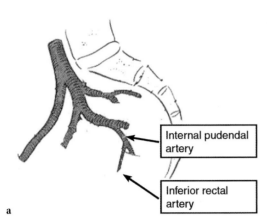

Internal pudendal artery

Inferior rectal artery

a

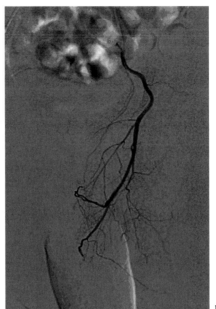

b

fistulas are bilateral we start with a 5 F sheath in both common femoral arteries. The internal iliac artery is selectively catheterized with a multi-purpose tip catheter. A firmer catheter allows a more stable position where a glide-catheter might not have enough stability to act as a guiding for a micro-catheter.

Diagnostic angiography is performed to establish the diagnosis and to guide the superselective embolization. A microcatheter 18" with a 14" floppy wire is used to position the tip of the microcatheter in/at the side of the fistula. The position has to be as selective as possible to warrant erectile function after the procedure (Fig. 13.3). Spasm might be a problem, therefore local spasmolytics, like nitroglycerin, can be applied before selective catheterization. Systemic spasmolytic support, such as ca-blockers, can also be helpful. If the patient is using anticoagulant medication, this should be stopped, but only after consultation of the primary physician.

Embolotherapy for high-flow priapism has been accomplished using a variety of agents including autologous clot, gelatin sponge pledgets, bucrylate and microcoils. It seems to be rational to advocate the use of temporary occlusive agents, such as autologous clot or gelatin sponge, to allow eventual recanalization and to preserve sexual function. However, in the literature it is shown that also more permanent agents show preservation of sexual function.

When the microcatheter tip has a superselective position in/at the fistula we prefer to use a microcoil because this allows the most precise local occlu-

sions without an inadvertent occlusion of nontarget branches. If we are not able to achieve this optimal position and stop in a more proximal position, we will use gelatin sponge but only with the catheter tip distally to the inferior rectal artery branch. We never use glue as, in our opinion, the delivery is

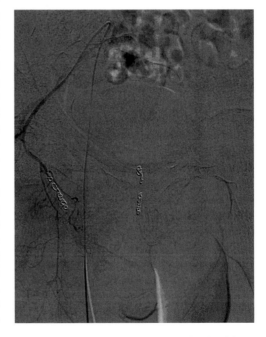

Fig. 13.3. Embolization of both internal pudendal arteries with coils in a patient with priapism and sickle cell disease. The aim of this treatment was to create permanent impotence and to prevent fibrosis

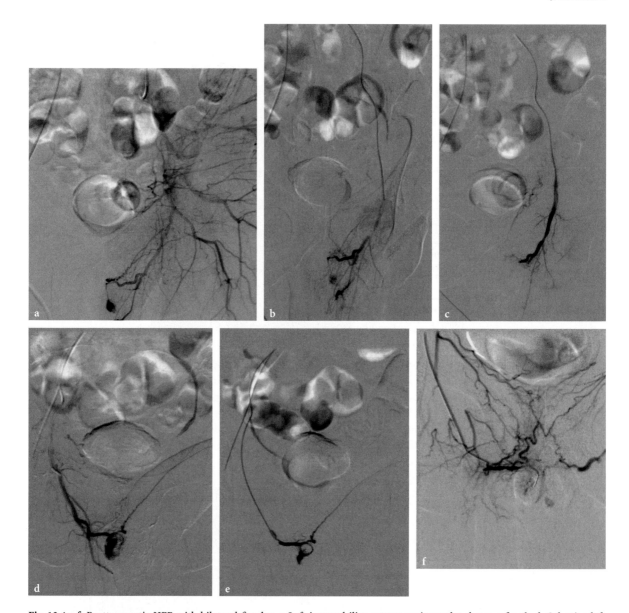

Fig. 13.4a–f. Posttraumatic HFP with bilateral fistulae. **a** Left internal iliac artery angiography shows a fistula. **b** Selective left IPA. **c** After closure of the fistula with gelatin sponge. **d** Selective right IPA shows a second fistula. **e** Microcatheter in superselective position. **f** End result after embolization with gelatin sponge. Patient had a full recovery and regained normal erectile function

never fully under control in this delicate area. Secondly, after glue delivery the microcatheter has to be removed and in case of a residual arteriovenous fistula selective catheterization has to be started again. However, successful glue embolization of HFP has already been reported [6].

After uni- or bilateral occlusion of all the fistula(s) has been achieved, the catheters and sheaths are removed. A color Doppler control after 24 h should be performed to document the local result. Although postembolization recurrence has been reported as high as 20%, it is lower in most publications, and not related to the embolic agent used [7].

13.7
Follow-up

Usually within hours after the embolization the priapism will be resolved. For normal erectile function to restore it might take up to 6–9 months [7]. As "normal" can be an subject of discussion an objective test like the International Index of Erectile Function (IIEF) should be used in follow-up. According to this test 80% of all patients will regain normal erectile function, while 20% will have a slight change in the quality of erection [7].

One of the concerns of embolization treatment is the local radiation of the gonads. Reduction of radiation can be achieved with the combined approach of X-ray and ultrasound imaging to facilitate the supraselective embolization of the arteriocavernous fistula reducing the radiation exposure and the applied dose of contrast medium [8]. It seems rational to advise refrainment from reproductive activity for a period of at least 3–6 months, although this recommendation is not supported in the literature.

13.8
Conclusion

Embolization for HFP is currently the treatment of choice if conservative therapy fails. It is safe and effective with a very high success rate and also a high recurrence of erectile function. Super-selective catheterization is mandatory. Microcoils and gelatin sponge are the embolic agents of choice.

Cookbook		
Introduction	5-F sheaths	Any
Guiding	Multipurpose 5-F (No glidecath)	Any
Guide wire	Terumo wire 35'	Terumo
Selective catherization	Microcatheter 18"+14' wire	Target (Boston Scientific)
Embolization material	Gelatin sponge or coils	Cordis/Boston Scientific/Cook

References

1. Eland IA, van der Lei j, Stricker BH, et al. (2001) Incidence of priapism in the general population. Urology 57:970
2. Kuefer R, Bartsch G Jr, Herkommer K, Kramer SC, Kleinschmidt K, Volkmer BG (2005) Changing diagnostic and therapeutic concepts in high-flow priapism. Int J Impot Res 17:109–113
3. Mentzel HJ, Kentouche K, Doerfel C, Vogt S, Zintl F, Kaiser WA High-flow priapism in acute lymphatic leukaemia. Pediatr Radiol 34:560-563
4. Gorich J, Ermis C, Kramer SC, Fleiter T, Wisianowsky C, Basche S, Gottfried HW, Volkmer BG (2002) Interventional treatment of traumatic priapism. J Endovasc Ther 9:614–617
5. Langenhuijsen JF, Reisman Y, Reekers JA, de Reijke Th M (2001) Highly selective embolization of bilateral cavernous arteries for post-traumatic penile arterial priapism. Int J Impot Res 13:354–356
6. Gandini R, Spinelli A, Konda D et al. (2004) Superselective embolization in posttraumatic priapism with Glubran 2 acrylic glue. Cardiovasc Intervent Radiol 27:544–548
7. Savoca G, Pietropaolo F, Scieri F, Bertolotto M, Mucelli FP, Belgrano E (2004) Sexual function after highly selective embolization of cavernous artery in patients with high flow priapism: long-term followup. J Urol 172:644–647
8. Bartsch G Jr, Kuefer R, Engel O, Volkmer BG (2004) Priapism: colour-Doppler ultrasound-guided supraselective embolization therapy. World J Urol 22:368–370

Aortic-Iliac

14 Endoleak: Definition, Diagnosis, and Management

David Valenti and Jafar Golzarian

CONTENTS

D. Valenti, MD
Royal Victoria Hospital, McGill University Health Centre,
McGill University, 687 Pine Avenue West, Suite A451,
Montreal, H3A 1A1, Canada
J. Golzarian, MD
Professor of Radiology, Director, Vascular and Interventional
Radiology, University of Iowa, Department of Radiology,
200 Hawkins Drive, 3957 JPP, Iowa City, IA 52242, USA

14.1 Introduction

Endoleak is defined as the persistent perfusion of the aneurysmal sac after endovascular aortic aneurysm repair (EVAR). A leak can appear during the first 30 days after implantation. This type of leak is called "primary endoleak". Secondary endoleak is one that occurs after 30 days. Leaks may also be classified as graft-related or non graft-related. The incidence of endoleak varies from 10% to 50% [1, 2]. In a report from EUROSTAR registry, the incidence of early endoleak was 18% [1]. A total of 69% of these leaks were graft related; 70% sealed spontaneously during the first 6 months without difference between graft-related and non graft-related endoleaks. There is not always a rational explanation of the cause of spontaneous resolution of some endoleaks and persistence or late occurrence of some others. The presence of outflow vessels (mainly lumbar arteries and inferior mesenteric artery) partially explains this phenomenon [3]. A leak communicating with these outflow vessels seldom disappears spontaneously [4]. Thus, these vessels should be identified. Whatever the cause of a persistent leak, it should be identified, monitored and treated. The details of EVAR will not be discussed here, except in relation to endoleaks.

This chapter will review classification and significance, diagnosis and treatment options for different types of endoleak.

14.2 Classification and Significance of Endoleaks

A generally accepted anatomic classification for endoleak has been developed over the years [5]. In this system, leaks are defined by their inflow source, regardless of the number and type of other vessels involved in the outflow (Table 14.1).

Table 14.1. Endoleak classification

Types	Mechanism
I	Flow originates from ineffective endograft seal at fixation zones
A	Proximal
B	Distal
C	Iliac occluder
II	Branch vessel retrograde flow
A	Single vessel (simple)
B	Two or more vessels creating a circuit (complex)
III	Flow results from structural endograft failure
A	Junctional separation (modular devices)
B	Endograft fracture or holes • Minor (<2 mm) • Major (≥2 mm)
IV	Endograft fabric porosity (<30 days after endograft implantation)
V	Endotension

14.2.1
Type I Endoleak

Type I endoleak is caused by failure to achieve a circumferential seal at either the proximal (type IA) or distal end (type IB) of the stentgraft. Type IC endoleak is due to non-occluded iliac artery in patients with aorto-mono-iliac stent and femoral–femoral bypass. With type I endoleak, the aneurysm is perfused directly from the aorta or the iliac arteries (inflows). The leak usually communicates through a channel (sometimes multiple channels) with the aneurysmal sac. There are several out-flow vessels, mainly lumbar arteries and inferior mesenteric artery (IMA) that communicate with the channel and or the sac (Figs. 14.1, 14.2). The pressure within a type I leak is systemic. The tension on the aortic wall remains high.

Causes of primary type I endoleak include inappropriate anatomy, with a significantly angulated neck, significant calcification/plaque at the proximal or distal landing zone, a non-circular landing zone, malpositioning of the stentgraft, type of endograft and under-dilation of the stentgraft. Secondary type I endoleak can be due to aneurysm re-modeling, resulting in stentgraft migration, progressive dilatation of the proximal neck, design and dimensions of stentgrafts or unfavourable infrarenal necks including the conically shaped neck and neck shorter than 15 mm. Grafts whose fixation relies on radial force are more prone to caudal migration and type I endoleak than grafts with hooks [6]. Endothelialization of bare stents at the landing zones may

contribute to a certain fixation, but endothelialization of the fabric itself does not occur. Proximal bare stent separation, as seen with the Vanguard device, and hook fractures, as seen with the EVT device, are also causes of delayed type I endoleak. Oversizing the graft by 20% is recommended to prevent a delayed endoleak. At the iliac level, type IB endoleak occurs when the limb of the graft is too short or migrates upward due to the sac's retraction pressure.

Although a type I endoleak can seal spontaneously, risk of rupture is high and intervention is indicated [4, 7, 8].

14.2.2
Type II Endoleak

A type II endoleak corresponds to the retrograde filling of the aneurysm mainly from lumbar arteries and/or IMA but also in rare situations from sacral, gonadal or accessory renal artery (Figs. 14.3, 14.4).

Type II endoleaks can be associated with aneurysmal expansion and rupture; however, this risk is much less than with the type I and III endoleaks (0.5 versus 3.4 %) [9, 10]. A leak in the setting of a shrinking aneurysm can generally be followed, without immediate intervention. It is well established that up to 40 % of type II endoleaks will seal spontaneously. Some have advocated intervening in all endoleaks persisting beyond 3–6 months, while other groups recommended observing leaks in the absence of aneurysm expansion. We favor the last approach. In our experience with biphasic helical CT follow-up of more than 300 patients treated by EVAR from 1994 to 1998, only three patients needed intervention for type II endoleak.

14.2.3
Type III Endoleak

Type III endoleaks are caused by a structural failure of the implanted device, including junctional separation of modular components, due to migration or changes in vessel morphology with aneurysm shrinkage, holes in the fabric, and fabric tears due to graft strut fracture or erosion (Figs. 14.5, 14.6). Graft disconnections were not infrequent with the first stentgraft generation due to a short overlap between the main body and the limb [11].

Type III leaks allow direct communication between the aorta and aneurysm sac. They have systemic arterial pressure. Similar to type I leak, type

III endoleak needs to be treated aggressively [10]. Type III endoleaks are considered to be the most dangerous, since there is an acute re-pressurization of the sac.

14.2.4
Type IV Endoleak

Type IV leaks are caused by porosity of the graft fabric. They are seen at the time of device implantation, as a faint blush on the post-implantation angiogram, when patients are fully anti-coagulated. It is important to rule out other types of endoleak before labeling a leak as type IV. They are rarely seen with current devices and will seal spontaneously. If a leak persists, other types should be excluded.

14.2.5
Type V Endoleak or Endotension

Endotension (or type V endoleak) corresponds to continued aneurysm expansion in the absence of a confirmed endoleak [12, 13]. The expansion of the aneurysm in a type V endoleak may be due to an undiagnosed endoleak, presumably with very slow flow and suboptimal imaging (e.g. no delayed helical CT acquisition). Endotension has been reported up to 18% in [14] a study evaluating the significance of endotension in 658 patients. The authors demonstrated that endotension is rare and concluded that it may represent missed endoleak rather than true aneurysm expansion in the absence of perigraft flow [15].

However, in most situations, endotension corresponds to an accumulation of yellowish fluid (seroma) [16]. Endotension is more common with ePTFE grafts due to ultra-filtration through graft pores.

14.3
Diagnosis of Endoleaks

14.3.1
Computed Tomography

Contrast enhanced helical computed tomography or CT angiography (CTA) is considered the imaging technique of choice for the detection of endoleak. CTA is reported to be superior to aortography for the demonstration of small leak [17]. The technique is also able to demonstrate the patency of lumbar arteries and IMA. However, selective aneurysmal angiography is superior to CTA for the detection of outflow vessels [4, 18].

The value of biphasic or triphasic CT scanning has been established for follow up of EVAR [19, 20]. Some authors favor obtaining an unenhanced helical CT series. ROZENBLIT at al. have demonstrated that the unenhanced series were helpful to diagnose an indeterminate endoleak in one patient [20]. Important mimickers of endoleak include calcification, contrast within the folds of unsupported portions of the graft and residual endosac contrast from the initial procedure when early CT follow-up is obtained at 1–3 days. This "pseudo-endoleak" was seen in up to 57% of patients [21].

It has been demonstrated that delayed acquisition uncovered up to 11% of endoleaks that were missed by arterial phase alone [19, 20]. An optimal CT protocol for the monitoring of the aorta after endoluminal therapy should include a delayed acquisition (Fig. 14.7).

14.3.2
Color Doppler Ultrasound

Color Doppler ultrasound (CDUS) is a noninvasive and cost-effective imaging modality. It is highly dependent on the operator and has limitations in obese patients and those with excessive bowel gas. Patients should be evaluated after 5–6 h fasting in supine and lateral position. The aorta is evaluated both transversally and longitudinally. Leak is suspected when a reproducible color and Doppler signal inside the aneurysm is visualized.

Variable success is reported for the detection and localization of the source of endoleaks with ultrasound, depending on technical factors, the imaging protocol, and the image quality. Reported sensitivities for overall endoleak detection range between 12% and 100%, with specificities of 74%–99% [22–26].

In a series of 55 patient with CDUS compared to biphasic CTA, CT was superior in detection of small leak. Discrepancies between helical CT and CDUS were observed in eight patients (14.5%). In five cases, a small perigraft leak that was clearly demonstrated by helical CT was not found on CDUS. All these leaks were small and disappeared during the follow-up. For the diagnosis of endoleak, the sensitivity, the specificity, the positive and negative pre-

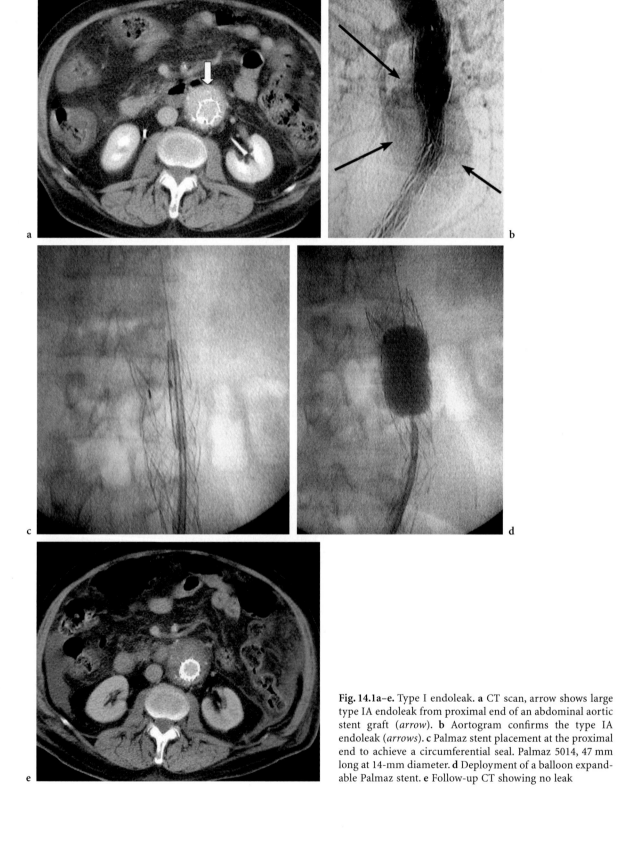

Fig. 14.1a–e. Type I endoleak. **a** CT scan, arrow shows large type IA endoleak from proximal end of an abdominal aortic stent graft (*arrow*). **b** Aortogram confirms the type IA endoleak (*arrows*). **c** Palmaz stent placement at the proximal end to achieve a circumferential seal. Palmaz 5014, 47 mm long at 14-mm diameter. **d** Deployment of a balloon expandable Palmaz stent. **e** Follow-up CT showing no leak

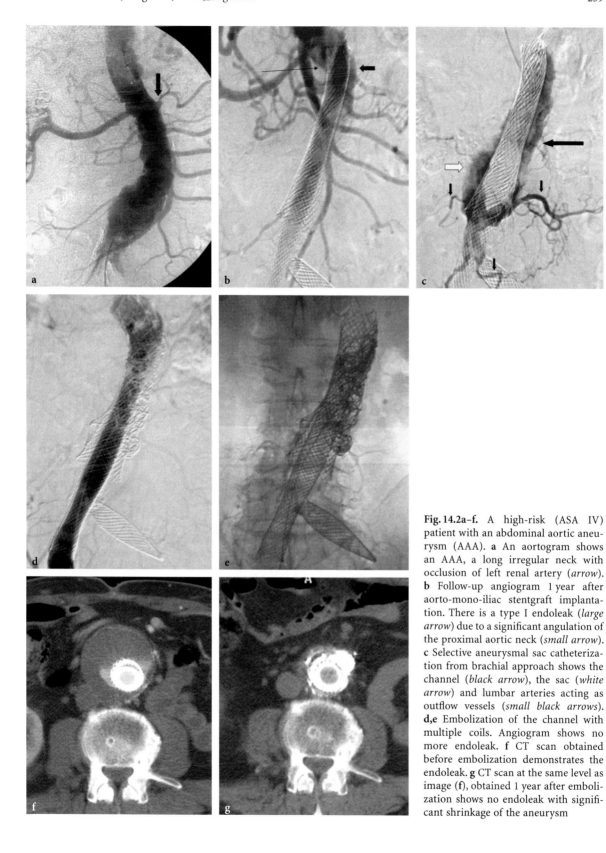

Fig. 14.2a–f. A high-risk (ASA IV) patient with an abdominal aortic aneurysm (AAA). **a** An aortogram shows an AAA, a long irregular neck with occlusion of left renal artery (*arrow*). **b** Follow-up angiogram 1 year after aorto-mono-iliac stentgraft implantation. There is a type I endoleak (*large arrow*) due to a significant angulation of the proximal aortic neck (*small arrow*). **c** Selective aneurysmal sac catheterization from brachial approach shows the channel (*black arrow*), the sac (*white arrow*) and lumbar arteries acting as outflow vessels (*small black arrows*). **d,e** Embolization of the channel with multiple coils. Angiogram shows no more endoleak. **f** CT scan obtained before embolization demonstrates the endoleak. **g** CT scan at the same level as image (**f**), obtained 1 year after embolization shows no endoleak with significant shrinkage of the aneurysm

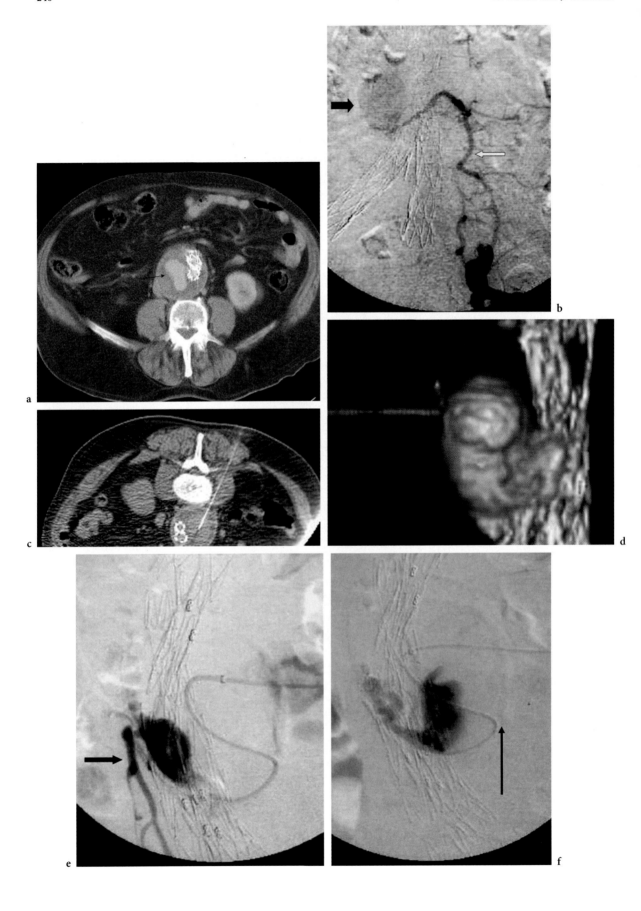

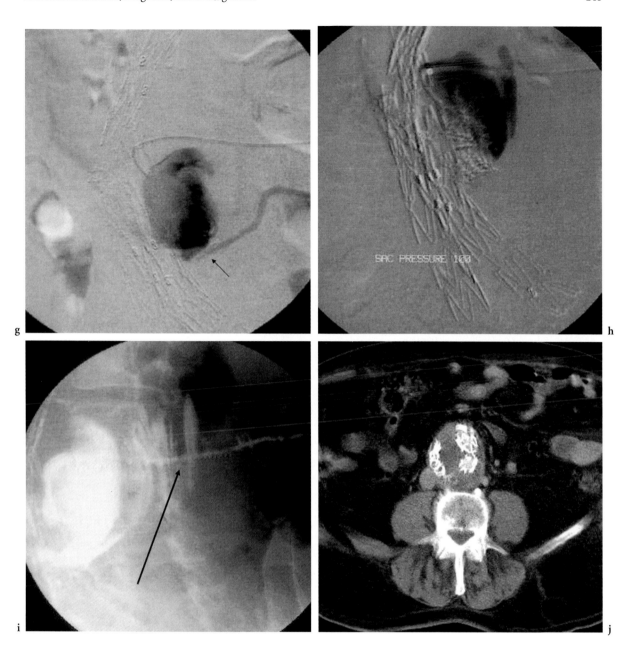

Fig. 14.3a–j. Type II endoleak. **a** Contrast enhanced CT shows an important peri-prosthetic leak (*arrow*). **b** Left internal iliac artery angiogram demonstrates a type II leak (*black arrow*) from iliolumbar artery (*white arrow*). **c,d** Translumbar approach has been used for the treatment of this endoleak. CT and volume rendering reconstruction shows the position of the needle and the aneurysmal sac. The pressure in the sac was then measured showing a systolic pressure of 180 mmHg. **e** Injection of the sac shows the involvement of the IMA (*black arrow*). **f** Embolization of the origin of the IMA. **g** After IMA embolization, the origin of the lumbar artery is embolized. *Arrow* shows the lumbar artery as the outflow vessel. **h** The aneurysmal sac is then embolized with coils. At this point, the systolic pressure in the sac drops to 100 mmHg. At the end of the procedure, the sac pressure was close to zero. **i** The tract (*arrow*) was then embolized with Gelfoam. **j** CT obtained 8 months after embolization shows no more endoleak

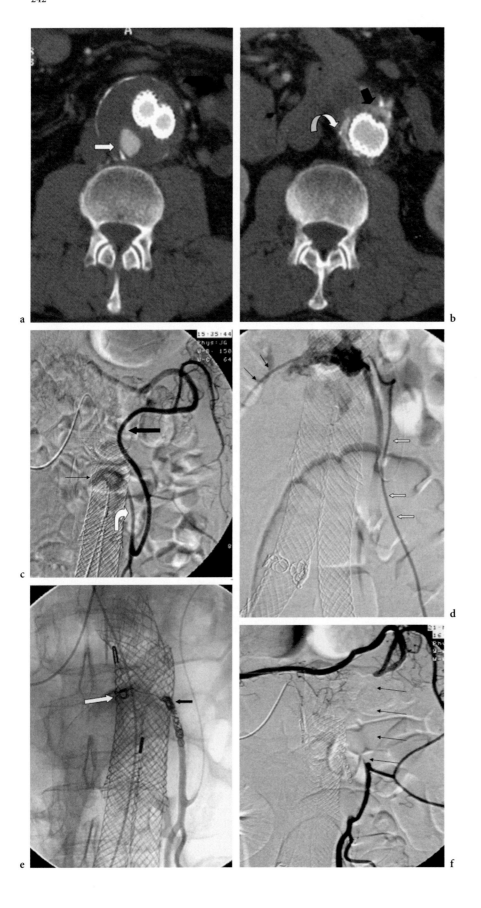

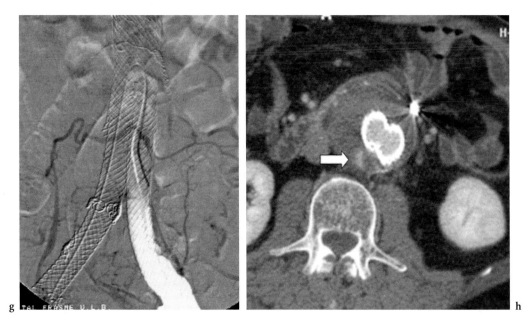

Fig. 14.4a–h. Type II endoleak. **a,b** CT scan demonstrates an endoleak involving both IMA and lumbar arteries. **a** Posterior endoleak (*white arrow*). **b** Right lateral (*curved arrow*) and anterior position of the endoleak (*black arrow*). **c** Superior mesenteric angiogram demonstrates the opacification of IMA (*curved arrow*) through arc of Riolan (*large black arrow*) and the endoleak cavity (*small black arrow*). **d** Selective microcatheter placement in the sac. Angiogram shows the aneurysm, one lumbar artery (*black arrows*) and spermatic artery (*white arrows*) acting as outflow. **e** Coil embolization at the origin of the lumbar artery (*white arrow*) was initiated however, the catheter was pushed back and the distal end of the coil released at the origin of the IMA (*black arrow*). The IMA was then embolized. **f** Angiogram shows no more endoleak with transient spasm of the arc of Riolan (*arrows*). **g** Left common iliac angiogram shows no endoleak from iliolumbar artery. **h** Enhanced CT obtained after embolization demonstrates a small endoleak from lumbar artery (*arrow*)

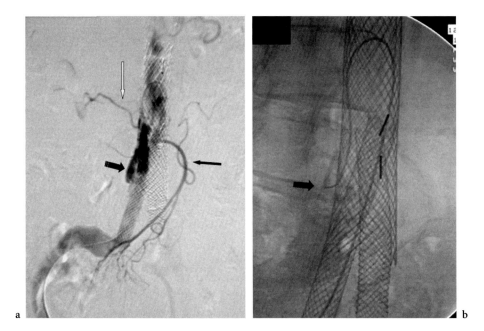

Fig. 14.5a,b. Type III endoleak due to a hole in the fabric. **a** Aortogram demonstrates the endoleak (*large black arrow*) with IMA (*small black arrow*) and a lumbar artery (*white arrow*) acting as an outflow vessel. **b** The wire is passed through the hole in the aortic aneurysm (*arrow*)

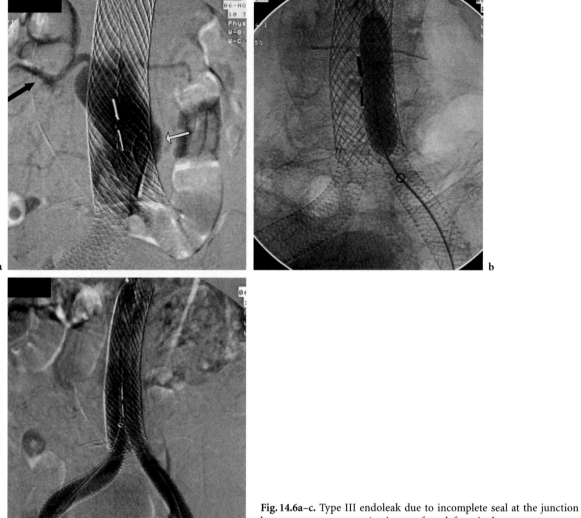

Fig. 14.6a–c. Type III endoleak due to incomplete seal at the junction between components. **a** Angiogram from left groin demonstrates a type III endoleak (*white arrow*) and a lumbar artery (*black arrow*). **b** Palmaz stent placement inflated to 12 mm. **c** Control angiogram shows no more endoleak

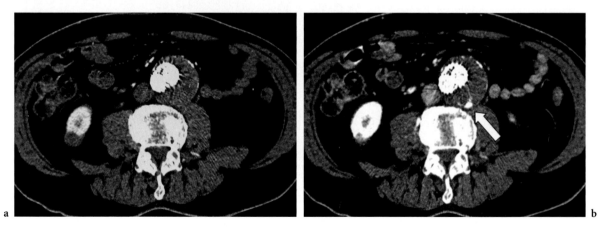

Fig. 14.7a,b. Biphasic helical CT. **a** Arterial phase demonstrates no endoleak. **b** Delayed phase showed a type II endoleak (*white arrow*)

dictive values CDUS as compared to helical CT were respectively 77%, 90%, 85%, and 85% [26].

Administration of an ultrasound contrast agent can increase the sensitivity for detecting endoleaks with color and power Doppler by 33%–300%; however, the specificity may decrease by 17% to 30% [27–31]. Utilizing an ultrasound contrast agent may also enable detection of endoleaks that are not seen by CT angiography [30, 31].

14.3.3
Magnetic Resonance Imaging (MRI)

MRI and MR angiography can provide all the information during EVAR follow-up for Nitinol based stentgrafts. As to detection of endoleaks, results are comparable to CT angiography for detecting type I and type III endoleaks. Depending on the CT section thickness and imaging protocol, MR angiography may yield a greater sensitivity to detect slow flow type II endoleaks [32–35]. Blood pool magnetic resonance angiography has been found useful in detecting small endoleaks. A study of six patients after EVAR using Ferumoxytol, a blood pool agent, showed four low flow endoleaks that were not detected by CT. Most importantly these patients also demonstrated no reduction in endograft size after EVAR [36]. Contrast enhanced MRA (CEMRA) with time-resolved (TR) technique provides dynamic angiographic information – similar to conventional angiography. TR-CEMRA affords a more comprehensive evaluation than standard MR angiography. The source and flow direction of endoleaks can be depicted, improving the characterization of the inflow and potential outflow of endoleaks. As this information impacts decision making for appropriate management, with advances in parallel imaging to reduce MR scan time, TR-CEMRA may become the routine method for post-EVAR MR angiography [37]. Phase contrast imaging can be applied to demonstrate endoleak direction and quantify flow and velocity [38].

Although all these non-invasive techniques are reliable to demonstrate an endoleak, the characterization and the type of endoleak can still be difficult.

14.3.4
Angiography

Digital subtraction angiography (DSA) remains the gold standard for characterization of the endoleaks and their endovascular treatment.

Angiographic examination should include a global pigtail injection of the aorta at the level of renal arteries and inside the stentgraft. A flush catheter is placed just above the proximal attachment site. A power injector is used to achieve an adequate flow rate, (10–15 ml/s for 2 s). Next, the catheter is withdrawn within the graft (to a level just above the flow divider in a bifurcated device). Frontal and/or bilateral oblique views are obtained, to search for distal type I and type III leaks. For these images the flow injection rate is decreased to 5–10 ml/s, to avoid reflux up to the level of the proximal attachment site, which could confuse the interpretation. Finally, selective arteriogram of the superior mesenteric artery (SMA) and both internal iliac arteries should be obtained, to hunt for type II leaks. On all the acquisitions it is important to carry the imaging out into the venous phase (i.e. 20–30 s) to search for slowly filling type II leaks. Images are acquired at 2–3 frames/s for the first 10 s, after this the frame rate can be lowered to 1.0–1.5 frames/s.

In case of type I endoleak, the origin of the sac is catheterized by placing the catheter between the stentgraft and aortic wall and intra-aneurysmal injection is performed for optimal evaluation of the outflow vessels.

14.4
Treatment of Endoleak

There is a consensus that type I and III leaks should be treated on a relatively urgent basis. There is still debate regarding the treatment of stable type II leaks. Multiple algorithms are proposed for the treatment of the endoleaks (Table 14.2). In this chapter, we will discuss the treatment options for each type of endoleak separately.

Table 14.2. Treatment algorithm

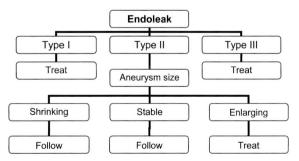

14.4.1
Type I Endoleak

Multiple modalities are available for the treatment of type I endoleak (Table 14.3). The choice of the optimal treatment is based on the source of the leak. Our policy in this matter is to use the least invasive yet the most durable treatment.

14.4.1.1
Type IA Endoleak

Placement of a proximal cuff or extension endograft is the most commonly used treatment in case of proximal endoleak associated with malpositioning, angulated neck or migration. This technique needs a new cut down and is not always feasible due to different anatomical and technical challenges.

In case of proximal endoleak associated with an irregular neck with no migration, simple balloon angioplasty with large balloons (25–30 mm) or large Palmaz stent placement could be sufficient to apply the stentgraft to the aortic wall. This procedure can be performed under local anesthesia using a long 12-F sheath that can allow the passage of a large Palmaz stent (Fig. 14.1).

Embolization and coiling of the aneurysmal sac and the outflow vessels has been proposed as an alternative treatment for type I endoleak in selected patients [4, 39–42]. Historically, this technique was used when proximal extension cuffs were not available. With current devices, proper size cuffs are generally always available. The majority of patients treated with this technique had extensive medical co-morbidities and short or highly angulated proximal neck. Although there have been concerns about the long-term efficacy of this technique, the results seem to be encouraging. GORICH et al. [40] have successfully treated 13 patients with embolization (mean follow-up: 6.8 months). SHEEHAN et al. [41] have reported a high clinical success rate in nine patients with type I endoleak treated just by coil embolization with a mean follow-up of 24 months. We have treated 32 patients with type I endoleak from 1996 to 2003. The majority of the patients received a Corvita stentgraft (n, 28), two Talent endografts and two AneuRx. All patients were considered high risk for surgery. Embolization was successful in 29 patients with the occlusion of the outflow vessels and the aortic channel and/or sac. Three patients with large neck had persistent endoleak after several procedures. Six patients were lost to follow-up. Among the remaining 26 patients, four died of cardiac disease between 7 to 90 days after the procedure. In all, 22 patients could be followed with a mean follow-up of 38.6 months. The aneurysm shrank in 15 patients and remained stable in five and increased in two patients with persistent endoleak. None of the patients with successful embolization has developed a new endoleak or an aneurysmal expansion (Fig. 14.2). This study confirms that upon achievement of thrombosis, embolization of the outflow vessels and the sac can be associated with long-term clinical success and freedom from endoleak.

Table 14.3. Treatment of persistent type I endoleak

Extension stentgraft or cuff
Balloon angioplasty
Bare stent
Embolization
Surgical conversion

14.4.1.1.1
Technique of Embolization

The key to success for type I endoleak is to disrupt the communications between the inflow and outflow vessels involved in the leak. Careful review of contrast enhanced CT scans will be helpful prior to the procedure, to select the best vascular access site (femoral or brachial). An aortogram is performed to more precisely define the entry site of the endoleak. Thereafter, the aneurysmal sac is selectively catheterised using either a 5-F multipurpose catheter or a 5-F cobra catheter by brachial or femoral access. In some situations a Side-winder II reverse curve catheter can be used. An intra-sac angiogram is then performed to better evaluate the outflow vessels. A selective occlusion of the outflow vessels is then performed (Fig. 14.2). If catheterization of the outflow vessels is difficult to achieve, coils can be placed in front of their origin. After outflow vessel embolization, the aneurysmal pouch and/or the leak channel are filled with additional segments of coil. Other embolic materials such as gelatin sponge fragments or thrombin can be used to induce the thrombosis, after extensive coil embolization of the channel or the sac and the collaterals. These agents may escape into the aorta more easily than coils during their injection and so should be infused with caution. The embolization endpoint is stasis within the sac or non-visualization of the endoleak on final aortogram.

14.4.1.2
Type IB Endoleak

All treatment options for the type IA endoleaks are valid for distal endoleak. In case of short landing or enlarged iliac artery, an extension endo-graft will be necessary. However most of type IB endoleaks can be treated with balloon angioplasty or bare stent implantation allowing the sealing of the stentgraft to the aortic wall. If the origin of internal iliac artery needs to be covered, it should be embolized to prevent from retrograde leak.

Embolization of the sac or the channel, although feasible, is usually not indicated in type I-B endoleak.

14.4.1.3
Type IC Endoleak

Type IC leaks occur in cases where an aorto-uni-iliac stentgraft has been deployed, in conjunction with a femoral-femoral bypass graft. An occluder device is then placed in the contra-lateral common iliac artery. Its function is to prevent back filling of the aneurysm from the excluded common iliac artery. The treatment of these leaks requires completion of the intended thrombosis of the common iliac artery. Embolization is the simplest way to complete this, either by passing the occluder and embolizing cranial to it, or, by placing a second occluder device caudal to the original device.

The occlusion of the iliac artery is usually sufficient to treat the leak. However, in cases of long-term type IC endoleak, many outflow vessels may have developed and the leak may communicate with multiple lumbar arteries and the IMA. These enlarged vessels might be source of late type II endoleak. Thus, we usually embolize both the outflow vessels and the sac before occluding the iliac artery. Another attractive technique to achieve the occlusion of the common iliac artery is to perform an endovascular internal to external iliac artery bypass using stentgraft. This technique can allow the exclusion of the common iliac preserving the internal iliac artery.

14.4.2
Type II Endoleak

Persistent type II endoleaks usually have a complex architecture. They have been compared to the arteriovenous malformation with the sac forming the 'nidus' of the lesion [43]. There are usually multiple inflow and outflow vessels. These vessels communicate most of the time through a channel. The channel is different from the endoleak sac that is generally seen during the angiogram and punctured in translumbar embolization. To achieve a successful embolization, the inflow vessels, the channel and/or the sac need to be embolized (Fig. 14.3). Like in embolization of type I endoleak, the key is to disrupt the communications between the vessels involved in the leak.

14.4.2.1
Transarterial Approach

A 5-F Cobra 2 catheter (0.038") is placed in the SMA. Once the diagnostic catheter is stable in the proximal SMA, a microcatheter is advanced to the IMA via the Arc of Riolan. It is prudent to inject 5000 units of heparin prior to attempting the cannulation of the Arc of Riolan. Similarly, vasodilators (Nitroglycerin, 100–200 μm) may be helpful to prevent spasm.

In some situations, the sac can be accessed from internal iliac artery through iliolumbar and lumbar arteries.

Regardless of the route chosen, the most important task is to access the channel or the sac. It is critical to disrupt the network between the involved vessels. This is more important than occluding any one vessel or even embolizing the endoleak sac (Figs. 14.3, 14.4). This explains the high rate of recurrence after IMA embolization alone (Fig. 14.4) compared to translumbar embolization for type II endoleak in one report [44].

There are many choices regarding embolic agent. Permanent agents, such as coils are preferred. When using coils the origins of all involved vessels are cannulated and embolized. However, getting into lumbar artery origins may be very challenging. In practice coils are deposited as close as possible to the origins of the involved vessels (coils of 2–3 mm diameter, 2–3 cm long). Once branch vessels are isolated then large coils can be used to fill the channel and/or the aneurysmal sac. In most situations, if the channel between the inflow and outflow vessels is interrupted, the sac does not need to be embolized. Thus, in case of complex type II endoleak, the filling of the endoleak cavity by translumbar approach, without treating the inflow or outflow channels. Some authors support the use of either a 5- to 10-ml solution of Gelfoam slurry, or a similar volume of saline mixed with 500–1000 units of thrombin.

Alternatively the coils can be soaked in a solution with a high thrombin concentration (20,000 units of thrombin in 20 ml of saline). The origin of the IMA has to be embolized with several coils adapted to its diameter.

14.4.2.2
Translumbar Approach

Previous experience with translumbar puncture of the aorta for diagnostic angiography showed that this puncture carries only minor risks, with a retroperitoneal hematoma rate of about 3% [45]. The aorta can be punctured under CT or fluoroscopic guidance.

Careful correlation with prior CT images will help plan the puncture in relation to the markers on the stent graft. Ideally the left side access is used to avoid IVC. However, if necessary the puncture can be done through the IVC. When performed under fluoroscopic guidance it is useful to frequently rotate the X-ray tube from the AP to the lateral projection, and in between, to help in assessing the needle track, and to avoid puncturing the stentgraft.

The translumbar puncture site is typically 8–10 cm from the midline. The access needle is angled at about 45°–60° anteromedially, aimed so as to pass just anterior to the vertebral body, avoiding the adjacent transverse process. As described for traditional translumbar aortography, it may be useful to actually aim for the vertebral body, then after bony contact, pull back 1 or 2 cm and aim more ventrally.

Using CT guidance the initial needle tip placement will be into the leak sac (Fig. 14.3). However, with fluoroscopic guidance and a relatively small leak, the initial puncture may end up in thrombus. In these cases, the leak sac can usually be found fairly easily using a hydrophilic guidewire and catheter.

Once in the angio-suite a proper angiogram of the sac is performed. Pressure measurements should be obtained within the sac. The measurement will show generally a systemic pressure. Coil embolization is then performed as for the arterial approach.

14.4.2.3
Other Embolic Materials

The use of several other agents has been reported with translumbar treatment of type II endoleaks, including Onyx, Ethibloc, thrombin, and Cyanoacrylate [46–50].

There are multiple reports of the use of thrombin in the percutaneous, translumbar embolization of type II leaks. Most authors report the use of 500–1500 units of thrombin [49]. The only reported serious complication occurred in a case where 8000 units were injected [50]. The complication was ischemic colitis in the recto-sigmoid region; the IMA was patent in this case. Despite the complication, the procedure was successful in sealing the endoleak.

Onyx, (Micro Therapeutics, Irvine, Ca), is a biocompatible liquid embolic agent. It is an ethylene vinyl alcohol copolymer dissolved in various concentrations of dimethyl sulfoxide (DMSO). Micronized tantalum powder is added to the solvent/polymer mixture at the time of production for radiopacity. When this mixture contacts aqueous media, such as blood, the DMSO rapidly diffuses away, with resulting in situ precipitation and solidification of the polymer. It forms a soft elastic embolus without adhesion to the vascular wall [51]. The polymerization process is time dependent and is mainly influenced by the amount of ethylene in the mixture; with less ethylene the polymer becomes softer. Onyx is available in several different concentrations; the higher concentration is more viscous. Using a higher concentration makes it easier to prevent the liquid from getting too far from the catheter tip. Since the polymer will solidify on contact with aqueous media the delivery catheter must be pre-flushed with DMSO. The embolization endpoint is stasis within the sac. A 'DMSO-compatible' catheter is required; DMSO will degrade most currently available catheters. Onyx is non-adhesive, allowing for easy removal of the delivery catheter, and of the polymer itself if the stentgraft is ever explanted. It is quite expensive. The reported success rate is high [46], and the results are durable (personal communication).

Ethibloc (Ethnor Laboratories/Ethicon Inc., Norderstedt, Germany) is a cornstarch product which polymerizes on contact with ionic fluids; it develops a consistency similar to chewing gum, and subsequently hardens further. It is an emulsion of zein (a water-insoluble prolamine derived from corn gluten), alcohol, poppy seed oil, propylene glycol and a contrast medium. It can be mixed with Lipiodol (Laboratoire Guerbet, Paris, France) to allow for improved visualization. Pump flushing through a three-way stopcock can emulsify the mixture; 10ml of Ethibloc are mixed with 0.5 ml of Lipiodol. This mixture does not dissolve catheters. The system must be primed with a non-ionic fluid, such as 50% glucose to prevent solidification in the delivery device. The embolization endpoint is stasis of the injected substance. It is important to slowly retract the delivery device while injecting the mixture.

NBCA (Trufill n-BCA, Cordis Neurovascular) is liquid glue. The manufacturer provides three components in the kit; NBCA monomer, (a free-flowing clear liquid), ethiodol and tantalum powder (to increase the radio-density of the glue). Polycarbonate syringes should not be used, only polyethylene or polypropylene are recommended by the manufacturer. NBCA polymerizes rapidly on contact with ionic fluids. The injection catheter must be rapidly removed from the embolization site to prevent the catheter itself from being glued in place. TL needles, even if adherent to the glue, can be easily removed. The volume of NBCA to be injected is determined by test injections of contrast; the volume should be sufficient to completely fill the aneurysm sac and to initiate reflux into the involved lumbar arteries. The spinal artery must be avoided, if visualized it should be protected with a coil. The reported success rate is very high, with durable results [52].

Surgical ligation of all relevant branches is a possible solution for type II leaks. However experience has shown that there are often more vessels involved in these lesions than is initially suspected, and unless they are all clipped the surgical route approach risks failure or recurrence. Ligation can be accomplished by laparoscopic or open technique.

14.4.3
Type III Endoleak

Angiography can confirm type III endoleak after placement of the pigtail catheter in the stent graft, just above the flow divider. If the cause is a separation of modular components there may be some difficulty in establishing guidewire access from one component to the next, but once this is accomplished deployment of a new extension is generally problem free. In some situations a new stentgraft needs to be implanted. When the leak is related to incomplete circumferential seal of different components, angioplasty or bare stent implantation can seal the leak (Fig. 14.6). In case of fabric tear, re-implantation of a new stentgraft or open conversion can be considered.

Embolization is almost never indicated in type III leaks.

14.4.4
Type V Endoleak – Endotension

There have been several reports of confirmed systemic pressurization within enlarging aneurysm sacs, despite the absence of visualized endoleak [12–16, 50]. Cases of sac enlargement and rupture have been recently reported even after treatment of AAA with open surgery. In one report, laparotomy demonstrated a seroma containing firm rubbery gelatinous materials [53]. Aortic puncture to analyze and empty the accumulated fluid is one way to treat this type of endoleak. However, the fluid often re-accumulates during follow-up. If the endotension is related to serous fluid accumulation, there is no need for a surgical treatment even in case of rupture [53]. Other treatment options include retroperitoneal drainage of the fluid, explantation of the graft with open surgery or insertion of a new stentgraft to reduce the porosity.

14.5
Conclusion

It seems certain that EVAR will continue to be a primary treatment for many years. Endoleak is an ongoing problem associated with EVAR. Imaging plays a critical role in detecting endoleak. CTA is the first line diagnostic modality. Optimal CTA protocol needs to include a delayed acquisition. There are many endovascular options available for treatment of persistent endoleaks. The optimal treatment depends on the type of the endoleak.

References

1. Cuypers P, Buth J, Harris PL, et al (1999) Realistic expectations for patients with stent-graft treatment of abdominal aortic aneurysms. Results of a European multicentre registry. Eur J Vasc Endovasc Surg 17:507–516
2. Parent FN, Meier GH, Godziachvili V et al (2002) The incidence and natural history of type I and II endoleak: a 5-year follow-up assessment with color duplex ultrasound scan. J Vasc Surg 35:474–81
3. Fan CM, Rafferty EA, Geller EC et al (2001) Endovascular stent-graft in abdominal aortic aneurysms: The relationship between patent vessels that arise from the aneurysmal sac and early endoleak. Radiology 218:176–182
4. Golzarian J, Struyven J, Abada HT, et al (1997) Endovascular aortic stent-grafts: transcatheter embolization of persistent perigraft leaks. Radiology 202:731–734

5. Veith FJ, Baum RA, Ohki T, et al (2002) Nature and significance of endoleaks and endotension: summary of opinions expressed at an international conference. J Vasc Surg 35:1029–1035

6. Malina M, Lindblad B, Ivancev K, et al (1998) Endovascular AAA exclusion: Will stents with hooks and barbs prevent stent-graft migration? J Endovasc Surg 5:310–317

7. White GH, Yu W, May J, et al (1997) Endoleak as a complication of endoluminal grafting of abdominal aortic aneurysms: classification, diagnosis, and management. J Endovasc Surg 4:152–168

8. Buth J, Harris PL, van Marrewijk C, Fransen G (2003) The significance and management of different types of endoleaks. Semin Vasc Surg 16:95–102

9. Zarins CK, White RA, Hodgson KJ, et al (2000) Endoleak as a predictor of outcome after endovascular aneurysm repair: AneuRx multicenter clinical trial. J Vasc Surg 32:90–107

10. van Marrewijk C, Buth J, Harris PL, et al (2002) Significance of endoleaks after endovascular repair of abdominal aortic aneurysms: the Eurostar experience. J Vasc Surg 35:461–473

11. Fransen GA, Vallabhaneni SR Sr, Van Marrewijk CJ, et al (2003) Rupture of infrarenal aortic aneurysm after endovascular repair: A series from EUROSTAR registry. Eur J Vasc Endovasc Surg 26:487–493

12. Gilling-Smith G, Brennan J, Harris P, Bakran A, Gould D, McWilliams R (1999) Endotension after endovascular aneurysm repair: definition, classification, and strategies for surveillance and intervention. J Endovasc Surg 6:305–307

13. White GH, May W, Petrasek P, Waugh R, Stephen M, Harris J (1999) Endotension: an explanation for continued AAA growth after successful endoluminal repair. J Endovasc Surg 6:308–315

14. Gilling-Smith GL, Martin J, Sudhindran S, et al (2000) Freedom from endoleak after endovascular aneurysm repair does not equal treatment success. Eur J Vasc Endovasc Surg 19:421–425

15. Meier GH, Parker FM, Godziachvili V, et al (2001) Endotension after endovascular aneurysm repair: The Ancure experience. Vasc Surg 34:421–427

16. Risberg B, Delle M, Lonn L, Syk I (2004) Management of aneurysm sac hygroma. J Endovasc Ther 11:191–5

17. Gorich J, Rilinger N, Sokiranski R et al (1999) Leakages after endovascular repair of aortic aneurysms: classification based on findings at CT, angiography, and radiography. Radiology 213:767–72

18. Gorich J, Rilinger N, Kramer S, et al (2000) Angiography of leaks after endovascular repair of infrarenal aortic aneurysms. AJR Am J Roentgenol 174:811–814

19. Golzarian J, Dussaussois L, Abada HT, et al (1998) Helical CT of aorta after endoluminal stent-graft therapy. AJR Am J Roentgenol 171:329–331

20. Rosenblit AM, Patlas M, Rosenbaum AT, et al (2003) Detection of endoleaks after endovascular repair of abdominal aortic aneurysms: value of unenhanced and delayed CT acquisitions. Radiology 227:426–433

21. Sawhney R, Kerlen RK, Wall SD et al (2001) Analysis of initial CT findings after endovascular repair of abdominal aortic aneurysm. Radiology 220:157–160

22. Elkouri S, Panneton JM, Andrews JC, et al (2004) Computed tomography and ultrasound in follow-up of patients after endovascular repair of abdominal aortic aneurysm. Ann Vasc Surg 18:271–279

23. Wolf YG, Johnson BL, Hill BB, et al (2000) Duplex ultrasound scanning versus computed tomographic angiography for post-operative evaluation of endovascular abdominal aortic aneurysm repair. J Vasc Surg 32:1142–8

24. Zannetti S, De Rango P, Parente B, et al (2000) Role of duplex scan in endoleak detection after endoluminal abdominal aortic aneurysm repair. Eur J Vasc Endovasc Surg 19:531–535

25. Pages, S, Favre JP, Cerisier A, et al (2001) Comparison of color duplex ultrasound and computed tomography scan for surveillance after aortic endografting. Ann Vasc Surg 15:155–162

26. Golzarian J, Murgo S, Dussaussois L, et al (2002) Evaluation of abdominal aortic aneurysm after endoluminal treatment: comparison of color Doppler sonography with biphasic helical CT. AJR Am J Roentgenol 178:623–628

27. McWilliams RG, Martin J, White D, et al (2002) Detection of endoleak with enhanced ultrasound imaging: comparison with biphasic computed tomography. J Endovasc Ther 9:170–179

28. McLafferty RB, McCrary BS, Mattos MA, et al (2002) The use of color-flow duplex scan for the detection of endoleaks. J Vasc Surg 36:100–104

29. Raman KG, Missing-Carroll N, Richardson T, et al (2003) Color-flow duplex ultrasound scan versus computed tomographic scan in the surveillance of endovascular aneurysm repair. J Vasc Surg 38:645–651

30. Bendick PJ, Bove PG, Long GW, et al (2003) Efficacy of ultrasound scan contrast agents in the noninvasive follow-up of aortic stent grafts. J Vasc Surg 37:381–385

31. Napoli V, Bargellini I, Sardella SG, et al (2004) Abdominal aortic aneurysm: contrast-enhanced US for missed endoleaks after endoluminal repair. Radiology 233:217–225

32. Haulon S, Lions C, McFadden EP, Koussa M, et al (1998) Prospective evaluation of magnetic resonance imaging after endovascular treatment of infrarenal aortic aneurysms. Eur J Endovasc Surg 22:62–69

33. Ayuso JR, de Caralt TM, Pages M, Riambau V, et al (2004) MRA is useful as a follow-up technique after endovascular repair of aortic aneurysms with nitinol endoprostheses. J Magn Reson Imaging 20:803–810

34. Cejna M, Loewe C, Schoder M, et al (2002) MR angiography vs CT angiography in the follow-up of Nitinol stent grafts in the endoluminally treated aortic aneurysms. Eur Radiology 12:2443–2450

35. Lutz AM, Willmann JK, Pfammatter T, Lachat M (2003) Evaluation of aortoiliac aneurysm before endovascular repair: comparison of contrast-enhanced magnetic resonance angiography with multidetector row computed tomographic angiography with an automated analysis software tool. J Vasc Surg 37:619–627

36. Ersoy H, Jacobs P, Kent KK, Prince MR (2004) Blood pool MR angiography of aortic stentgraft endoleak. AJR Am J Roentgenol 182:1181–1186

37. Lookstein RA, Goldman J, Pukin L, Marin ML (2004) Time-resolved magnetic resonance angiography as a noninvasive method to characterize endoleaks: initial results compared with conventional angiography. J Vasc Surg 39:27–33

38. Hellinger JC, Draney M, Markl M, Pelc NJ, et al (2003) Appli-

cation of cine phase contrast magnetic resonance imaging and SPAMM-tagging for assessment of endoleaks and aneurysm sac motion. Radiology 229:SS573, (Abstract)

39. Amesur NB, Zajko AB, Orons PD, Makaroun MS (1999) Embolotherapy of persistent endoleaks after endovascular repair of abdominal aortic aneurysm with the ancure-endovascular technologies endograft system. J Vasc Interv Radiol 10:1175–82

40. Gorich J, Rilinger N, Sokiranski R et al (2000) Treatment of leaks after endovascular repair of aortic aneurysms. Radiology 215:414–420

41. Faries PL, Cadot H, Agarwal G et al (2003) Management of endoleak after endovascular aneurysm repair: cuffs, coils, and conversion. J Vasc Surg 37:1155–1161

42. Sheehan M, Barbato J, Compton NC et al (20004) Effectiveness of coiling in the treatment of endoleak after endovascular repair. J Vasc Surg 40:430–434

43. Baum RA, Stavropoulos SW, Fairman RM, Carpenter JP (2003) Endoleaks after endovascular repair of abdominal aortic aneurysms. J Vasc Interv Radiol 14:1111–1117

44. Baum RA, Carpenter JP, Golden MA et al (2002) Treatment of type 2 endoleaks after endovascular repair of abdominal aortic aneurysms: comparison of transarterial and translumbar techniques. J Vasc Surg 35:23–29

45. Hessel SJ, Adams DF, Abrams HL (1981) Complications of angiography. Radiology 138:273–281

46. Martin ML, Dolmatch BL, Fry PD, Machan LS (2001) Treatment of Type II endoleaks with Onyx. J Vasc Interv Radiol 2:629–632

47. Schmid R, Gurke L, Aschwanden M, et al (2002) CT-guided percutaneous embolization of a lumbar artery maintaining a Type II endoleak. J Endovasc Ther 9:198–202

48. van den Berg JC, Nolthenius RP, Casparie JW et al (2001) CT-guided thrombin injection into aneurysm sac in a patient with endoleak after endovascular abdominal aortic aneurysm repair. AJR Am J Roentgenol 175:1649–1651

49. Ellis PK, Kennedy PT, Collins AJ, Blair PH (2003) The use of direct thrombin injection to treat a Type II endoleak following endovascular repair of abdominal aortic aneurysm. Cardiovasc Intervent Radiol 26:482–484

50. Gambaro E, Abou-Zamzam AM Jr, Teruya TH et al (2004) Ischemic colitis following translumbar thrombin injection for treatment of endoleak. Ann Vasc Surg 18:74–78

51. Numan F, Omeroglu A, Kara B, Cantasdemir M, Adaletli I, Kantarci F (2004) Embolization of peripheral vascular malformations with ethylene vinyl alcohol copolymer (Onyx). J Vasc Interv Radiol 15:939–946

52. Steinmetz E, Rubin BG, Sanchez LA, et al (2004) Type II endoleak after endovascular abdominal aortic aneurysm repair: a conservative approach with selective intervention is safe and cost-effective. J Vasc Surg 39:306–313

53. Thoo CHC, Bourke BM, May J (2004) Symptomatic sac enlargement and rupture due to seroma after open abdominal aortic aneurysm repair with polytetrafluoroethylene graft: Implications for endovascular repair and Endotension. J Vasc Surg 40:1089–1094

15 Internal Iliac Artery Embolization in the Stent-Graft Treatment of Aortoiliac Aneurysms

Mahmood K. Razavi

CONTENTS

embolization of previously patent vessel where no collateral supply has been established. Review of the surgical literature indicates that the claudication of the buttocks and sexual dysfunction are the two most common symptoms. More serious but less commonly observed findings include bowel ischemia/necrosis [5–8], lumbosacral plexopathy [8–11], bladder or rectal sphincter dysfunction [8], and buttock or perineal necrosis in susceptible individuals [8, 11]. These complications have also been reported after IIA embolization associated with EVAR and will be further examined in this chapter.

15.1 Introduction

Endoluminal placement of stent-grafts for the repair of aortoiliac aneurysmal disease is an accepted alternative to open surgical repair. According to various reports, approximately 25%–50% of these patients will develop endoleak. The incidence of endoleak varies according to the patient's anatomy, device used, and method of post procedural surveillance. As described elsewhere in this book, the most common endoleak is type II. To reduce the risks of both type I and II endoleaks, occasionally it is necessary to embolize the internal iliac artery (IIA) to prevent retrograde flow into the aneurysm. Studies suggest that between 24% and 45% of patients undergoing endovascular aortoiliac aneurysm repair of (EVAR) will need IIA embolization [1–4]. Although the utility of this approach has been questioned [4], IIA embolization remains a common practice.

Loss or reduction of flow in IIAs is not completely benign and can be associated with various clinical symptoms. These are more likely to occur in the setting of acute IIA occlusion such as intentional

15.2 Embolization of the Internal Iliac Artery

As mentioned above, status of the internal iliac arteries is an important anatomic consideration in the treatment of aortoiliac aneurysms. Indications for embolization of IIA in association with EVAR include aneurysm of the IIA or ectatic or aneurysmal common iliac artery (CIA) involving the origin of IIA. Additionally, extension of stent-graft into the external iliac artery (EIA) may become necessary if the CIA is judged to be too short for adequate or safe anchoring of the device or if there is a distal type-I endoleak. This will lead to loss of antegrade flow in the IIA.

Occasionally, communications between branches of an uninvolved IIA and distal lumbar arteries can create type-II endoleaks (Fig. 15.1). This can be a more technically challenging situation and embolization of the distal branches should be attempted only if growth of the aneurysm sac has been documented (see Sect. 15.2.1).

15.2.1 Technical Considerations

As a general rule, the most proximal non-aneurysmal segment(s) of IIA is embolized with coils to pre-

M. K. Razavi, MD
Director, Center for Research and Clinical Trials, St. Joseph Vascular Institute, Orange, CA 92868, USA

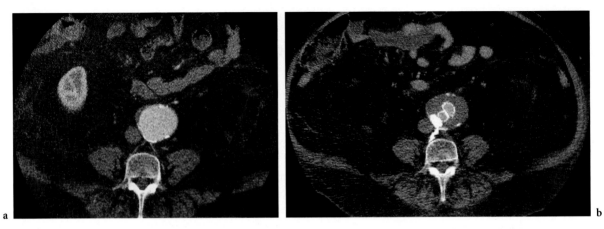

Fig. 15.1. a Contrast-enhanced CT of abdomen shows an abdominal aortic aneurysm with patent lumbar and inferior mesenteric arteries. Patient developed a type II endoleak after endograft placement. **b** Non-contrast CT shows glue embolization of the lumbar arteries and the sac through a branch of the internal iliac artery

vent retrograde flow into the aneurysm (Fig. 15.2). Attempts should be made not to interrupt the communication between the anterior and posterior trunks of the IIA when possible. This practice has been observed to reduce the complications associated with IIA embolization [12, 13].

In the setting of EVAR, coils are the embolic agents of choice. Particle or liquid agents may flow into the distal branches of IIA and cause serious complications such as perineal necrosis or ischemic radiculopathy. It has been suggested that complete cessation of antegrade flow in the target IIA during embolization is not necessary to prevent late endoleaks [12, 14]. Heye et al. embolized 53 IIAs in 45 patients prior to EVAR [14]. In 30 of these patients, antegrade flow was still present at the end of the embolization procedure. No significant difference was observed in the rate of type-II endoleaks among those patients who had complete versus partial embolization of the IIA. Similarly, Cynamon et al. observed only one retrograde leak among the 13 patients with incomplete embolization of IIAs [12]. While complete stasis of flow in the IIA may not be necessary, coil embolization should slow the flow sufficiently to cause thrombosis of the vessel after the deployment of the stent-graft. Obtaining access into the IIA after covering its origin may prove difficult if a type-II leak develops.

To achieve safe embolization, it is important to use accurately sized coils. Selection of a coil too small for the intended artery leads to its distal migration and occlusion of the non-target distal branches. Conversely, proximal dislodgement can occur in a short target area during the delivery of a coil that is either too large and/or too long. This scenario may be encountered in patients with patent proximal IIA branches such as iliolumbar or lateral sacral arteries in which coils need to be extended proximal to their origin. To reduce the risk of proximal coil dislodgment, a coaxial system can be employed for better control over the delivery. Use of detachable coils can also reduce the risk of coil misplacement when accurate deposition is necessary.

Occasionally, communications between various branches of the IIA and the lumbar arteries may cause retrograde flow into the sac of an aortic aneurysm creating a type-II endoleak. Microcatheter traversal of the entire length of these communications may not always be possible. Under such circumstances, liquid embolic agents have been employed to occlude the feeder arteries. As mentioned above, this practice may cause ischemic radiculopathy if the targeted vessels are either lateral sacral or iliolumbar arteries. It may be more prudent to coil embolize these arteries and use alternative approaches to deal with the possible residual type-II endoleak (see Chap. 14).

Manipulation of bulky devices in tortuous iliac arteries in the presence of atherosclerotic plaques or large amount of mural thrombus increases the risk of atherothrombotic embolization into the IIA or lower extremity circulations. Atherothrombotic macro or micro-embolization into the IIA may cause serious complications such as bladder, buttock, or colon infarction (see Sect. 15.2.2). Care must be taken to minimize excessive manipulation during EVAR or coil embolization of the IIAs.

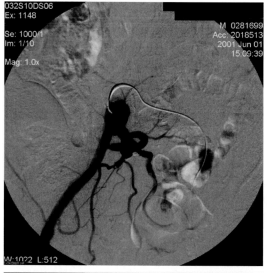
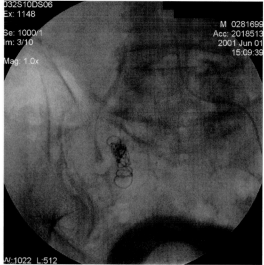
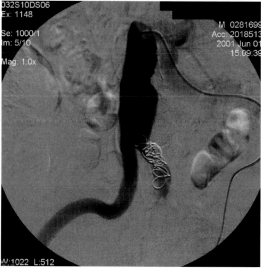

Fig. 15.2a–c. Embolization of IIA before aortic stent graft implantation (courtesy of Dr Luc Stockx). **a** Right common iliac angiogram demonstrating the internal and external iliac arteries. **b,c** Coil embolization of the proximal IIA. Note the extension of the aneurysm to the level of iliac bifurcation

15.2.1.1
Sequential vs Simultaneous Embolization of IIAs

Loss of flow in bilateral IIAs has been correlated with higher incidence of ischemic complications after EVAR [2, 15]. It has been suggested that a staged approach to IIA embolization may reduce the risks of developing symptoms [16]. This practice would presumably allow for the development of collateral circulation prior to the interruption of flow in the contralateral IIA. Although this logic appears to make intuitive sense, ENGELKE and colleagues have made the opposite observation [17]. Among 16 patients who underwent bilateral IIA embolization, eight had simultaneous occlu-

sion of IIAs and eight had sequential embolization. Patients with simultaneous embolization had a lower complication rate than those with staged embolization (12.5% vs 50%, respectively). Based on the available data, however, it is unclear if there are any advantages to staged versus simultaneous IIA embolization.

15.2.2
Complications

The need to prevent endoleaks must be balanced against the necessity to preserve the blood supply to the pelvic structures. Although the majority of patients will remain asymptomatic after the loss of IIA, maintenance of adequate pelvic blood flow has been a management problem in the open surgical treatment of patients with AAA or aortoiliac disease. Occlusion of IIAs during or after such operations has been associated with rare but serious and often life-threatening complications such as spinal cord or lumbosacral plexus ischemia, buttock necrosis, or colorectal infarction [8–11]. Such complications have also been observed in the setting of EVAR and IIA embolization (Table 15.1). These complications are discussed in more detail below.

15.2.2.1
Buttock Claudication

This is the most common sequela of the reduction or loss of flow in the IIAs. The incidence varies from 10%–50% depending on the quality of collateral circulation, location of coil deposition and whether communications between anterior and posterior divisions of IIA have been interrupted. Review of the available literature on this issue suggests that those with embolization of bilateral IIAs have a higher chance of becoming symptomatic as compared with those who had unilateral embolization [2]. Despite this finding, status of the contralateral IIA at the time of unilateral embolization does not appear to affect the outcome [1]. This conclusion is consistent with the results of ILIOPOULUS et al. concluding that the branches of the ipsilateral external iliac and femoral arterial system provide a more significant collateral pathway than the contralateral IIA [18].

Claudication is a transient condition in the majority of these patients and tends to improve or resolve over time. Thigh and buttock claudication can last anywhere from a few weeks to few years. Resolution occurs in 41%–77% of patients depending on the patients' level of activity and status of collateral circulation [1, 13, 19, 20].

15.2.2.2
Sexual Dysfunction

Another common complication of the embolization of IIA is sexual dysfunction. In the surgical literature, interruption of flow in the IIAs bilaterally has been shown to be associated with a higher rate of impotence as compared to the unilateral IIA [21–23]. This observation has also been made

in patients undergoing endovascular treatment of AAA. LIN et al. in a prospective evaluation of penile brachial index (PBI) in 12 patients undergoing either unilateral ($n=8$) or bilateral ($n=4$) IIA embolization reported a significantly higher drop in PBI in those who had bilateral IIA occlusion [15]. Patients with unilateral IIA embolization experienced 13%±14% reduction in PBI (NS). Conversely, those with bilateral IIA occlusion had 39%±14% drop in their PBI ($p<0.05$).

The reported incidence of sexual dysfunction varies between 2.5% to 36% after IIA flow interruption (Table 15.1). The true risk of sexual dysfunction may be higher than reported. The high rate of pre-existing sexual dysfunction among this patient population may mask the true incidence of this complication. Furthermore, the inherent inaccuracy of personal interviews and questionnaires in establishing the diagnosis and causes of sexual dysfunction introduces an unknown risk of error in results obtained in this fashion [24, 25].

15.2.2.3
Colon Ischemia

Ischemic colitis is a rare but serious complication after loss of flow in IIAs. Acute mesenteric ischemia develops in 1%–3% of the patients undergoing surgery for AAA repair [7, 26]. The risk factors for the development of mesenteric ischemia in such patients include ruptured AAA and shock, prolonged operating and cross-clamping times, and ligation of one or both IIAs [5, 7, 27]. It appears that the ligation or loss of the IMA does not significantly enhance the risk of colon ischemia in the presence of a normal SMA. This is due to the existence of collaterals between the two arteries. Prior bowel resection, however, may interrupt these collaterals and predispose the patient to the risk of complications.

Colon ischemia has also been reported after IIA embolization [20, 28]. KARCH et al. reported this complication in three of their 22 patients (14%) who had undergone IIA embolization [28]. All three patients had either accidental or intentional occlusion of bilateral IIAs during EVAR. The true risk of colon ischemia after IIA embolization, however, is difficult to quantify. This is due to the small number of reported cases and is likely to be substantially less than what was observed by KARCH et al. and similar to that of the open surgical AAA repair.

Although confounding risk factors for bowel ischemia such as significant blood loss, aortic

Table 15.1. Summary of studies reporting embolization of internal iliac arteries in association with endovascular treatment of aortoiliac aneurysms

Author/year of publication	Patients with IIA emboliza- tion	Unilateral/ bilateral emboliza- tion	Percentage of patients developing symptoms			Comments
			Claudi- cation	Sexual dysfunction	Other	
Razavi/2000 [1]	32	25/7	28%	16%[a]	3%	Sx more common among those with IA than AAA
Lee/2000 [19]	28	NR	18%	4%	4%	
Cynamon/2000 [12]	32	NR	40%	NR	NR	
Criado/2000 [3]	39	28/11	13%	2.5%	NR	
Karch/2000 [28]	22		32%	NR	13.5%	Three patients developed colon ischemia
Yano/2001 [20]	103	92/11	11.5%	8.5%	1%	One patient developed colon ischemia
Wolpert/2001 [35]	18	11/7	50%	11%	0	
Mehta/2001 [36]	154	134/20	11%	6%	1%	47 Patients had open repair
Schoder/2001 [2]	55	46/9	45%	25%[b]	NR	Sx more common among those with bilateral IIA embolization
Lin/2002 [15]	12	8/4	50%	36%	16%	Prospective study; two patients developed peri- neal necrosis
Heye/2005 [14]	45	37/8	35%	NR	4.5%	Two patients developed ischemic neuropathy

[a] This refers to the percentage of patients without prior sexual dysfunction who developed new symptoms.
[b] Five of 20 men in this study developed erectile dysfunction.
AAA, Abdominal aortic aneurysm; *IIA*, internal iliac aneurysm; *NR*, not reported; *Sx*, symptoms.

cross-clamping, bowel retraction, and procedural circulatory instability are not typical features of an endovascular approach, microembolization into the colonic vasculature can occur as a result of excessive endovascular manipulation causing bowel infarction. Dadian et al. [29] reported overt colon ischemia in eight (2.9%) of their patients after EVAR without IIA embolization. Pathologic examination revealed evidence of atheroemboli in the colonic vasculature. Geraghty et al. made a similar observation in four patients (1.7%) with bilaterally patent IIAs [30]. These observations underscores the importance of preservation of distal IIA flow when possible.

We should emphasize, however, that the IMA exclusion or embolization in patients with SMA stenosis or prior partial colectomy where the collateral pathways between the IMA and SMA have been interrupted, is not advised [31].

15.2.2.4
Perineal Ischemia/Necrosis

Perineal skin necrosis is another rare complications of IIA devascularization and has been reported after IIA embolization [15]. This serious complication is associated more frequently with bilateral IIA occlusion. The major predisposing factor appears to be poor collateral circulation in chronically bed-ridden patients.

15.2.2.5
Lumbosacral Plexus Ischemia

Embolization of the IIA or its branches (lumbosacral or lateral sacral arteries) may cause ischemia of the lumbosacral nerve roots. The pain associated with this condition resembles nerve root compression and can be mistaken for buttock and thigh claudication. The pain and discomfort is usually more intense, lasts longer, and may be associated with ipsilateral weakness. This condition can be precipitated by unilateral IIA embolization and should be considered in patients with persistent symptoms.

15.2.3
Prevention

Preventive measures such as surgical or endovascular revascularization of IIA may become necessary in patients who are at high risk of developing complications after IIA embolization (Table 15.2). Surgical bypass to IIA has been reported with good outcome in this setting [32]. Use of endografts with fenestrated iliac limbs is another alternative in such individuals.

A patient's ability to tolerate IIA embolization may be tested by temporary balloon occlusion of the target artery and measurement of the penile brachial index (PBI) pre and post IIA balloon occlusion. This can assess the risk of post procedure impotence. A

Table 15.2. Factors predisposing to development of symptoms after IIA embolization

1. Poor quantity or quality of collateral circulation
   a. > 70% Stenosis of the patent IIA
   b. Diseased ipsilateral profunda or its superior branches
   c. Absent ipsilateral circumflex iliac
   d. Absence of a complete arc of Riolan
2. Isolated iliac aneurysms
3. Embolization of bilateral IIAs
4. Embolization distal to the division of anterior and posterior trunks of IIA
5. Age > 75 years
6. Atherothrombotic embolization during EVAR

PBI of less than 0.7 may indicate vasculogenic impotence. Similarly, monitoring the superior rectal arterial signal using a transrectal Doppler probe during balloon occlusion of IIA will test the adequacy of mesenteric collaterals. Disappearance of the signal that does not reappear within 15 min may signal poor collateral circulation and a high risk of colonic ischemia [33].

Another reliable measure of poor circulation to colon is the direct quantification of mucosal oxygenation by a rectal probe [34]. A small disposable rectal probe with an atraumatic tip is inserted into the rectum and oxygenation of the mucosa measured. If the levels drop below a certain critical level after balloon occlusion of the IIA, that patient is not a candidate for IIA embolization.

15.2.4
Conclusion

Although the incidence of serious complications such as colonic, lumbosacral plexus, or buttock necrosis is low after IIA embolization, the incidence of claudication and sexual dysfunction is high enough to warrant preservation of the IIA circulation if possible. In final analysis, the decision whether to embolize an IIA or not should be weighed against the potential risks and benefits of the other therapeutic alternatives. The risk of development of such symptoms as claudication or sexual dysfunction may outweigh the hazards of IIA revascularization or aneurysm rupture and death if no action is taken.

References

1. Razavi M, DeGroot M, Olcott C, Sze D, Kee S, Semba C, Dake M (2000) Embolization of the internal iliac artery in stent-graft treatment of aorto-iliac aneurysms: Analysis of complications and outcome. J Vasc Interv Radiol 11:561–566
2. Schoder M, Zaunbauer L, Holzenbein T et al. (2001) Internal iliac artery embolization before endovascular repair of abdominal aortic aneurysms: frequency, efficacy, and clinical results. Am J Roentgenol 177:599–605
3. Criado FJ, Wilson EP, Velazquez OC et al. (2000) Safety of coil embolization of the internal iliac artery in endovascular grafting of abdominal aortic aneurysms. J Vasc Surg 32:684–688
4. Tefera G, turnipseed WD, Carr SC et al. (2004) Is coil embolization of hypogastric artery necessary during endovascular treatment of aortoiliac aneurysms? Ann Vasc Surg 18:143–146
5. Jarvinen O, Laurikka J, Sisto T, Tarkka MR (1996) Intestinal ischemia following surgery for aorto-iliac disease. A review of 502 consecutive aortic reconstructions. Vasa 25:148–155
6. Pittaluga P, Batt M, Hassen-Khodja R, Declemy S, Le Bas P (1998) Revascularization of internal iliac arteries during aortoiliac surgery: a multicenter study. Ann Vasc Surg 12:537–543
7. Bjorck M, Troeng T, Bergqvist D (1997) Risk factors for intestinal ischaemia after aortoiliac surgery: a combined cohort and case-control study of 2824 operations. Eur J Vasc Endovasc Surg 13:531–539
8. Iliopoulos JI, Howanitz PE, Pierce GE, Kueshkerian SM, Thomas JH, Hermreck AS (1987) The critical hypogastric circulation. Am J Surg 154:671–675
9. Gloviczki P, Cross SA, Stanson AW, Carmichael SW, Bower TC, Pairolero PC, Hallett JW, Jr, Toomey BJ, Cherry KJ Jr. (1991) Ischemic injury to the spinal cord or lumbosacral plexus after aorto-iliac reconstruction. Am J Surg 162:131–136
10. Hefty TR, Nelson KA, Hatch TR, Barry JM (1990) Acute lumbosacral plexopathy in diabetic women after renal transplantation. J Urol 143:107–109
11. Picone AL, Green RM, Ricotta JR, May AG, DeWeese JA (1986) Spinal cord ischemia following operations on the abdominal aorta. Vasc Surg 3:94–103
12. Cynamon J, Lerer D, Veith F et al. (2000) Hypogastric artery coil embolization prior to endoluminal repair of aneurysms and fistulas: buttock claudication, a recognized but possibly preventable complication. J Vasc Interv radiol 11:543–545
13. Kritpracha B, Pigott JP, Price CI et al. (2003) Distal internal iliac artery embolization: a procedure to avoid. J Vasc Surg 37:943–948
14. Heye S, Nevelsteen A, Maleux G (2005) Internal iliac artery coil embolization in the prevention of potential type-2 endoleak after endovascular repair of abdominal aortic

and iliac aneurysms: effect of total occlusion versus residual flow. J Vasc Interv Radiol 16:235–239

15. Lin PH, Bush RL, Chaikof EL et al. (2002) A prospective evaluation of hypogastric artery embolization in endovascular aortoiliac aneurysm repair. J Vasc Surg 36:500–506

16. Mehta M, Veith FJ, Darling RC et al. (2004) Effects of bilateral hypogastric artery interruption during endovascular and open aortoiliac aneurysm repair. J Vasc Surg 40:698–702

17. Engelke C, Elford J, Morgan RA, Belli AM (2002) Internal iliac artery embolization with bilateral occlusion before endovascular aortoiliac aneurysm repair- clinical outcome of simultaneous and sequential intervention. J Vasc Interv Radiol 13:667–676

18. Iliopoulos JI, Hermreck AS, Thomas JH, Pierce GE (1989) Hemodynamics of the hypogastric arterial circulation. J Vasc Surg 9:637–641; discussion 641–642

19. Lee CW, Kaufman JA, Fan CM et al. (2000) Clinical outcome of internal iliac artery occlusions during endovascular treatment of aortoiliac aneurysmal diseases. J Vasc Interv Radiol 11:543–545

20. Yano OJ, Morrissey N, Eisen L et al. (2001) Intentional internal iliac artery occlusion to facilitate endovascular repair of aortoiliac aneurysms. J Vasc Surg 34:204–211

21. Burns JR, Houttuin E, Gregory JG, Hawatmeh IS, Sullivan TR (1979) Vascular-induced erectile impotence in renal transplant recipients. J Urol 121:721–723

22. Gittes RF, Waters WB (1979) Sexual impotence: the overlooked complication of a second renal transplant. J Urol 121:719–720

23. Billet A, Davis A, Linhardt GE Jr, Queral LA, Dagher FJ, Williams GM (1984) The effects of bilateral renal transplantation on pelvic hemodynamics and sexual function. Surgery. 95:415–419

24. Brannen GE, Peters TG, Hambidge KM, Kumpe DA, Kempczinski RF, Schroter GP, Weil R (1980) Impotence after kidney transplantation. Urology 15:138–146

25. Levy NB (1973) Sexual adjustment to maintenance hemodialysis and renal transplantation: national survey by questionnaire: preliminary report. Trans Am Soc Artif Intern Organs 19:138–143

26. Brewster DC, Franklin DP, Cambria RP, Darling RC, Moncure AC, Lamuraglia GM, Stone WM, Abbott WM (1991) Intestinal ischemia complicating abdominal aortic surgery. Surgery 109:447–454

27. Kim MW, Hundahl SA, Dang CR, McNamara JJ, Straehley CJ, Whelan TJ Jr. (1983) Ischemic colitis after aortic aneurysmectomy. Am J Surg 145:392–394

28. Karch LA, Hodgson KJ, Mattos MA et al. (2000) Adverse consequences of internal iliac artery occlusion during endovascular repair of abdominal aortic aneurysm. J Vasc Surg 32:676–683

29. Dadian N, Ohki T, Veith FJ et al. (2001) Overt colon ischemia after endovascular repair: the importance of microembolization as an etiology. J Vasc Surg 34:986–996

30. Geraghty PJ, Sanchez LA, Rubin BG et al. (2004) Overt ischemic colitis after endovascular repair of aortoiliac aneurysms. J Vasc Surg 40:413–418

31. Crawford ES, Morris GC, Myhre HO, Roehm JO (1977) Celiac axis, superior mesenteric artery, and inferior mesenteric artery occlusion: surgical considerations. Surgery 82:856–866

32. Faries PL, Morrissey N, Burks JA et al. (2001) Internal iliac artery revascularization as an adjunct to endovascular repair of aortoiliac aneurysms. J Vasc Surg 34:892–899

33. Iwai T, Sakurazawa K, Sata S, Muraoka Y, Inoue Y, Endo M (1991) Intra-operative monitoring of the pelvic circulation using a transanal Doppler probe. Eur J Vasc Surg 5:71–74

34. Benaron DA, Parachikov IH, Friedland S, Soetikno R, Brock-Utne J, van der Starre PJ, Nezhat C, Terris MK, Maxim PG, Carson JJ, Razavi MK, Gladstone HB, Fincher EF, Hsu CP, Clark FL, Cheong WF, Duckworth JL, Stevenson DK (2004) Continuous, noninvasive, and localized microvascular tissue oximetry using visible light spectroscopy. Anesthesiology 100:1469–1475

35. Wolpert LM, Dittrich KP, Hallisey MJ, et al. (2001) Hypogasteric artery embolization in endovascular AAA repait. J Vasc Surg 33:1193–8

36. Mehta M, Veith FJ, Ohki T, et al. (2001) Unilateral and bilateral hypogasteric artery interruption during aortoiliac aneurysm repair in 154 patients: a relatively innocuous procedure. J Vasc Surg 33(suppl):S27–32

Respiratory System

16 Bronchial Artery Embolization

JOS C. VAN DEN BERG

16.1
Introduction

Massive hemoptysis represents a major medical emergency that is associated with a high mortality.

Bronchial artery embolization was first described in the literature in the 1970s by REMY [1], and over time it has become a well established treatment for patients with (massive) hemoptysis [2–5]. Technical improvements in both catheters and embolizing agents have attributed to the increase of the safety of the procedure and it's applicability.

In this chapter the pathophysiology and etiology of hemoptysis will be discussed, as well as the diagnostic work-up of patients suffering from severe bronchial bleeding. Anatomy of bronchial arterial supply will be described. The techniques, pitfalls, complications and results of bronchial artery embolization will be discussed.

J. C. VAN DEN BERG, MD, PhD
Head of the Service of Interventional Radiology, Ospedale Regionale di Lugano, sede Civico, Via Tesserete 46, 6900 Lugano, Switzerland

16.2
Pathophysiology and Etiology

Expectoration of blood, or hemoptysis, is a potentially life threatening condition. Massive hemoptysis in non-trauma patients is reported to carry 35%–85% mortality. Death from hemoptysis is rarely caused by exsanguination, but rather by asphyxia that results from flooding of the airways and alveoli with blood [6]. Hemoptysis is considered severe or massive when the total amount of blood expectorated exceeds 300–600 mL over a 24-h period [7–9]. Hemoptysis is defined to be trivial when only drops of blood or bloody sputum are present, and moderate with a blood loss of less then 200 mL/24 h [7].

Hemoptysis has a propensity to recur if definitive therapy is not instituted. Patients presenting with massive hemoptysis who underwent medical therapy alone, had recurrence within 6 months after discharge, with a fatal outcome in about half of the patients [10].

In the vast majority (90%) of cases the source of the bleeding is the bronchial circulation. Bleeding from the pulmonary circulation (e.g. pulmonary arteriovenous malformation, pulmonary endometriosis, pulmonary aneurysm, injury from Swan-Ganz catheter [11, 12]) and hemorrhage directly from the aorta (e.g. aortobronchial fistula and ruptured thoracic aneurysm) or non-bronchial systemic arterial supply to the lungs each account for 5% of the cases. Hemoptysis of pulmonary and direct aortic origin will not be discussed in this chapter.

In most patients with hemoptysis the underlying cause is chronic or acute inflammatory lung disease, including pulmonary tuberculosis, bronchiectasis, cystic fibrosis and aspergilloma. All possible causes of hemoptysis are listed in Table 16.1.

In patients with acute or chronic lung diseases (who constitute the majority of those presenting with hemoptysis) pulmonary circulation is reduced or completely blocked due to hypoxic vasoconstriction, thrombosis and vasculitis at the level of the

Table 16.1. List of causes of hemoptysis

Infectious

    Bronchiectasis
    (Necrotizing) pneumonia
    Chronic bronchitis
    Lung abscess
    Aspergillosis/mycetoma
    Tuberculosis
    Nontuberculous mycobacterial infection
    Cystic fibrosis

Neoplasm

    Carcinoma
    Bronchial adenoma
    Bronchial carcinoid
    Metastatic disease
    Endometriosis

Cardiovascular

    Severe left ventricular heart failure
    Mitral stenosis
    Pulmonary embolism or infarction
    Aortic aneurysm
    Pulmonary aneurysm
    Bronchovascular fistula
    AV-malformation
    Iatrogenic lesions (e.g. Swann-Ganz)

Vasculitic

    Wegener's granulomatosis
    Systemic lupus erythematosus
    Goodpasture's syndrome

Miscellaneous

    Idiopathic pulmonary hemosiderosis
    Aspirated foreign body
    Pulmonary trauma or contusion
    Post-biopsy (transthoracic/transbronchial)
    Use of anticoagulants/fibrinolytics

pulmonary arterioles. This leads to proliferation and enlargement of the bronchial arteries in an attempt to compensate for the reduced pulmonary circulation. In patients with bronchiectasis blood circulation can increase and may represent as much as 30% of cardiac output [13]. In the inflamed surroundings the bronchial arteries are prone to rupture due to direct erosion by a bacterial agent in combination with the presence of a locally elevated blood pressure. The bronchial arteries being part of the systemic circulation implies that extravasation of blood into the bronchial tree occurs under sys-

temic arterial pressure, and thus results in massive bleeding [8, 14].

16.3
Diagnostic Work-Up

The most commonly used diagnostic modalities to find the cause of the hemoptysis and to identify the pulmonary lobes in which the bleeding is localized are conventional radiography, fiberoptic bronchoscopy and CT. Knowledge of the localization of the bleeding is of importance for the interventionalist in order to facilitate the subsequent embolization procedure.

16.3.1
Conventional Radiography

Although frequently performed because of its availability, the diagnostic yield of conventional radiography is low. In 17%–81% of patients with hemoptysis radiographic findings are normal, or do not help in localizing the bleeding source. Overall chest radiographs are diagnostic in about half of the cases [7, 8, 15].

16.3.2
Fiberoptic Bronchoscopy

Bronchoscopy is generally considered the modality of choice in the diagnosis and management of patients with hemoptysis. It has the advantage that it can identify central bronchial lesions, such as carcinoma, that generally are not considered candidates for bronchial artery embolization. Furthermore fiberoptic bronchoscopy can be used to administer vasoconstrictive drugs to control bleeding. Bronchoscopy can localize the bleeding site in up to 93% of cases, but the diagnostic accuracy of fiberoptic bronchoscopy drops considerably in patients who have a normal chest radiograph (range 0%–31%). The overall diagnostic accuracy of bronchoscopy in all patients with hemoptysis (irrespective of findings at conventional radiography) is reported to be 10%–43% [7, 16, 17]. Major source of difficulty is in patients with massive bleeding where blood may fill up all ipsilateral lobar bronchi and even the contralateral main stem bronchus. In patients with known causation of hemoptysis, in which the site of bleeding can be determined from conventional radiographs fiberoptic bronchoscopy has been demonstrated to be of little added value [15].

16.3.3
CT

CT offers the possibility to demonstrate both airway and vascular pathology (e.g. bronchiectasis, bronchogenic carcinoma, aneurysmal disease of the thoracic aorta), and has been reported to be the modality of first choice in patients with hemoptysis [18]. In patients who have a non-diagnostic fiberoptic bronchoscopy, CT can provide a diagnosis in half of the cases, while in patients with non-conclusive chest radiography this rate varies from 39% to 88% [16, 17]. Localization of the bleeding site can be achieved in 63%–100% of all cases [7, 15]. Current multidetector CT scanners also allow visualization of bronchial and non-bronchial systemic artery anatomy, and may thus be of help for the interventionalist to plan the procedure [8, 13, 19, 20].

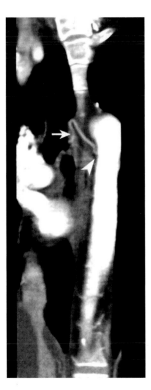

Fig. 16.1. Curved multiplanar reconstruction of CT of the thoracic aorta, clearly demonstrating the origin (*arrowhead*) and bifurcation into intercostal branches and bronchial artery (*arrow*) of right intercostobronchial trunk

16.4
Anatomy

16.4.1
Bronchial Artery Anatomy

Almost all bronchial arteries originate from the thoracic aorta between the level of T4 and T7 [21, 22], with 90% originating between the upper border of T5 and the lower border of T6 [23]. There are usually two bronchial arteries supplying the right. The first commonly arises from the descending aorta as a common intercostobronchial trunk with the third right posterior intercostal artery, and has a posterolaterally lying orifice. This right intercostobronchial artery commonly has an initial vertical or oblique course upward. On CT it can be identified to the right of the retroesophageal space (Fig. 16.1) [13]. The second important artery is the common right and left bronchial artery that arises from the anterior surface and supplies both lungs. On the left side a separate left bronchial artery is usually present, and arises from the anterolateral surface of the aorta. In a cadaveric study the right intercostobronchial trunk was present in 97.5% of cases, with an associated accessory right bronchial artery in 7.5% of cases. A common bronchial trunk was present in half of the cases, and

the left bronchial arterial system was characterized by the presence of a direct left bronchial artery in 76% of cases and a double left bronchial artery in 20% (Fig. 16.2) [23]. It is extremely rare that a left bronchial artery arises from a common trunk of an intercostobronchial artery.

At fluoroscopy in the AP-projection, the vast majority of the bronchial arteries have their origin at the level where the left main stem bronchus overlies the aorta, slightly below the level of the tracheal carina (Fig. 16.3) [19, 24].

Four classical bronchial artery patterns have been identified [8]:

- Type I: two bronchial arteries on the left, and one on the right (intercostobronchial trunk); present in 40% of cases.
- Type II: one bronchial artery on the left and one intercostobronchial artery on the right; present in 20% of cases.
- Type III: two bronchial arteries on the left, and a bronchial artery and an intercostobronchial artery on the right; present in 20% of cases.
- Type IV: one bronchial artery on the left, and a bronchial artery and an intercostobronchial artery on the right; present in 10% of cases.

In real terms, it is not uncommon among the western population that left and right bronchial

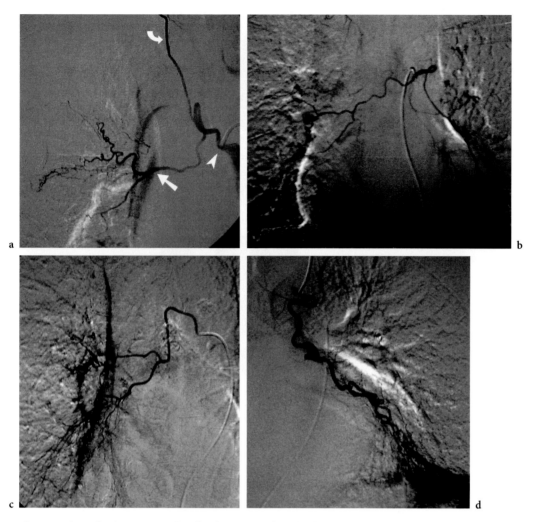

Fig. 16.2a–d. a Selective angiography of right intercostobronchial trunk: catheter tip at level of ostium (*arrowhead*); representation of right bronchial artery (*arrow*) and intercostal branch (*curved arrow*). **b** Selective angiography of common bronchial trunk; division into left and right bronchial artery. **c** Selective angiography of right bronchial artery, originating directly from the aorta. **d** Selective angiography of left bronchial artery, originating directly from the aorta

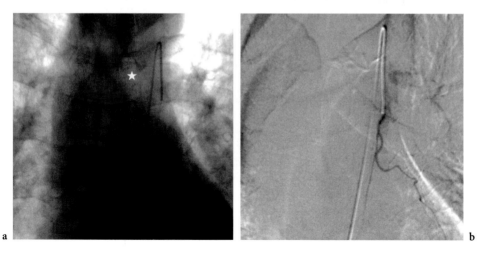

Fig. 16.3. a Fluoroscopic image demonstrating relationship of catheter tip with respect to left main stem bronchus (*asterisk*). **b** Selective angiography in same patient as (**a**): visualization of left bronchial artery

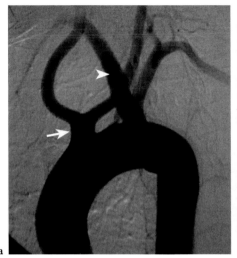
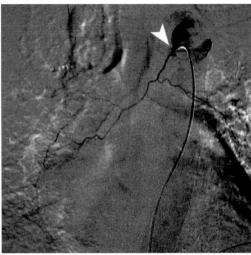

a   b

Fig. 16.4. a Aortic arch angiography in patient with common origin of right and left common carotid artery (*arrow*), and right subclavian artery (*arrow head*) with origin at he level of the proximal descending thoracic aorta (arteria lusoria). b Selective angiography demonstrating common bronchial trunk with origin at the level of the aortic arch (*arrowhead*)

arteries arise from the aorta as a common trunk (up to 48%).

The bronchial arteries supply the trachea, pulmonary airways (both intra- and extrapulmonary), regional lymph nodes, (visceral) pleura, esophagus, and vasa vasorum of aorta and pulmonary artery and vein.

Many variations occur, and bronchial arteries may have their origins from the aortic arch (Fig. 16.4), internal thoracic or mammary artery (Fig. 16.5), thyrocervical and costocervical trunk, innominate artery, left subclavian artery and inferior thyroid artery, inferior phrenic artery or abdominal aorta [22]. A key finding in aberrant bronchial arteries, that distinguishes them anatomically and angiographically from non-bronchial systemic collateral vessels, is their course following the branching of the major bronchi [22]. Non-bronchial systemic collateral circulation (that can develop after successful embolization of bronchial arterial supply) usually enter the lung parenchyma through adjacent pleura or the pulmonary ligament, and have a typical course that does not parallel the bronchial tree.

Communications between bronchial arteries and systemic vessels are ubiquitous, and can sometimes complicate an embolization procedure. The most commonly seen communication is that of a right intercostobronchial trunk with an anterior medullary artery that contributes to the vascular supply of the spinal cord through the anterior spinal artery. The anterior medullary arteries have a characteristic 'hairpin' configuration, and follow a course

parallel to the spinal cord (Fig. 16.6) [25]. Other less commonly seen communications are with the left or right subclavian artery (Fig. 16.7) [26, 27], and right coronary artery (Fig. 16.8) [28].

Normal bronchial arteries have a diameter of less then 1.5 mm at their origin, and 0.5 mm at the level of the entrance into a bronchopulmonary segment. Pathologic features of the bronchial artery are

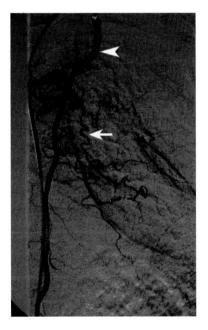

Fig. 16.5. Selective angiography of the left internal mammary artery (*arrowhead*), giving off bronchial arterial branches (*arrow*)

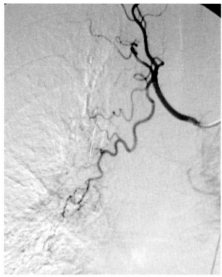

a

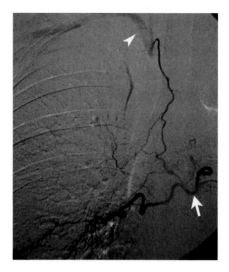

Fig. 16.7. Selective angiography of right intercostobronchial trunk (*arrow*), demonstrating connection with the right subclavian artery (*arrowhead*)

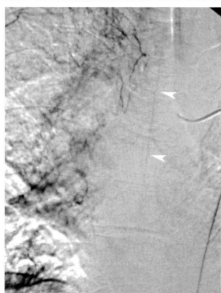

b

Fig. 16.6. **a** Selective angiography of right intercostobronchial trunk, early phase. **b** Selective angiography of right intercostobronchial trunk, late phase demonstrating thin arterial structure, with course parallel to vertebral column: anterior spinal artery (*arrowheads*)

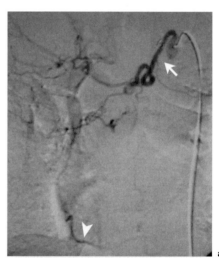

a

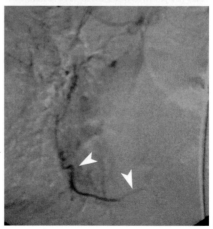

b

Fig. 16.8. **a** Selective angiography of right bronchial artery (*arrow*), early phase, demonstrating connection with a vessel overlying the heart (*arrowhead*). **b** Selective angiography of right bronchial artery, late phase: typical filling pattern distally of right coronary artery (*arrowheads*)

hypertrophy (in a study comparing multi-detector row CT and selective angiography an average of one-third of the bronchial arteries showed dilatation over 1.5 mm [19]) and tortuosity (Fig. 16.9), neo- and hypervascularity, vascular blush, dense soft tissue staining (Fig. 16.10), shunting into the pulmonary vascular system (arterial or venous; Figs. 16.10 and 16.11), extravasation of contrast medium into the alveoli or bronchial tree (Fig. 16.12) and formation of bronchial artery aneurysm/pseudoaneurysm [9, 15, 29–31].

16.4.2
Non-bronchial Systemic Artery Anatomy

Several non-bronchial systemic arteries have been identified as possible sources of hemoptysis, especially in patients after repeat bronchial artery embolization, and in patients who have concomitant pleural involvement of disease. In one-third to 45% of patients a significant blood supply from non-bronchial arteries contributes to the hemoptysis [32, 33]. Pathologic vessels may originate from intercostals arteries, branches of subclavian and axillary arteries (e.g. thyrocervical trunk; Fig. 16.13), internal mammary artery (Fig. 16.14), phrenic arteries (Fig. 16.15) and left gastric artery [34]. CT angiography can be useful in identifying pathologic vasculature in patients with pleural thickening and hemoptysis [8].

16.5
Technique of Bronchial Artery Embolization

The first priority in treating patients with life-threatening hemoptysis is to maintain the airway, optimize oxygenation and stabilize the hemody-

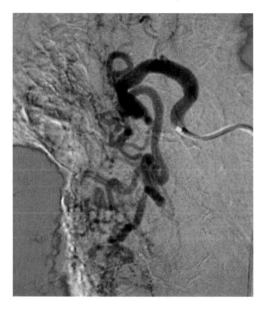

Fig. 16.9. Selective angiography of right bronchial artery, demonstrating hypertrophy and tortuosity

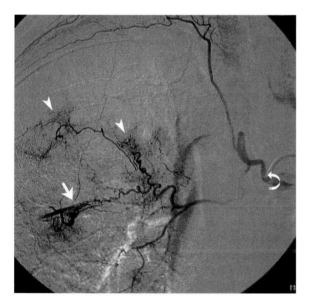

Fig. 16.10. Selective angiography of right intercostobronchial trunk (*curved arrow*), depicting pathologic blush (*arrowheads*), and shunting to pulmonary circulation (*arrow*)

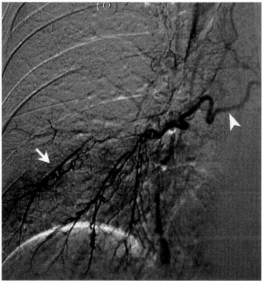

Fig. 16.11. Selective angiography of right intercostobronchial trunk (*arrowhead*), depicting shunting to pulmonary circulation (*arrow*)

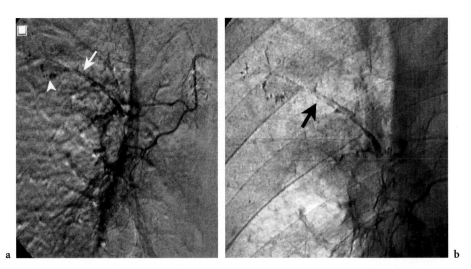

Fig. 16.12. a Superselective angiography of bronchial branch of right intercostobronchial artery, demonstrating extravasation of contrast into alveoli (*arrowhead*) and bronchi (*arrow*). **b** Non-subtracted image, depicting to advantage presence of contrast medium in the bronchus (*arrow*)

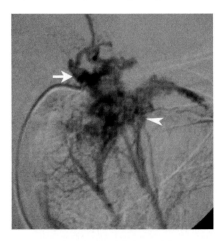

Fig. 16.13. Selective catheterization of thyrocervical trunk (*arrow*), demonstrating pathologic enhancement of left apical region and pulmonary shunting (*arrowhead*)

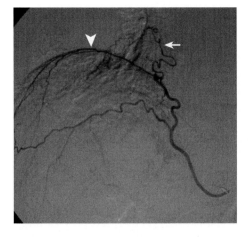

Fig. 16.15. Selective angiography of right phrenic artery (*arrowhead*), connection with pathologic intrapulmonary vessels is clearly depicted (*arrow*)

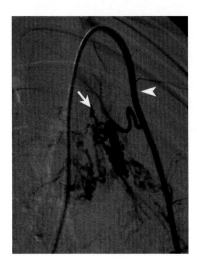

Fig. 16.14. Selective angiography of left internal mammary artery (*arrowhead*), with pleural connections supplying intrapulmonary pathologic vasculature (*arrow*)

namic status, followed by the embolization procedure [6, 35].

After standard preparation the common femoral artery is punctured, an introduction sheath (4 F or 5 F), and a flush catheter is advanced into the upper part of the descending thoracic aorta. A diagnostic angiography is performed in an AP projection. The flush aortogram is used to identify any pathologic bronchial artery [36]. The injection rate is no less than 25 ml/s and lasts at least 2 s. The flush catheter is then exchanged for a selective diagnostic catheter that needs to have a minimum length of 100 cm, a lumen of 0.038" and should not have side holes. The latter is of utmost importance since in some cases the selective catheter can not be advanced into the target vessel beyond a point at which the side holes are still at the level of the aorta (a position that would lead to inadvertent spill of embolic agents into the aorta). The most commonly used selective catheters are cobra-curved or Simmons-type catheters. The Simmons catheter can be used with the tip of the catheter pointing cranially in the descending thoracic aorta (i.e. without reforming it's shape in the aortic arch; Fig. 16.16a), or in the classical way (after re-shaping in the arch). In the former configuration bronchial arteries that have an origin with an upward oriented, acute angle with respect to the aorta can be cannulated. Given the large variety in anatomy a range of diagnostic catheters should be at hand, and should include mammary catheters, multi-purpose and specific bronchial artery catheters.

Selective angiography is then performed using hand-injection (frame rate 3/s). The selective angiography serves to establish the presence of pathologic vasculature and to demonstrate any connections to other vascular territories (e.g. anterior spinal artery). If any side branches of importance are present attempts should be made to advance the tip of the catheter beyond the point of the origin of these branches. This super-selective catheterization can be performed by advancing the 4-F catheter using a Glidewire where care should be taken not to create spasm or dissection. As an alternative a microcatheter can be used, that is placed through the diagnostic catheter (co-axial system; Figs. 16.16b,c, Fig. 16.17) and that is fixed to the diagnostic catheter with a

Y-connector (Fig. 16.18). The latter also allows for continuous flushing of the guiding catheter. Alternatively, a side hole can be created in a diagnostic catheter (at a distance from the tip as determined by the operator), which can serve as an exit for a microcatheter. This technique has been described to be helpful in the embolization of proximal subclavian arterial branches, when stable catheter position cannot be achieved in other ways [21]. In a similar fashion catheters with pre-fabricated side holes can be used in difficult anatomical situations [37].

Finally a microcatheter can be used as a "tapered" extension of a 4-F diagnostic catheter, in cases where the diameter of the ostium of the target vessel is smaller than the outer diameter of the diagnostic catheter (Fig. 16.19).

Before proceeding to the embolization of the target vessel, stability of the catheter tip and absence of backflow into the descending thoracic aorta should be confirmed by means of a test-injection using contrast medium.

The embolic agents of choice are non-absorbable particles (see below). These particles are administered through a three-way stopcock with small tubing that is connected to either the 4-F diagnostic catheter or microcatheter (Fig. 16.20). The embolic particles should be dispersed into contrast medium, in order to allow visualization of any backflow and to monitor for slowing of flow, which is indicative of progression of distal embolization. Preferably 1-ml syringes are used. Advantages of the three-

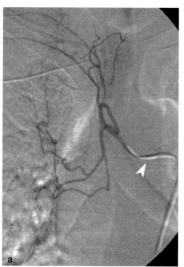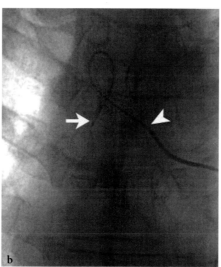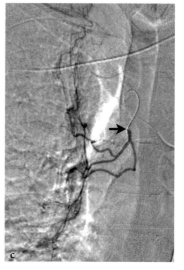

Fig. 16.16a–c. a Selective catherization of right intercostobronchial trunk with Simmons type 1 catheter; notice non-reformed shape, with point of catheter pointing upwards (*arrowhead*); filling of both intercostal and bronchial branches. **b** Same patient as in (**a**), after advancement of microcatheter (*arrow*) through 4-F diagnostic catheter (*arrowhead*). **c** Superselective angiography through microcatheter; no flow into intercostal branches is seen, with clear depiction of bronchial vasculature (*arrow*)

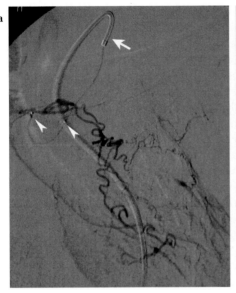
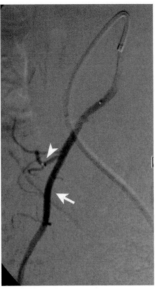

Fig. 16.17. a Superselective angiography of bronchial artery originating from left internal mammary artery (same patient as Fig. 16.5); diagnostic 5-F mammary catheter (*arrow*) and markers on microcatheter (*arrowheads*) are clearly seen. **b** Control angiography after embolization performed through diagnostic catheter demonstrates absence of filling of pathologic vasculature (*arrowhead*) and patency of distal internal mammary artery (*arrow*)

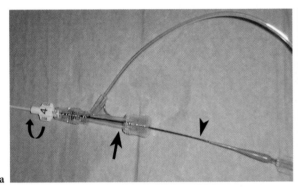
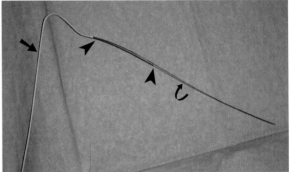

Fig. 16.18. a Microcatheter (*arrowhead*) introduced through Y-connector (*arrow*) that is connected to 4-F diagnostic catheter (*curved arrow*). **b** Microcatheter (*arrowheads*), with accompanying guidewire (*curved arrow*), protruding from diagnostic catheter (*arrow*); this allows for superselective catheterization

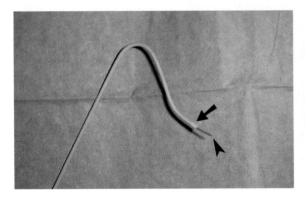
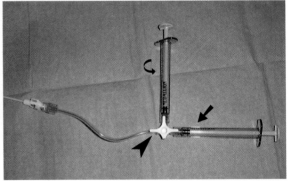

Fig. 16.19. Microcatheter (*arrowhead*) protruding several millimeters from the tip of diagnostic catheter (*arrow*); this allows for cannulation of small diameter ostia of bronchial arteries

Fig. 16.20. Three-way stopcock with tubing (*arrowhead*), connected to two 1-ml syringes; one syringe is used for administration of the embolic agent mixed with contrast (*arrow*), while the other syringe is used for flushing with saline

way stopcock are that frequent solution exchanges between two syringes can be performed to maintain the particles in a suspended condition, and that the catheter can be flushed easily with saline, without disconnecting the syringe filled with the mixture of contrast and microparticles. Care should be taken to keep only one syringe reserved for the embolic agent, in order to avoid inadvertent injection of embolic particles (e.g. during control angiography). Throughout the procedure regular angiographic controls should be performed, in order to detect appearance of previously not visible connections to other vascular territories such as the anterior spinal artery. After occlusion of peripheral bronchial artery branches, which leads to an increase of resistance both distally and centrally, particles may reflux into side branches not detected initially [38, 39]. After successful embolization of all pathologic bronchial arteries as visualized on the flush angiography in the above-described manner, it is recommended to perform another aortic angiography in order to scrutinize for any pathologic vessels previously not visible. When present, these vessels should also be embolized. This approach helps in reducing the number of recurrences.

In the future the need for flush aortography prior to and after embolization may be obviated, when the use of multi-detector row CT becomes more and more common. There are indications that the use of thin-section CT scanning reduces procedural time, as well as the potential iatrogenic risks of a selective search for ectopic bronchial or abnormal non-bronchial systemic arteries [19].

Table 16.2 lists the materials most commonly used for bronchial artery embolization.

16.5.1
Embolic Agents

Various embolic agents can be employed for bronchial artery embolization, and include gelatin sponge, microspheres and coils.

Absorbable gelatin sponge is readily available, inexpensive and easy to handle. Disadvantage is the fact that it is not radiopaque, and absorbable. The latter may lead to recanalization of the vessel treated, and thus to recurrences. Therefore gelatin sponge is not the embolic agent of first choice, although it can be used as an efficient temporary embolic agent.

The most commonly used embolic agents are polyvinyl alcohol particles. Polyvinyl alcohol particles are biocompatible and non-biodegradable and are

Table 16.1. Cookbook:

Diagnostic catheters
  Flush (pigtail, universal flush)
  Selective: Cobra (C2 and C3)
                Simmons (type 1 and type 2)
                Mammary
  Multipurpose
  Bronchial
Microcatheter (Progreat, Tracker, Transend, Prowler)
Y-connector
Pressurized saline flush
Three-way stopcock with tube
1 ml Syringes
Embolic agents
Microspheres (size range 100 µm–1000 µm; Embosphere, Bead Block, Ivalon, Contour)
Coils (pushable, fibred coils)

considered to be a permanent embolic agent and the agent of first choice [38]. More recently tris-acryl gelatin microspheres have become available. Use of these particles has been mainly in uterine fibroid embolization, and experience in bronchial artery embolization is limited [40]. Tris-acryl gelatin particles can be administered more smoothly through micro-catheters, without the risk of plug-formation as can occur with the (older generation) polyvinyl alcohol particles, and better penetration characteristics [41]. Both polyvinyl alcohol and tris-acryl gelatin particles are available in various diameters, ranging from 75 ìm to 1000 ìm. Particles smaller than 350 ìm should be used with extreme caution, since particles smaller than this size may pass bronchopulmonary anastomoses, or may cause a very distal occlusion in normal peripheral branches, that provide vascular supply to bronchi, esophagus etc. Occlusion of these branches may lead to bronchial or esophageal necrosis [25, 42].

Stainless steel or platinum coils and detachable balloons are rarely used as a primary embolic agent in bronchial artery embolization. Although these can be used to occlude a pathologic bronchial artery efficiently, use of coils precludes repeat embolization, which is often needed as patients are prone to distal collateralization (Fig. 16.21) [43, 44]. The primary indication for use of coils is in patients with a bronchial artery aneurysm. Secondly, in cases where a superselective position of a (micro) catheter cannot be reached, coils can be used to protect a normal distal vascular territory against inadvertent embolization [25].

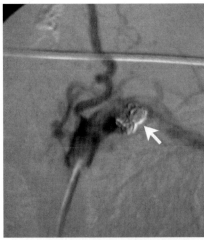

Fig. 16.21a–c. a Same patient as Fig. 16.13; 1 month after coil embolization of the thyrocervical trunk presenting with recurrent hemoptysis; notice presence of coils (*arrow*). **b** Late phase of selective angiography of the left subclavian artery: recurrence of pathologic enhancement (*arrow*) and pulmonary shunting (*arrowhead*). **c** Selective angiography of left subclavian artery showing filling of pathologic area of apical vessels through vertebral artery (*arrowhead*), C2–C3 collaterals (*arrow*) and lateral cervical branches (*curved arrow*); this situation precludes repeat embolization

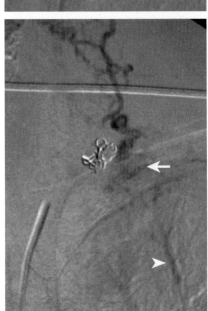

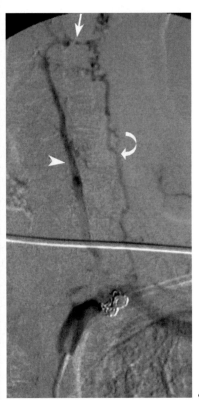

Thrombin injection into the bronchial artery has been described, and has a theoretical advantage in patients where tortuosity of the target artery precludes superselective catheterization [45]. However, given the rather unpredictable behavior, and risk of peripheral embolization, this agent has not gained wide acceptance, the same as using absolute alcohol as an embolic agent.

16.6
Results

Bronchial artery embolization is highly effective in the treatment of acute hemoptysis. Short-term non-recurrence rates (with follow-up up to 1 month) range from 73% to 98% [1, 46, 47]. Technical success rates have increased by development of a more meticulous technique, using superselective embolization, and performing control thoracic aortography as described above [14, 48]. Procedural failures are usually caused by inability to achieve a stable catheter position, or a position beyond the origin of spinal cord branches [38]. Recurrences at long-term follow-up can be as high as 52%, however, success rates of 100% can be achieved using repeat embolization and control of underlying disease either pharmacologically or surgically [25, 38, 47, 49–51]. Recurrence of hemoptysis may occur due to recanalization of embolized vessels, incomplete embolization, revascularization by means of development of new collateral pathways, including development of contribution of non-bronchial systemic arterial supply [25]. The presence of anomalous bronchial arteries may also contribute to occurrence of recurrences [52, 53].

The underlying disease is also of importance: patients with chronic tuberculosis more frequently suffer from recurrent hemoptysis, since the development of non-bronchial systemic collaterals is more extensive [33, 54]. However, repeat embolization in such patients, including treatment of non-bronchial collaterals often leads to satisfactory results [32, 55–57].

Finally, operator experience in bronchial artery embolization is of crucial importance in achieving high success and low complication rates. Given the low incidence of acute massive hemoptysis, the risk that each patient represents a new "learning" experience is not unimaginable [38], and therefore bronchial artery embolization should only be performed by skilled operators (at least five to ten cases a year).

16.7
Complications

The most commonly occurring complication encountered after bronchial artery embolization is (transient) chest pain, being reported in 24% up to 91% of cases. This is probably related to ischemia of embolized branches, and can be severe when intercostal branches are inadvertently embolized. Pleural pain can be avoided by using superselective embolization techniques, with or without the use of large particles. The second most common complication is dysphagia, caused by embolization of esophageal branches, with a reported occurrence from 0.7% to 18.2% [30]. Spontaneous resolution of symptoms usually occurs.

Incidentally subintimal dissection or perforation of the bronchial artery (caution with use of glide-wire-type guidewires) or dissection of the aorta may occur [29].

The most devastating complication is spinal cord ischemia, that has been reported to occur in 1.4%–6.5% of patients treated with bronchial artery embolization [9, 30, 39]. The occurrence of this complication can be reduced by using a superselective embolization technique, performing regular control angiograms before and after administration of embolic agents as has been described above.

Rare complications as have been reported in literature are aortic and bronchial necrosis [58], bronchial stenosis [59], unilateral diaphragmatic paralysis [60], pulmonary infarction (especially in patients who have suffered pulmonary artery embolism), left main bronchial-esophageal fistula [61], and non-target embolization (colon, coronary and cerebral circulation) [62]. Especially the newer spherical embolic materials (tris-acryl gelatin) can traverse from the bronchial into the pulmonary circulation, and then through unoccluded pulmonary arteriovenous malformations into the systemic circulation [41].

16.8
Conclusion

Bronchial artery embolization is the treatment of choice in acute hemoptysis.

Knowledge of bronchial and non-bronchial systemic circulation is mandatory to reduce complications and to increase technical success.

References

1. Remy J, Arnaud A, Fardou H, Giraud R, Voisin C (1977) Treatment of hemoptysis by embolization of bronchial arteries. Radiology 122:33–37
2. Haponik EF, Fein A, Chin R (2000) Managing life-threatening hemoptysis: has anything really changed? Chest 118:1431–1435
3. Johnson JL (2002) Manifestations of hemoptysis. How to manage minor, moderate, and massive bleeding. Postgrad Med 112:101–109, 113
4. Jougon J, Ballester M, Delcambre F, Mac BT, Valat P, Gomez F et al. (2002) Massive hemoptysis: what place for medical and surgical treatment. Eur J Cardiothorac Surg 22:345–351
5. Marshall TJ, Flower CD, Jackson JE (1996) The role of radiology in the investigation and management of patients with haemoptysis. Clin Radiol 51:391–400
6. Hakanson E, Konstantinov IE, Fransson SG, Svedjeholm R (2002) Management of life-threatening haemoptysis. Br J Anaesth 88:291–295
7. Hirshberg B, Biran I, Glazer M, Kramer MR (1997) Hemoptysis: etiology, evaluation, and outcome in a tertiary referral hospital. Chest 112:440–444
8. Yoon W, Kim JK, Kim YH, Chung TW, Kang HK (2002) Bronchial and nonbronchial systemic artery embolization for life-threatening hemoptysis: a comprehensive review. Radiographics 22:1395–1409
9. Wong ML, Szkup P, Hopley MJ (2002) Percutaneous embolotherapy for life-threatening hemoptysis. Chest 121:95–102

10. Knott-Craig CJ, Oostuizen JG, Rossouw G, Joubert JR, Barnard PM (1993) Management and prognosis of massive hemoptysis. Recent experience with 120 patients. J Thorac Cardiovasc Surg 105:394–397

11. Foster DC, Stern JL, Buscema J, Rock JA, Woodruff JD (1981) Pleural and parenchymal pulmonary endometriosis. Obstet Gynecol 58:552–556

12. DeLima LG, Wynands JE, Bourke ME, Walley VM (1994) Catheter-induced pulmonary artery false aneurysm and rupture: case report and review. J Cardiothorac Vasc Anesth 8:70–75

13. Do KH, Goo JM, Im JG, Kim KW, Chung JW, Park JH (2001) Systemic arterial supply to the lungs in adults: spiral CT findings. Radiographics 21:387–402

14. Chun HJ, Byun JY, Yoo SS, Choi BG (2003) Added benefit of thoracic aortography after transarterial embolization in patients with hemoptysis. AJR Am J Roentgenol 180:1577–1581

15. Hsiao EI, Kirsch CM, Kagawa FT, Wehner JH, Jensen WA, Baxter RB (2001) Utility of fiberoptic bronchoscopy before bronchial artery embolization for massive hemoptysis. AJR Am J Roentgenol 177:861–867

16. Naidich DP, Funt S, Ettenger NA, Arranda C (1990) Hemoptysis: CT-bronchoscopic correlations in 58 cases. Radiology 177:357–362

17. McGuinness G, Beacher JR, Harkin TJ, Garay SM, Rom WN, Naidich DP (1994) Hemoptysis: prospective high-resolution CT/bronchoscopic correlation. Chest 105:1155–1162

18. Vernhet H, Dogas G, Bousquet C, Durand G, Godard P, Senac JP (2003) [Value of thoracic CT in the management of severe hemoptysis]. J Radiol 84:685–691

19. Remy-Jardin M, Bouaziz N, Dumont P, Brillet PY, Bruzzi J, Remy J (2004) Bronchial and nonbronchial systemic arteries at multi-detector row CT angiography: comparison with conventional angiography. Radiology 233:741–749

20. Ko SF, Ng SH, Lee TY, Wan YL, Lee CM, Hsieh MJ et al. (2000) Anomalous systemic arterialization to normal basal segments of the left lower lobe: helical CT and CTA findings. J Comput Assist Tomogr 24:971–976

21. Won JH, Park SI, Park KJ, Oh YJ, Hwang SC (2004) Microcatheter placement through a side hole created in a 5-F catheter into proximal subclavian arterial branches causing hemoptysis. J Vasc Interv Radiol 15:881–884

22. Sancho C, Escalante E, Dominguez J, Vidal J, Lopez E, Valldeperas J et al. (1998) Embolization of bronchial arteries of anomalous origin. Cardiovasc Intervent Radiol 21:300–304

23. Carles J, Clerc F, Dubrez J, Couraud L, Drouillard J, Videau J (1995) The bronchial arteries: anatomic study and application to lung transplantation. Surg Radiol Anat 17:293–299

24. Tanomkiat W, Tanisaro K 8 (2003) Radiographic relationship of the origin of the bronchial arteries to the left main bronchus. J Thorac Imaging 18:27–33

25. Marshall TJ, Jackson JE (1997) Vascular intervention in the thorax: bronchial artery embolization for haemoptysis. Eur Radiol 7:1221–1227

26. Cowling MG, Belli AM (1995) A potential pitfall in bronchial artery embolization. Clin Radiol 50:105–107

27. Furnari ML, Salerno S, Rabiolo A, Caravello V, Pardo F (2003) Bronchial to subclavian shunt in a CF patient. A potential pitfall for embolization. J Cyst Fibros 2:217–219

28. Van den Berg JC, Overtoom TT, De Valois JC (1996) Case report: bronchial to coronary artery anastomosis – a potential hazard in bronchial artery embolization. Br J Radiol 69:570–572

29. Swanson KL, Johnson CM, Prakash UB, McKusick MA, Andrews JC, Stanson AW (2002) Bronchial artery embolization : experience with 54 patients. Chest 121:789–795

30. Ramakantan R, Bandekar VG, Gandhi MS, Aulakh BG, Deshmukh HL (1996) Massive hemoptysis due to pulmonary tuberculosis: control with bronchial artery embolization. Radiology 200:691–694

31. Zhang JS, Cui ZP, Wang MQ, Yang L (1994) Bronchial arteriography and transcatheter embolization in the management of hemoptysis. Cardiovasc Intervent Radiol 17:276–279

32. Keller FS, Rosch J, Loflin TG, Nath PH, McElvein RB (1987) Nonbronchial systemic collateral arteries: significance in percutaneous embolotherapy for hemoptysis. Radiology 164:687–692

33. Yu-Tang GP, Lin M, Teo N, En Shen WD (2002) Embolization for hemoptysis: a six -year review. Cardiovasc Intervent Radiol 25:17–25

34. Sellars N, Belli AM (2001) Non-bronchial collateral supply from the left gastric artery in massive haemoptysis. Eur Radiol 11:76–79

35. Cahill BC, Ingbar DH (1994) Massive hemoptysis. Assessment and management. Clin Chest Med 15:147–167

36. Phillips S, Ruttley MS (2000) Bronchial artery embolization: the importance of preliminary thoracic aortography. Clin Radiol 55:317–319

37. Miyayama S, Matsui O, Akakura Y, Yamamoto T, Fujinaga Y, Koda W et al. (2001) Use of a catheter with a large side hole for selective catheterization of the inferior phrenic artery. J Vasc Interv Radiol 12:497–499

38. White RI, Jr (1999) Bronchial artery embolotherapy for control of acute hemoptysis: analysis of outcome. Chest 115:912–915

39. Mal H, Rullon I, Mellot F, Brugiere O, Sleiman C, Menu Y et al. (1999) Immediate and long-term results of bronchial artery embolization for life-threatening hemoptysis. Chest 115:996–1001

40. Yoon W (2004) Embolic agents used for bronchial artery embolisation in massive haemoptysis. Expert Opin Pharmacother 5:361–367

41. Vinaya KN, White RI, Jr, Sloan JM (2004) Reassessing bronchial artery embolotherapy with newer spherical embolic materials. J Vasc Interv Radiol 15:304–305

42. Bookstein JJ, Moser KM, Kalafer ME, Higgins CB, Davis GB, James WS (1977) The role of bronchial arteriography and therapeutic embolization in hemoptysis. Chest 72:658–661

43. Barben J, Robertson D, Olinsky A, Ditchfield M (2002) Bronchial artery embolization for hemoptysis in young patients with cystic fibrosis. Radiology 224:124–130

44. Saluja S, Henderson KJ, White RI, Jr (2000) Embolotherapy in the bronchial and pulmonary circulations. Radiol Clin North Am 38:425–48, ix

45. Vrachliotis T, Sheiman RG (2002) Treatment of massive hemoptysis with intraarterial thrombin injection of a bronchial artery. AJR Am J Roentgenol 179:113–114

46. Uflacker R, Kaemmerer A, Picon PD, Rizzon CF, Neves CM, Oliveira ES et al. (1985) Bronchial artery embolization in

the management of hemoptysis: technical aspects and long-term results. Radiology 157:637–644

47. Lampmann LE, Tjan TG (1994) Embolization therapy in haemoptysis. Eur J Radiol 18:15–19

48. Tanaka N, Yamakado K, Murashima S, Takeda K, Matsumura K, Nakagawa T et al. (1997) Superselective bronchial artery embolization for hemoptysis with a coaxial microcatheter system. J Vasc Interv Radiol 8(1 Pt 1):65–70

49. Cremaschi P, Nascimbene C, Vitulo P, Catanese C, Rota L, Barazzoni GC et al. Therapeutic embolization of bronchial artery: a successful treatment in 209 cases of relapse hemoptysis. Angiology 1993; 44(4):295–299.

50. Endo S, Otani S, Saito N, Hasegawa T, Kanai Y, Sato Y et al. (2003) Management of massive hemoptysis in a thoracic surgical unit. Eur J Cardiothorac Surg 23:467–472

51. Kato A, Kudo S, Matsumoto K, Fukahori T, Shimizu T, Uchino A et al. (2000) Bronchial artery embolization for hemoptysis due to benign diseases: immediate and long-term results. Cardiovasc Intervent Radiol 23:351–357

52. McPherson S, Routh WD, Nath H, Keller FS (1990) Anomalous origin of bronchial arteries: potential pitfall of embolotherapy for hemoptysis. J Vasc Interv Radiol 1:86–88

53. Cohen AM, Antoun BW, Stern RC (1992) Left thyrocervical trunk bronchial artery supplying right lung: source of recurrent hemoptysis in cystic fibrosis. AJR Am J Roentgenol 158:1131–1133

54. Mossi F, Maroldi R, Battaglia G, Pinotti G, Tassi G (2003) Indicators predictive of success of embolisation: analysis of 88 patients with haemoptysis. Radiol Med (Torino) 105:48–55

55. Antonelli M, Midulla F, Tancredi G, Salvatori FM, Bonci E, Cimino G et al. (2002) Bronchial artery embolization for the management of nonmassive hemoptysis in cystic fibrosis. Chest 121:796–801

56. Brinson GM, Noone PG, Mauro MA, Knowles MR, Yankaskas JR, Sandhu JS et al. (1998) Bronchial artery embolization for the treatment of hemoptysis in patients with cystic fibrosis. Am J Respir Crit Care Med 157(6 Pt 1):1951–1958

57. Osaki S, Nakanishi Y, Wataya H, Takayama K, Inoue K, Takaki Y et al. (2000) Prognosis of bronchial artery embolization in the management of hemoptysis. Respiration 67:412–416

58. Ivanick MJ, Thorwarth W, Donohue J, Mandell V, Delany D, Jaques PF (1983) Infarction of the left main-stem bronchus: a complication of bronchial artery embolization. AJR Am J Roentgenol 141:535–537

59. Girard P, Baldeyrou P, Lemoine G, Grunewald D (1990) Left main-stem bronchial stenosis complicating bronchial artery embolization. Chest 97:1246–1248

60. Chapman SA, Holmes MD, Taylor DJ (2000) Unilateral diaphragmatic paralysis following bronchial artery embolization for hemoptysis. Chest 118:269–270

61. Munk PL, Morris DC, Nelems B (1990) Left main bronchial-esophageal fistula: a complication of bronchial artery embolization. Cardiovasc Intervent Radiol 13:95–97

62. Lemoigne F, Rampal P, Petersen R (1983) [Fatal ischemic colitis after bronchial artery embolization]. Presse Med 12:2056–2057

17 Pulmonary Arteriovenous Malformations

JEAN-PIERRE PELAGE, PASCAL LACOMBE, ROBERT I. WHITE JR., and JEFFRAY S. POLLAK

CONTENTS

J.-P. PELAGE, MD, PhD; P. LACOMBE, MD
Department of Radiology Hôpital Ambroise Pare, 9, Avenue Charles De Gaulle, 92104 Boulogne Cedex, France
R. I. WHITE, Jr., MD
Yale University School of Medicine, Department of Diagnostic Radiology, 333 Cedar Street, Room 5039 LMP, New Haven, CT 06520, USA
J. S. POLLAK, MD
Yale University School of Medicine, Department of Diagnostic Radiology, PO Box 20842, New Haven, CT 06504-8042, USA

17.1 Introduction

Pulmonary arteriovenous malformations are caused by abnormal communications between pulmonary arteries and pulmonary veins, which are most commonly congenital in nature [4, 20]. Although these lesions are uncommon, they are an important part of the differential diagnosis of common pulmonary problems such as hypoxemia and pulmonary nodules. These abnormal communications have been given various names including pulmonary arteriovenous fistulas, pulmonary telangiectases, and pulmonary arteriovenous malformations [20, 66].

Between 60% and 90% of patients with PAVM have hereditary hemorrhagic telangiectasia (HHT) but abnormal communications between blood vessels of the lung may also be found in a variety of acquired conditions [4, 20]. Right-to-left shunting as a result of communications between pulmonary arteries and pulmonary veins has been reported in hepatic cirrhosis, mitral stenosis, trauma and Fanconi's syndrome [4, 35, 52, 70].

PAVMs provide a direct capillary-free communication between the pulmonary and systemic circulations with three main clinical consequences: (1) pulmonary arterial blood passing through these right-to-left shunts cannot be oxygenated which may lead to hypoxemia, (2) the absence of normal filtering capillary bed allows particulate material (air bubbles or clots) to reach directly the systemic circulation (paradoxical embolism) with potential clinical sequelae in the cerebral circulation (transient ischemic attack, stroke, brain abscess), and (3) these abnormal vessels may rupture into the bronchus (hemoptysis) or the pleural cavity (hemothorax) particularly during pregnancy.

Hereditary hemorrhagic telangiectasia (HHT) is a genetic disorder of blood vessels [21, 63]. Also known as Rendu-Osler-Weber syndrome, HHT is a condition which is transmitted in an autosomal dominant pattern, and characterized by arteriovenous malformations (AVM) in the skin, mucous membranes and visceral organs [4]. There are two types of HHT, type l and 2, caused by mutations in the endoglin and ALK-1 genes, respectively [20, 63, 64]. The endoglin and ALK-1 genes code for proteins that are involved in proper blood vessel development. HHT has variable expression in each affected member of a family [21]. Mild to moderate epistaxis is the most common symptom of HHT [20, 21, 48]. To permit a high degree of clinical suspicion, recent international consensus diagnostic criteria have developed based on the four criteria of spontaneous recurrent epistaxis, mucocutaneous telangiectasia, visceral involvement (including PAVMs, hepatic, cerebral or spinal arteriovenous malformations) and an affected first degree relative [64]. The most common serious symptoms in adults are ischemic stroke, transient ischemic attack or brain abscess, due to PAVMs or hemorrhagic stroke or seizure due to cerebral arteriovenous malformation [20, 21, 26, 41, 44]. Unfortunately, the underlying disorder, HHT, is rarely identified by the family physician, neurology specialist or diagnostic radiologist. The implications of the underlying disorder are not clearly presented to the family and as a result affected relatives may develop sudden catastrophic symptoms instead of receiving counseling, screening, and treatment before complications occur. A crucial issue for families is that no child of a patient with HHT can be informed they do not have HHT unless they have had a molecular diagnosis. Penetrance is age-related and is nearly complete by the age of 40 [4, 49]. Other common symptoms in older adults include frequent nosebleeds and less commonly, gastrointestinal bleeding [20, 21, 48]. A smaller number of patients with HHT are affected by liver malformations, which can cause symptoms such as heart failure, abdominal pain, abnormal liver function tests or even cirrhosis [17, 20, 38].

The focus of this chapter will be mainly congenital PAVM. We will discuss HHT predominantly as it relates to PAVMs.

17.2
Epidemiology

PAVMs are not a common clinical problem. In an autopsy study, only three cases of PAVM were detected in 15,000 consecutive autopsies [20]. Around 10% of cases of PAVMs are identified in infancy or childhood, followed by a gradual increase in the incidence through the fifth and sixth decades [20]. Approximately 60%–90% of the cases of PAVM are associated

with HHT [20, 29, 65, 77]. Conversely, approximately 15%–35% of patients with HHT have PAVMs [22, 31, 42, 78]. PAVMs were found in only 4.6% of 324 patients with HHT from an endemic region in France but chest radiographs were not routinely performed [49].

With the onset of asymptomatic screening programs in the United States and most European countries, a much higher frequency of involvement is seen. It has been estimated that at least 30% of HHT patients have PAVMs, 30% have hepatic involvement and 10% cerebral involvement [14, 17, 22, 31].

About 10% of people with HHT die prematurely or are disabled due to complications of their vascular malformations. These "events" are preventable by early diagnosis, treatment, and follow-up. Most patients are largely asymptomatic before their first serious complication. Approximately 50% of patients with HHT will have an arteriovenous malformation of the brain, lung, or liver, or a combination of two or three and will require therapy usually by a pluridisciplinary team consisting of internists and interventional radiologists with special expertise in this disorder.

Because catastrophic cerebral events such as cerebral abscess, transient ischemic attack or embolic stroke occur in patients with PAVMs regardless of the degree of respiratory symptoms, it is of paramount importance to diagnose PAVMs to offer embolization as a means of prevention.

17.3
Clinical Manifestations of PAVMs

Up to 55% of PAVMs are asymptomatic and those that are symptomatic can present in a remarkable variety of ways [4]. Most of these clinical manifestations can be attributed to right-to-left shunting. Symptoms in early life may vary from being totally absent to severe [20]. In recent studies, about 70% of patients have symptoms referable to the PAVMs or underlying HHT [29, 65, 77]. Symptoms related to PAVM often develop between the fourth and sixth decades [20]. It is usually considered that the incidence of symptoms is higher in patients with multiple PAVMs rather than a single PAVM [20]. In the Mayo Clinic study, symptoms were seen in 37% of patients with a single PAVM and in 59% of patients with bilateral PAVM [67]. In addition, patients with diffuse PAVMs are almost always symptomatic [12, 20]. The most common complaint in symptomatic patients with PAVMs is epistaxis, caused by bleeding from mucosal telangiectases and reflects the high incidence of HHT in patients with PAVMs [20]. Dyspnea is the second most common complaint in patients with PAVMs particularly in those with large or diffuse PAVM. Dyspnea is seen in almost all patients who have associated cyanosis, clubbing, easy fatigability, or polycythemia [3, 4, 20]. Hemoptysis and hemothorax occur in roughly 10% of patients [1, 13, 77]. Less common complaints include chest pain, cough and migraine headaches [4, 20, 53]. Many of these symptoms are not specific and may be related to hypoxemia or cerebrovascular complications. Thus, the classic triad of dyspnea, cyanosis, and clubbing which is suggestive of PAVM was present in only 10% of patients with PAVM in one study [54]. It is estimated that 25% of patients with PAVMs experience transient ischemic attack or stroke and 10% experience cerebral abscess on presentation of PAVMs [64, 77].

Since patients with clinically silent PAVMs are still at risk of hemorrhage and more commonly neurological sequelae due to paradoxical embolism, screening of asymptomatic patients should be performed. Neurologic complications in patients with untreated PAVMs are common and the incidence of stroke has been reported to be as high as 40% and brain abscess 20% with a mortality of up to 40% [8, 73]. These data illustrate the need for aggressive screening and treatment for PAVMS in patient with HHT. Complications associated with PAVMs can be limited if the condition is recognized and treated, with transcatheter embolization offering the safest method of treatment [20, 73].

17.4
Pulmonary Function Tests

Oxygenation is commonly affected in patients with PAVMs. In recent studies, 80%–100% of patients with PAVMs had either a Pao2 < 80 mm Hg or a SaO2 < 97%–98% on room air [8, 20, 45]. Orthodeoxia which is the laboratory correlate of platypnea (represents a decrease in PaO2 or SaO2 when going from the recumbent to the seated or upright position) is present in most patients with PAVMs [11, 20, 71].

17.5
Imaging

Different imaging techniques can be used to confirm the diagnosis of PAVMs but also for treatment planning particularly before embolization. Screening methods vary between centers but are based on noninvasive methods to image the PAVMs or to detect the right-to-left shunt. Contrast-enhanced echocardiography is often used as the first line test in screening patients with HHT for intrapulmonary shunting because of its sensitivity greater than 95% [2, 43]. PAVMs may also be directly diagnosed using a variety of noninvasive imaging modalities including chest radiography, computed tomography (CT) and magnetic resonance imaging (MRI) [2, 4, 10, 30, 43, 47, 56, 73]. Pulmonary angiography is still used for treatment planning in some centers [78].

17.5.1
Contrast Material-Enhanced Echocardiography

Contrast echocardiography is an excellent tool for evaluation of cardiac and intrapulmonary shunts and is able to identify small right-to-left shunts [2, 43, 61]. The technique (the so-called bubble study) consists in injecting 5–10 cc of agitated saline into a peripheral vein while simultaneously imaging the right and left atria [61]. In patients without right-to-left shunting, the contrast is visualized in the right atrium as a cloud of echoes and gradually dissipates as the bubbles become trapped in the pulmonary circulation [61]. In patients with intracardiac shunting, the contrast is visible in the left atrium within one cardiac cycle following its appearance in the right atrium. Conversely in patients with PAVMs, there is usually a delay of between three and eight cardiac cycles before contrast is visualized in the left atrium [2]. Diagnosis of PAVMs can be made with a high sensitivity probably close to 95%–100% for detecting clinically important (i.e., large) PAVMs [2, 46]. Contrast echocardiography detects the presence of PAVMs with a high sensitivity but is not correlated with the size, location, or number of PAVMs [2, 37, 43]. Overdetection of clinically unimportant PAVM not requiring embolization may limit the use of contrast echocardiography as the exclusive screening test for PAVM [2, 20].

17.5.2
Chest Radiography

Diagnosis of PAVMs may be suspected on chest radiographs because abnormal findings have been described in the majority of patients with PAVMs [56, 65]. The most common findings are peripheral circumscribed, noncalcified oval or round lesions connected by blood vessels to the hilum or the presence of nodules often described as coin lesions (Fig. 17.1). However, chest radiography can be normal in 20% of patients with small PAVMs [73]. In addition, PAVMs can be obscured by hemorrhage or atelectasis [20, 45].

17.5.3
Pulmonary Angiography

In some centers, a complete diagnostic pulmonary angiography is performed prior to embolotherapy [78]. Selective injections in right and left pulmonary arteries in standard, oblique, and lateral projections are obtained. Outpatient pulmonary angiography in patients with diffuse PAVMs provides a basis for deciding which side to occlude first, to detail the anatomy, determine the best projection for occluding the PAVMs, and measure the feeding pedicles which helps to select the occlusion technique [76, 78].

17.5.4
Computed Tomography

When contrast echocardiography often used as a screening tool is positive, indicating a PAVM, thin section spiral chest CT should be performed to confirm the diagnosis and evaluate if treatment is necessary [56]. The characteristic appearance of a PAVM on CT scans is the presence of a homogeneous, well-circumscribed, noncalcified nodule measuring up to several centimeters in diameter or the presence of a serpiginous mass connected with blood vessels (Fig. 17.2) [56]. The use of contrast-material is still a matter of debate because spiral CT and multiplanar reconstructions allows easy identification of the feeding artery, aneurysm sac, and efferent veins without contrast injection [57]. Multiplanar

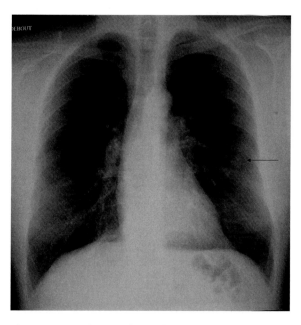

Fig. 17.1. PAVM diagnosed on a chest radiograph. Plain chest radiograph showing a single PAVM with smooth borders of the left lung (*arrow*)

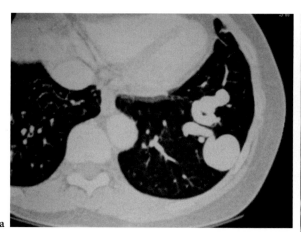

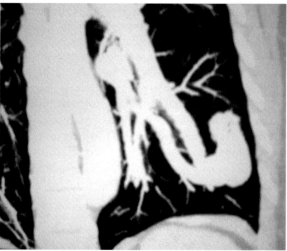

Fig. 17.2a,b. PAVM diagnosed using CT with multiplanar reconstructions. CT obtained in axial view (**a**) and coronal maximum intensity projection view (**b**) shows a single PAVM of the left lower lobe. The feeding artery, aneurysmal sac and draining vein are easily identified

and three-dimensional reconstructions, potentially useful to obtain precise angioarchitecture of PAVMs before embolization, may replace diagnostic pulmonary angiography (Fig. 17.2) [56, 57].

17.5.5
Magnetic Resonance Imaging

MRI of PAVMs has been evaluated less than CT. Conventional spin-echo MRI of pulmonary nodules or vascular lesions shows lesions with high signal intensity on T2-weighted images. Several techniques have been recently developed to improve sensitivity to flow [10, 30, 58]. The use of gradient-refocused echo MRI technique or MR angiography with venous or arterial signal elimination or contrast injection has been reported with a high sensitivity [10, 30, 58]. The obvious advantage of MRI over CT is the absence of radiation exposure but its main limitations include expense and limited availability [20].

17.5.6
Which Diagnostic Approach to Suspected PAVMs?

Based on current scientific data, it seems that contrast echocardiography is the best initial screening tool in patients with suspected PAVMs due to its excellent sensitivity and availability [19]. If the result is negative, the likelihood of significant PAVMs (i.e. requiring embolization) is low. The value of spiral CT in a screening algorithm is still considered low [53]. Conversely, all patients with positive echocardiography should be evaluated using spiral CT in order to identify PAVMs amenable to embolization. In addition, initial CT will be used as a baseline study that can be compared with postembolization examinations [53, 56].

Treatment of PAVMs consists of transcatheter embolization performed by interventional radiologists who are specially trained. Fibered platinum coils and in some instances balloons are placed in the feeding artery to the PAVM.

Follow-up of patients with treated PAVM is critical. By 3–6 months after treatment, the PAVM should be markedly reduced in size leaving a residual scar. Spiral chest CT should be repeated every 5 years in order to identify recanalization of embolized PAVMs and assess growth of any small AVM, until the threshold size (3-mm diameter feeding artery) is reached.

17.6
Classification of PAVMs

A classification of PAVMs based on segmental pulmonary artery anatomy was proposed by WHITE et al. in 1983 [76]. PAVMs can be classified as either simple or complex [76]. In the initial classification, the simple type was defined as having a single segmental artery and draining vein [76]. The complex type of PAVM was defined as having two or more arteries supplying the PAVM and one or two draining veins [76]. Based on CT findings, this classification has been modified subsequently [78]. A simple PAVM consists in single or multiple feeding arteries originating from a single segmental artery (Fig. 17.3) [78]. Conversely, in complex PAVMs, feeding arteries always originate from two or more segmental arteries (Fig. 17.4) [78]. Simple PAVMs usually account for 80%–90% of PAVMs but simple and complex PAVMs are frequently seen in the same patient [76]. The majority of PAVMs are located in the lower lobes [20, 77]. In some patients with simple and/or complex PAVMs, a diffuse pattern of PAVMs can be present. WHITE et al. have described diffuse PAVMs when almost all segmental arteries have small PAVMs arising from subsegmental branches (Fig. 17.5) [76]. Patients with diffuse PAVMs usually have a more severe clinical presentation with exercise intolerance and profound cyanosis [12]. They are also at higher risk of neurologic complications [12].

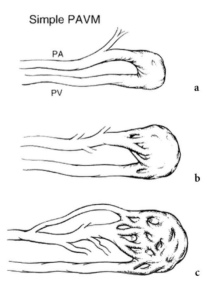

Fig. 17.3a–c. Simple form of PAVM. The simple PAVM is supplied by one segmental artery. The artery to the aneurysmal sac may consist of a single branch (**a**), multiple branches (**b**) or multiple branches arising proximally from the same segmental artery (**c**). (Reproduced from [76], with permission)

Complex PAVM

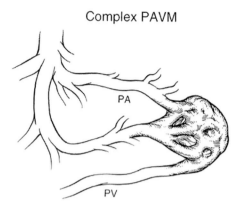

Fig. 17.4. Complex form of PAVM. The complex PAVM is supplied by two or more segmental arteries. (Reproduced from [76], with permission)

17.7
Therapeutic Options and Rationale for Treatment

17.7.1
Treatment Options

The current preferred treatment for PAVMs consists of embolization using coils or other intravascular devices [28]. Surgical resection used to be the only method of treatment before 1977 [8,28,54,65,66]. Vascular ligations, local resection, segmentectomy, lobectomy, or pneumonectomy were performed [20]. Properly performed in well-selected patients, surgery is associated with minimal morbidity and mortality but carries at least the same risks as any other

thoracic surgery [8, 65, 66]. Perioperative mortality varied from 0% to 9% [8, 54, 65, 66]. Postoperative follow-up is associated with 0%–10% recurrence rate in treated patients [8, 54, 65, 66]. Thus the disadvantages of surgery are the morbidity associated with a thoracotomy, the potential loss of normal pulmonary parenchyma surrounding the PAVM particularly in case of lobectomy or segmentectomy and the long hospital stay [54]. The first successful case of embolization of PAVMs was reported by PORSTMANN in 1977. Since that time embolization has become the first line treatment and surgery is rarely indicated since embolization results in permanent occlusion of PAVMs in a vast majority of patients with minimal complications in experienced hands [20].

17.7.2
Rationale for Treatment

Indications for treatment of PAVMs include three broad categories: prevention of hemorrhage, improvement of hypoxemia in patients with exercise intolerance, and, most importantly, prevention of the complications associated with paradoxical embolism. Exercise intolerance consisting of dyspnea and fatigue is difficult to quantify because most patients tolerate quite well significant hypoxemia. In most centers, the primary indication for embolization of PAVMs is prevention of neurologic complications.

It is usually considered that PAVMs with feeding arteries (i.e. the artery leading to the malforma-

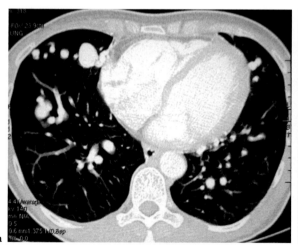
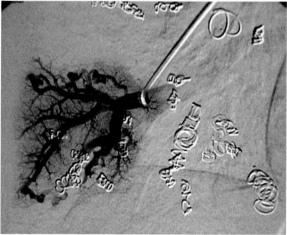

Fig. 17.5a,b. Diffuse PAVMs. **a** CT obtained at the level of both lower lobes shows multiple PAVMs involving both lungs. **b** Selective injection of pulmonary artery to the middle lobe confirms that all segmental arteries supply small PAVMs. Note that multiple large PAVMs have already been embolization with coils

tion) that are 3 mm or greater in diameter, should be treated to prevent complications [20, 26, 77, 78]. The reason is that individuals with PAVM of this size or larger are at risk of stroke or transient ischemic attack due to passage of small clots through the malformation [73, 77]. The potential for brain abscess is reduced by treating all identified 3 mm diameter arteries leading to PAVMs, but not eliminated, hence the need for continued antibiotic prophylaxis before dental work [20]. Of interest, a recent case of neurological complication in a patient with two small PAVMs < 3 mm has been reported [72].

In patients with diffuse PAVMs, depending on the patient tolerance and the amount of iodinated contrast used, multiple PAVMs can be embolized during the same session. However, additional sessions are usually necessary to treat all the visible PAVMs. In these patients, embolotherapy may result in partial improvement of dyspnea, oxygenation, and shunt fraction.

Finally, emergent embolization of PAVMs in patients with life-threatening complication such as pulmonary hemorrhage, hemothorax or hemoptysis can be discussed [1, 13, 18].

Women should be informed that PAVMs may enlarge during pregnancy and fatal hemorrhage from maternal PAVMs has been described [16, 20]. Altered hemodynamics and hormones found in pregnancy likely cause changes in PAVMs that predispose them to deterioration [13, 18]. Most cases of PAVM deterioration seem to occur during the second or third trimester when blood volume and cardiac output are at their maximum [18]. The use of embolization in pregnant women has been reported in case of complications [18]. However, because of concerns about fetal radiation exposure; it is desirable to screen women with HHT or previous PAVMs before pregnancy [13]. PAVMs should therefore be treated maximally before pregnancy [3, 20].

17.8
Procedure

17.8.1
Preparation

Unilateral femoral vein puncture is performed under local anesthesia and a 7- or 8-F introducer sheath is placed. Mild sedation is usually used. Prophylactic antibiotics are given at the beginning of the procedure. Intravenous heparin (5000 IU) is given

preprocedurally supplemented with 1000–2500 IU hourly during catheterization. Continuous EKG, arterial pressure and SaO2 monitoring are obtained. Diagnostic angiography is still used by some interventionalists to obtain precise segmental anatomy, to measure arterial diameter and to choose the projection that best displays the PAVM [78]. A baseline pulmonary artery pressure is usually obtained at the beginning of the procedure.

17.8.2
Technique of Catheterization

The method of catheterization has been extensively described by WHITE et al. [77, 78]. The procedure first involves localization of the PAVM by angiography followed by catheterization of the feeding artery, advancement of the catheter tip to a point beyond any branches to normal lung and immediately proximal to the dilated venous portion and arterial occlusion using coils or balloons [77]. The development of 6- and 7-F guide catheters (Gonadal, Cordis; Lumax, Cook) has greatly simplified access to PAVMs and stability of catheters when introducing balloons or standard pushable fibered coils (Fig. 17.6). Guide catheters stabilize one's position proximally in the feeding artery, in order to provide a controlled and precise delivery of coils through a coaxially placed 4- or 5-F catheters (Fig. 17.6). Multipurpose catheters (Cordis), Cobra catheters (Terumo) or Judkins right coronary catheters (Cook) are particularly suitable for catheterizing most PAVMs. For the right middle lobe or lingula, a Judkins Left coronary catheters may be useful to get access to the feeding artery (Fig. 17.6). Selective catheter positioning is achieved by advancing the catheter either directly or over a wire under fluoroscopic guidance. Once a segmental artery has been selected, it is mandatory to aspirate blood through the catheter to prevent air or clot injections that may pass through the PAVM or enter the coronary circulation causing angina, bradycardia or electrocardiographic ST segment wave changes. If blood return is not obtained during aspiration, the catheter must be gently removed. The catheter must be carefully flushed using a heparinized solution before injection of iodinated contrast material. An underwater technique must also be used for exchanges of wires to prevent air from going through the PAVM [40, 78].

The use of a coaxial microcatheter for catheterization and embolization may be needed to increase stability or to embolize the venous sac [9, 79]. In addition, the use of a microcatheter avoids

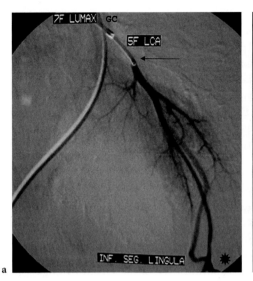
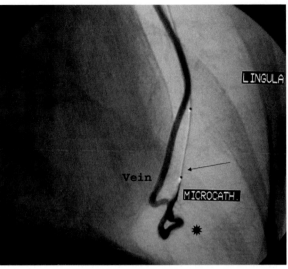

Fig. 17.6a,b. Embolization of a lingular PAVM. **a** The feeding artery to a lingular PAVM (*asterisk*) is selectively catheterized using a left Judkins 5-F catheter (*arrow*) which is stabilized using a 7-F guiding catheter (*GC*). **b** A 3-F microcatheter is then carefully advanced in the feeding artery close to the aneurysmal sac (*asterisk*)

the risk that the catheter may be dislocated during the advancement of macrocoils or balloons and the subsequent problem of coil deployment in inappropriate vascular territory [9]. The risk of perforating the aneurysmal sac when superselective peripheral catheterization is performed is reduced when microcatheters are used. Finally, a microcatheter is extremely helpful when a Judkins left coronary catheter is required to get access to the right middle lobe or lingula (Fig. 17.6).

17.8.3
Embolization Materials

Embolization needs to be carried out with devices large enough to occlude the feeding artery securely. In the first case reported by PORSTMANN in 1977 [51], the PAVM was embolized using hand-made steel coil. WHITE et al. performed most of the early cases using different types of detachable balloon systems [75]. These devices initially developed for neurovascular and cardiovascular large-vessel occlusion are no longer available in most countries [27, 50, 75]. Balloons had the advantage of providing total cross-sectional artery occlusion and recanalization due to early deflation was a rare event [50]. In the long-term, most of these balloons deflated but occlusion time was sufficient to obtain thrombosis of the PAVM. Experience with detachable balloons as well as newer occlusion devices, like the "Amplatzer",

vascular plugs and the "Gianturco-Grifka vascular occlusion device" suggested that cross sectional occlusion should be the goal for embolotherapy of PAVMs [15].

Nowadays, most groups favor the use of coils as the primary embolization agent. Initially only stainless steel coils such as the Gianturco-Anderson-Wallace were available [11, 23, 55, 78]. More recently platinum coils available in fibered and nonfibered variants have become available (Fig. 17.7) [40]. The choice of a coil of a correct size is critical: too small, the coil may pass through the venous portion of the PAVM into the systemic circulation with potential disastrous consequences [78]. Too large, the coil may cause occlusion of proximal normal pulmonary arterial branches or may elongate leading to recanalization [33, 78]. After placement of the first coil, additional coils must be positioned until blood flow to the PAVM has ceased [78]. Packing of smaller coils in the center of the first placed coil is mandatory to obtain complete cross-sectional occlusion and prevent recanalization (Fig. 17.8). If the number of coils is not sufficient recanalization may also occur because of insufficient thrombosis formation [33, 78].

The role of venous sac embolization remains unclear [79]. Venous sac closure is usually necessary in less than 1% of PAVMs when the artery to the PAVM is short (2 cm or less) and has high flow or uneven diameter and there is a risk of paradoxical embolization [6, 9, 78].

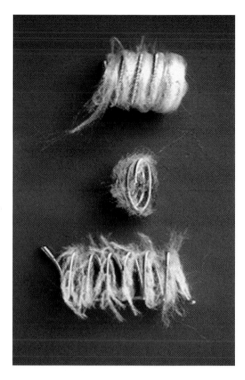

Fig. 17.7. Different types of coils that can be used for embolization of PAVMs

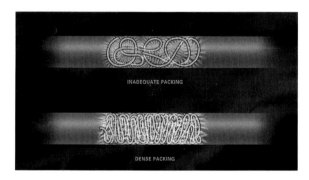

Fig. 17.8. Packing technique. Inadequate packing of coils may be associated with central recanalization of the embolized PAVM. Adequate packing consists of complete cross-sectional occlusion

Detachable coils such as the Guglielmi coils (GDCs) have been occasionally used to perform embolization of the venous sac [9, 32]. A less expensive alternative to GDCs when repositioning or controlled placement is required is interlocking detachable coils [68]. The specific advantages of detachable coils is that they can be retracted if placed in undesired position. They can also be helpful to treat large high-flow fistulas that lack venous component [9]. The disadvantage of occluding the venous sac is the increased number of coils needed to pack the sac compared with the

number of coils used in the occlusion of the feeding artery alone [9, 68]. Another approach to the embolization of the venous sac is the use of a temporary occlusion balloon catheter with a microcatheter placed into the aneurysm, the so-called vein of Galen technique (Fig. 17.9) [69]. Microcoils equivalent to the diameter of the aneurysmal sac and exceeding the diameter of the draining vein are placed.

17.8.4
Embolization Techniques

Different techniques for using pushable fibered coils have been developed. In general, these techniques for closing vessels 3–15 mm in diameter are equally applicable for all arterial occlusions in the systemic circulation as well. It is of paramount importance to achieve cross sectional occlusion at the time of initial therapy in order to reduce the risk of recanalization. The majority of arterial and venous occlusions can be performed using "current generation" 0.035 or 0.038-in. pushable fibered coils which produce reliable cross sectional occlusion, providing they are placed coaxially through a guide catheter and deployed into a dense mass of fibered coils. Rarely microcoils or detachable coils are required [79].

17.8.4.1
Anchor Technique

This technique is used for closing high-flow feeding arteries. It is also useful for routine occlusion if there is any concern about movement of the coil after deployment. The first centimeters of a long coil are anchored in a side branch immediately proximal to the site to be occluded (Fig. 17.10). The remaining coil is tightly packed into a "nest" and additional coils are added and packed until cross sectional occlusion of the artery is achieved (Fig. 17.11).

17.8.4.2
Scaffold Technique

Using stainless steel or inconnel (European equivalent of stainless steel) high radial force coils, an "endoskeleton" is constructed within the artery to be occluded (Fig. 17.12). Usually the first high radial force coil should have a diameter 2 mm larger than the artery to be occluded. The occlusion is finished

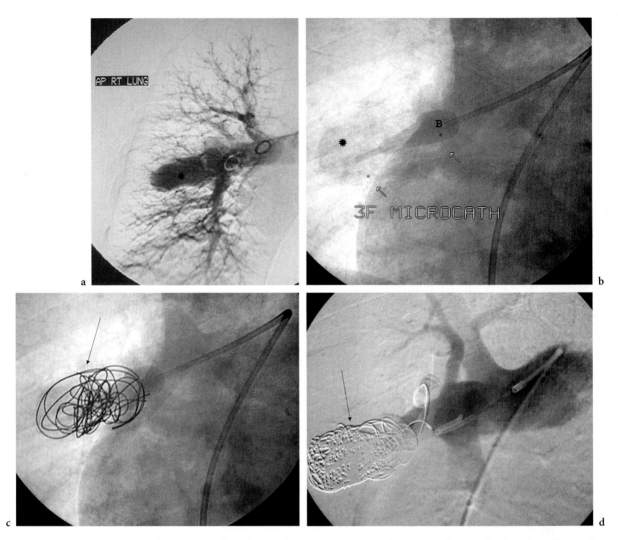

Fig. 17.9a–d. Vein of Galen technique. **a** Right pulmonary artery angiogram: a large central PAVM (*star*) with a short and high-flow feeding artery is identified. **b** a temporary occlusion balloon catheter (B) is inflated occluding the feeding artery. A 3-F microcatheter is placed in the aneurysmal sac (*arrows*). **c** a total of 12 vein of Galen and complex helical coils have been deployed into the aneurysmal sac (*arrow*). **d** additional coils with a maximum diameter of 12 mm have been placed to obtain complete occlusion of the sac (*arrow*) (Reproduced from [69], with permission)

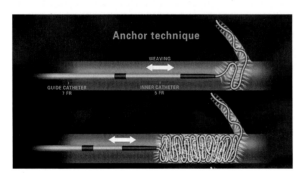

Fig. 17.10. Anchor technique. The first centimeters of a long coil are carefully placed in a side branch immediately proximal to the site to be occluded. This technique prevents coil migration at the time of placing additional coils to obtain complete cross-sectional occlusion

by "packing" long fibered coils to achieve cross sectional occlusion (Fig. 17.12).

17.8.4.3
Occlusion Balloon Assisted Technique

This technique is often utilized in a high-flow PAVM or if the feeding artery is large (>12 mm). A temporary occlusion balloon catheter is placed to occlude the PAVM. The initial coils are placed through the balloon occlusion catheter are high radial force stainless or inconnel coils and they may also be "anchored" in a side branch proximal to the site to be occluded. After placing between

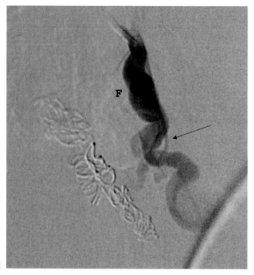
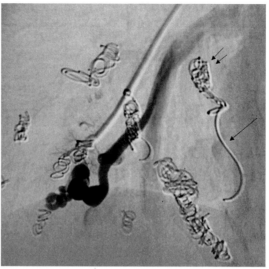

Fig. 17.11a,b. Anchor technique. **a** A small side branch (*arrow*) immediately proximal to the site to be occluded (*F*) is identified. **b** The first centimeters of a long coil are anchored in the side branch (*arrow*)

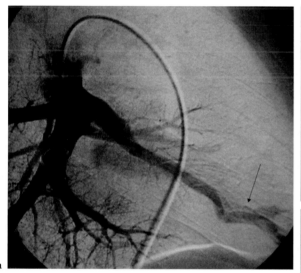

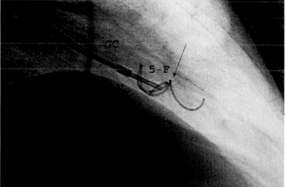

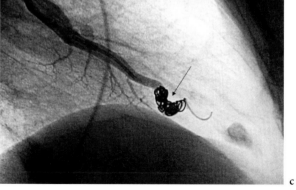

Fig. 17.12a–c. Scaffold technique. **a** A large PAVM of the left lower lobe is identified (*arrow*). **b** With the use of a 7-F guiding catheter (*GC*) and a 5-F catheter, an "endoskeleton" is constructed within the artery to be occluded using a high radial force coil (*arrow*). The first coil should have a diameter 2 mm larger than the artery to be occluded. **c** The occlusion is finished by "packing" long fibered coils to achieve cross sectional occlusion (*arrow*)

two and three high radial force coils, the balloon occlusion catheter is deflated and a standard coaxial guide catheter substituted. Embolization is then finished by "packing" long fibered coils to achieve cross sectional occlusion as previously described.

17.8.4.4
Vein of Galen Technique

This technique is used for occluding the aneurysmal sac of short and/or high-flow PAVMs. Oversized microcoils are injected through microcatheters directly in the aneurysm of the PAVM [69]. The interventional radiologist should be aware of this technique even if it is not commonly used. In a recent study, the vein of Galen technique was used in six out of 650 consecutive patients only [69]. However, it is particularly recommended in case of a short artery, usually less than 1–2 cm in length or when it is difficult to place safely standard fibered coils, because of high flow to the PAVM (Fig. 17.9).

17.8.4.5
Squirt Technique

This technique is suitable for all fibered pushable microcoils (0.018-in.) through microcatheters. The microcoil is loaded into the microcatheter and a 1-ml luer lock syringe with saline flush is attached to the hub of the microcatheter. Under fluoroscopic guidance the microcoil is delivered with small boluses of flush. Final adjustment of the microcoil can be done by moving the microcatheter before final delivery of the complete coil, if the initial deployment of the coil is distal to the site for deployment.

17.8.4.6
Wire Push Technique

For large lumen microcatheters, it is necessary to use a 0.021 or 0.025-in. pusher wire to avoid catheter occlusion. In the newer microcatheters (Renegade Hi-Flo, Boston Scientific; Progeat 2.7, Terumo or Embocath, Biosphere Medical), the use of standard 0.016-in. pusher wires will cause trapping of microcoils between the inner diameter of the microcatheter and the microcoil. To avoid this the "squirt technique" is utilized or a larger pusher wire is required.

17.8.4.7
Pulmonary Flow Redistribution

This technique has been developed as an approach to improve hypoxemia in patients with a diffuse pattern of disease [62]. A temporary occlusion of lobar arteries of the most affected lobes (usually both lower lobes) is performed to determine if there is any improvement in oxygenation. In the patients whose PaO2 increases by at least 10 mm Hg, a permanent lobar artery embolization is performed in order to obtain flow redistribution in the remaining (less affected) lobes [12].

17.9
Results

Long-term follow-up is indicated in all patients with PAVMs even after a successful therapy because of the risks of serial growth of small lesions and reperfusion of embolized PAVMs [20, 33]. Clinical and imaging follow-up of patients treated with embolization has been published in several studies originating from a limited number of centers [11, 25, 40, 50, 55].

17.9.1
Clinical Follow-up

Long-term follow-up of patients treated with embolization has been reported in several studies [11, 40, 55, 60, 71, 77]. In a recent study, the long-term outcomes of embolization (mean follow-up 62 months), were successful in 83% of 112 treated patients overall and in 96% of patients in whom all angiographically visible PAVMs were embolized [40]. During the follow-up after embolization major neurological complications such as cerebral abscess, transient ischemic attack, or stroke related to reperfused treated or new PAVMs have been reported [11, 25, 40, 77]. The long-term morbidity of reperfused PAVMs is unknown but some patients have already suffered from stroke because of recanalized PAVMs [40].

Repeat treatment is therefore indicated during the follow-up because of recanalization of previously embolized PAVMs or enlargement of untreated PAVMs may be seen in up to 13% of treated patients (Fig. 17.13) [33, 40]. Simple PAVMs are usually easy to occlude without risk of recanalization (Fig. 17.14). Different mechanisms accounting for reperfusion of embolized PAVMs have been described with follow-up CT [33]. These include recanalization of embolized PAVMs due to insufficient packing, recruitment of adjacent normal branches and rarely systemic supply to the embolized PAVM (Fig. 17.15) [33, 59].

In most patients with diffuse PAVMs, improvement of dyspnea, oxygenation, and shunt fraction is not complete [12]. The residual shunt is believed to represent the shunt through small PAVMs [12]. Even if clinical and radiological evaluation is necessary, oxygen saturation tests are equally important to predict recurrence. It is recommended that patients with diffuse or non treated PAVMs be given antibiotic prophylaxis before dental and surgical procedures to avoid seeding of PAVMs and subsequent development of brain abscess.

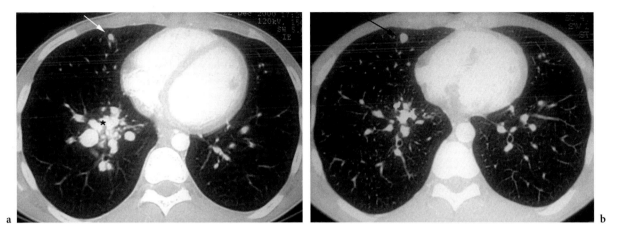

Fig. 17.13a,b. Enlargement of small PAVMs. **a** CT performed before embolization a large PAVM (*asterisk*) of the right lower lobe. A small PAVM of the right middle lobe is seen (*arrow*). **b** At 1 year later, there is significant enlargement of the PAVM (*arrow*). Good retraction of the treated PAVM is seen

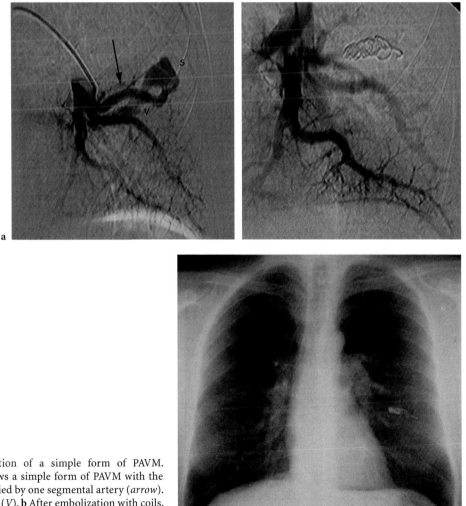

Fig. 17.14a–c. Embolization of a simple form of PAVM. **a** Selective injection shows a simple form of PAVM with the aneurysmal sac (*S*) supplied by one segmental artery (*arrow*). The draining vein is seen (*V*). **b** After embolization with coils, complete occlusion is seen. **c** Chest radiograph obtained 6 months after embolization shows retraction of the PAVM

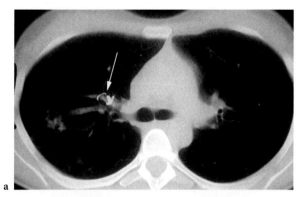

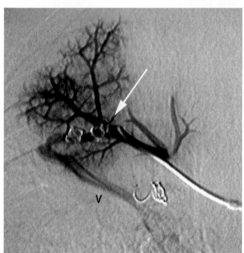

Fig. 17.15. a CT performed 6 months after embolization of a complex PAVM of the right upper lobe shows recanalization of the feeding artery (*arrow*) due to insufficient packing. The draining vein is still opacified (*V*). **b** Selective injection of the feeding artery confirms recanalization (*arrow*). Additional embolization has been performed to obtain complete cross-sectional occlusion

Rare reports of pulmonary hypertension following embolization have been published [24].

17.9.2
Imaging Follow-Up

Imaging follow-up of treated patients in conjunction with clinical and physiological evaluation should be performed in order to document involution or reperfusion of embolized PAVMs but also to detect growth or enlargement of small PAVMs [5, 33, 57]. Small PAVMs can over time reach the threshold size for complications (Fig. 17.13). In one study of patients who underwent embolization of large PAVMs, 91% of treated PAVMs disappeared on chest radiograph at a mean follow-up of over 4 years (Fig. 17.14) [36]. In one large study, follow-up with CT scan 1 or more years after embolization showed that 96% of treated PAVMs were either undetectable or reduced in size [56]. This phenomenon is believed to be the result of thrombosis and retraction of the aneurysmal sac following embolization (Figs. 17.13, 17.14) [56]. Reperfusion of accurately embolized PAVMs is considered as a rare event, predominantly affecting large and/or complex PAVMs [36, 40]. As previously mentioned, reperfusion may be due to several mechanisms. Insufficient cross-sectionnal occlusion (coil packing) at the time of embolization is an obvious cause of recanalization (Fig. 17.14) [7, 33, 59]. Small accessory branches to the PAVM may be missed during the initial embolization or recruitment of initially normal branches adjacent to the PAVM may occur [33]. Small branches supplying the embolized PAVM may also be missed during follow-up CT evaluation particularly in the absence of contrast enhancement or because of coil-related artifacts [33, 59, 74]. Bronchial artery hypertrophy has been identified as a cause of reperfusion of small residual aneurysm after embolization [34]. Bronchial-to-pulmonary artery anastomoses may enter the pulmonary circulation distally to the embolized artery supplying the scarred region of the obliterated PAVM and may lead to future recanalization [7]. It is not known if the formation of systemic collaterals may place patients at risk for future hemoptysis [33].

Contrast echocardiography and MR perfusion imaging are probably too sensitive and remain positive in the majority of patients even after successful occlusion of all angiographically visible PAVMs [37, 47].

17.10
Complications: Description and Prevention

Complications following embolization of PAVMs have in general been infrequent and self-limited, particularly in experienced hands [20, 40]. Most of the reported complications are minor and self-limited, most of these only require symptomatic treatment [20]. Pleuritic chest pain occurring in the first 24 h after embolization is the most frequent complication encountered in up to 13% of treated patients [11, 20, 40, 55, 77]. The incidence seems higher in patients presenting with large PAVMs [20, 36]. Pleural effusion has been reported in up to 12% of patients [40]. Pulmonary infarction has been observed in 3% of patients and most likely was related to occlusion of normal pulmonary arterial branches [55, 71, 76]. The catheter tip should therefore be advanced distal to any arterial branch supplying normal lung parenchyma as close as possible to the neck of the PAVM. Air embolism during embolization has been reported in up to 4% of patients who developed transient symptoms such as angina, bradycardia or perioral paresthesia [11, 50, 71, 77]. Careful flushing of the catheters and observation of back bleeding before injection make this complication completely avoidable.

Major complications such as paradoxical embolization of a device and stroke are extremely rare. Device migration has been reported in about 1% of cases mainly with coils [11, 23, 40, 50, 55, 71]. Rare reports of balloon migrations have been published [11, 23, 40, 50, 54]. Coil migration is more likely to occur in case of large (> 8 mm) or high-flow PAVMs and during the learning curve of the interventional radiologist [40, 77]. These migrations may require additional intervention using an intravascular retrieval device. The use of occlusion balloon-assisted or vein of Galen techniques for short, large, or high-flow PAVMs may reduce the risk of coil migration [69]. In all cases the first coil should be oversized in order to form a nest and prevent further coil migration.

One report of cerebral infarction occurring 1 week after coil embolization of a single PAVM has been recently published [39]. Clot migration from the embolized PAVM partially reperfused via a previously embolized feeding pulmonary artery and a bronchial artery was the supposed mechanism accounting for this stroke [39].

17.11
Conclusion and Perspectives

Although embolization is a safe and effective treatment in the management of PAVMs, long-term follow-up of patients is mandatory to document aneurysmal retraction or reperfusion of treated lesions and to detect growth of small PAVMs reaching the threshold size for neurologic emboli. From a technical point of view, it is important to perform the embolization with coils placed as distally as possible in the feeding vessel to a PAVM close to the venous sac. This technique avoids the occlusion of branches to normal lung and reduces the rate of reperfusion and the risk of pleurisy or pulmonary infarction. In patients with localized PAVMs, prevention of neurological complications can be achieved in almost all cases if all PAVMs are occluded. Conversely in patients with diffuse PAVMs, multiple procedures will be necessary to improve the profound hypoxia, decrease the risks of neurological events and obtain an acceptable quality-of-life.

Embolization of PAVMs requires a specific expertise and should be performed by specially-trained interventional radiologists only. Pluridisciplinary management of PAVMs in HHT is mandatory in order to apply the appropriate treatment and to fully educate the patients and their family about the diagnosis, its clinical implications, and its hereditary nature.

Cookbook:

1. Technique of catheterization of PAVMs

Indication	First choice	Second choice
Simple or complex PAVM	5-F Judkins right catheter	5-F Cobra-shaped catheter
		5-F Multipurpose catheter
PAVM of the right middle lobe or lingula	5-F Judkins left catheter	3-F Microcatheter
Embolization of the venous sac	3-F Microcatheter	

2. Technique of embolization of PAVMs

Indication	First choice	Second choice
PAVM with normal flow	Scaffold technique	Anchor technique
PAVM with high flow	Anchor technique	Vein of Galen technique
PAVM with large feeding artery	Anchor technique	Occlusion balloon-assisted technique

References

1. Adegboyega PA, Yuoh G, Adesokan A (1996) Recurrent massive hemothorax in Rendu-Osler-Weber. South Med J 89:1193–1196

2. Barzilai B, Waggoner AD, Spessert C, Picus D, Goodenberger (1991) Two-dimensional contrast echocardiography in the detection and follow-up of congenital pulmonary arteriovenous malformations. Am J Cardiol 68:1507–1510

3. Begbie ME, Wallace GMF, Shovlin CL (2003) Hereditary hemorrhagic telangiectasia (Osler-Weber-Rendu syndrome): a view from the 21st century. Postgrad Med 79:18–24

4. Burke CM, Safai C, Nelson DP, Raffin TA (1986) Pulmonary arteriovenous malformations: a critical update. Am Rev Respir Dis 134:334–339

5. Clark JA, Pugash RA (1998) Recanalization after coil embolization of pulmonary arteriovenous malformations (letter). Am J Roentgenol 171:142

6. Coley SC, Jackson JE (1996) Venous sac embolization of pulmonary arteriovenous malformations in two patients. Am J Roentgenol 167:452–454

7. De Wispelaere JF, Trigaux JP, Weynants P, Delos M, de Coene B (1996) Systemic supply to a pulmonary arteriovenous malformation: potential explanation for recurrence. Cardiovasc Intervent Radiol 19:285–287

8. Dines DE, Arms RA, Bernatz PE, Gomes MR (1974) Pulmonary arteriovenous fistulas. Mayo Clin Proc 49:460–465

9. Dinkel HP, Triller J (2002) Pulmonary arteriovenous malformations: embolotherapy with superselective coaxial catheter placement and filling of venous sac with Guglielmi detachable coils. Radiology 223:709–714

10. Dinsmore BJ, Gefter WB, Hatabu H, Kresel HY (1990) Pulmonary arteriovenous malformations: diagnosis by gradient-refocused MR imaging. J Comput Assist Tomogr 14:918–923

11. Dutton JAE, Jackson JE, Hugues JMB, Whyte MKB, Peters AM, Ussov W, Allison DJ (1995) Pulmonary arteriovenous malformations: results of treatment with coil embolization in 53 patients. Am J Roentgenol 165:1119–1125

12. Faughnan ME, Lui YW, Wirth JA, Pugash RA, Redelmeier DA, Hyland RH, White Jr RI (2000) Diffuse pulmonary arteriovenous malformations: characteristics and prognosis. Chest 117:31–38

13. Ference BA, Shannon TM, White RI Jr, Zavin M, Burdge CM (1994) Life-threatening pulmonary hemorrhage with pulmonary arteriovenous malformations and hereditary hemorrhagic telangiectasia. Chest 106:1387–1390

14. Fulbright RK, Chaloupka JC, Putman CM, Sze GK, Merriam MM, Lee GK, Fayad PB, Awad IA, White Jr RI (1998) MR of hereditary hemorrhagic telangiectasi: prevalence and spectrum of cerebrovascular malformations. Am J Neuroradiol 19:477–484

15. Gamillscheg A, Schuchlenz H, Stein JI, Beitzke A (2003) Interventional occlusion of a large pulmonary arteriovenous malformation with an Amplatzer septal occuder. J Interv Cardiol 16:335–339

16. Gamon RB, Miksa AK, Keller FS (1990) Osler-Weber-Rendu disease and pulmonary arteriovenous fistulas. Deterioration and embolotherapy during pregnancy. Chest 98:1522–1524

17. Garcia-Tsao G, Korzenik JR, Young L, Henderson KJ, Jain D, Byrd B, Pollak JS, White Jr RI (2000) Liver disease in patients with hereditary hemorrhagic telangiectasia. N Engl J Med 343:931–936

18. Gershon AS, Faughnan ME, Chon KS, Pugash RA, Clark JA, Bohan MJ, Henderson KJ, Hyland RH, White RI Jr (2001) Transcatheter embolotherapy of maternal pulmonary arteriovenous malformations during pregnancy. Chest 119:470–477

19. Gossage JR (2003) The role of echocardiography in screening for pulmonary arteriovenous malformations. Chest 123:320–322

20. Gossage JR, Kanj G (1998) Pulmonary arteriovenous malformations: a state of the art review. Am J Respir Crit Care Med 158:643–661

21. Guttmacher AE, Marchuk DA, White RI (1995) Hereditary hemorrhagic telangiectasia. N Engl J Med 333:918–924

22. Haitjema TJ, Disch F, Overtoom TC, Westermann JJ, Lammers JW (1995a) Screening family members of patients with hereditary hemorrhagic telangiectasia. Am J Med 99:519–524

23. Haitjema TJ, Overtoom TT, Westerman CJ, Lammers JW (1995b) Embolisation of pulmonary arteriovenous malformations: results and follow-up in 32 patients. Thorax 50:719–723

24. Haitjema TJ, Ten Berg JM, Overtoom TT, Ernst JM, Westermann CJ (1996) Unusual complications after embolization of a pulmonary arteriovenous malformation. Chest 109:1401–1404

25. Hartnell GG, Jackson JE, Allison DJ (1990) Coil embolizationof pulmonary arteriovenous malformations. CardioVasc Intervent Radiol 13:347–350

26. Hewes RC, Auster M, White RI (1985) Cerebral embolism: first manifestation of pulmonary arteriovenous malformations in patients with hereditary hemorrhagic telangiectasia. CardioVasc Intervent Radiol 8:151–155

27. Hieshima GB, Grinnel VS, Mehringer CM (1981) A detachable balloon for therapeutic transcatheter occlusions. Radiology 138:227–228

28. Hugues JMB, Allison DJ (1990) Pulmonary arteriovenous malformations: the radiologist replaces the surgeon. Clin Radiol 41:297–298

29. Jackson JE, Whyte MKB, Allison DJ, Hugues JMB (1990) Coil embolization of pulmonary arteriovenous malformations. Cor Vasa 32:191–196

30. Khalil A, Farres MT, Mangiapan G, Tassart M, Bigot JM, Carette MF (2000) Pulmonary arteriovenous malformations: diagnosis by contrast-enhanced magnetic resonance angiography. Chest 117:1399–1403

31. Kjeldsen AD, Oxhoj H, Andersen PE, Elle B, Jacobsen JP, Vase P (1999) Pulmonary arteriovenous malformations: screening procedures and pulmonary angiography in patients with hereditary hemorrhagic telangiectasia. Chest 116:432–439

32. Klein GE, Szolar DH, Karaic R, Stein JK, Hausegger KA, Schreyer HH (1996) Extracranial aneurysm and arteriovenous fistula: embolization with the guglielmi detachable coil. Radiology 201:489–494

33. Lacombe P, Lagrange C, El-Hajjam M, Chinet T, Pelage JP (2005) Reperfusion of complex large pulmonary arteriovenous malformations after embolization: report of three cases. CardioVasc Intervent Radiol 28:30–35

34. Laffey KJ, Thomashow B, Jaretzki A III, Martin EC (1985)

Systemic supply to a pulmonary arteriovenous malformation: a relative contraindication to surgery. Am J Roentgenol 145:720–722

35. Lange PA, Stoller JK (1995) The hepatopulmonary syndrome. Ann Intern Med 122:521–529

36. Lee DW, White RI Jr, Egglin TK, Pollak JS, Fayad PB, Wirth JA, Rosenblatt MM, Dickey KW, Burdge CM (1997) Embolotherapy of large pulmonary arteriovenous malformations: long-term results. Ann Thorac Surg 64: 930–940

37. Lee WL, Graham AF, Pugash RA, Hutchinson SJ, Grande P, Hyland RH, Faughnan ME (2003) Contrast echocardiography remains positive after treatment of pulmonary arteriovenous malformations. Chest 123:351–358

38. Longacre AV, Gross CP, Gallitelli M, Henderson KJ, White RI Jr, Proctor DD (2003) Diagnosis and management of gastrointestinal bleeding in patients with hereditary hemorrhagic telangiectasia. Am J Gastroenterol 98:59–65

39. Mager HJ, Overtoom TT, Mauser HW, Westermann KJJ (2001) Early cerebral infarction after embolotherapy of a pulmonary arteriovenous malformation (letter). J Vasc Interv Radiol 12:122–123

40. Mager JJ, Overtoom TT, Blauw H, Lammers JWJ, Westermann CJJ (2004) Embolotherapy of pulmonary arteriovenous malformations: long-term results in 112 patients. J Vasc Interv Radiol 15:451–456

41. Maher CO, Piepgras DG, Brown Jr RD, Friedman JA, Pollock BE (2001) Cerebrovascular manifestations in 321 cases of hereditary hemorrhagic telangiectasia. Stroke 32:877–882

42. McAllister KA, Lennon F, Bowles-Biesecker B, Mc Kinnon WC, Helmbold EA, Markel DS, Jackson CE, Guttmacher AE, Pericak-Vance MA, Marchuk DA (1994) Genetic heterogeneity in hereditary hemorrhagic telangiectasia: possible correlation with clinical phenotype. J Med Genet 31:927–932

43. Moser RJ, Tenholder MF (1986) Diagnostic imaging of pulmonary arteriovenous malformations. Chest 89:586–589

44. Moussoutas M, Fayad P, Rosenblatt M, Hashimoto M, Pollak J, Henderson K, Ma TY, White RI Jr (2000) Pulmonary arteriovenous malformation: cerebral ischemia and neurological manifestations. Neurology 55:959–964

45. Moyer JH, Glantz G, Brest AN (1962) Pulmonary arteriovenous fistulas: physiologic and clinical considerations. Am J Med 32:417–435

46. Nanthakumar K, Graham AT, Robinson TI, Grande P, Pugash RA, Clarke JA, Hutchison SJ, Mandzia JL, Hyland RH, Faughnan ME (2001) Contrast echocardiography for detection of pulmonary arteriovenous malformations. Am Heart J 141:243–246

47. Ohno Y, Hatabu H, Takenaka D, Adachi S, Hirota S, Sugimura K (2002) contrast-enhanced MR perfusion imaging and MR angiography: utility for management of pulmonary arteriovenous malformations for embolotherapy. Eur J Radiol 41:136–146

48. Peery WH (1987) Clinical spectrum of hereditary hemorrhagic telangiectasia (Osler-Weber-Rendu disease). Am J Med 82:989–998

49. Plauchu H, de Chadarevian JP, Bideau A, Robert JM (1989) Age-related clinical profile of hereditary hemorrhagic telangiectasia in an epidemiologically recruited population. Am J Med Genet 32:291–297

50. Pollak JS, Egglin TK, Rosenblatt MM, Dickey KW, White RI Jr (1994) Clinical results transvenous systemic embolotherapy with a neuroradiologic detachable balloon. Radiology 191:477–482

51. Porstmann W (1977) Therapeutic embolization of arteriovenous pulmonary fistula by catheter technique. In: Kelop O (ed) Current concepts in pediatric radiology. Springer, Berlin Heidelberg New York, pp 23–31

52. Prager RL, Laws KH, Bender HW Jr (1983) Arteriovenous fistula of the lungs. Ann Thorac Surg 36:231–235

53. Pugash RA (2001) Pulmonary arteriovenous malformations: overview and transcatheter embolotherapy. Can Assoc Radiol 52:92–102

54. Puskas JD, Allen MS, Moncure AC, Wain JC Jr, Hilgenberg AD, Wright C, Grillo HC, Mathisen DJ (1993) Pulmonary arteriovenous malformations: therapeutic options. Ann Thorac Surg 56:253–258

55. Remy-Jardin M, Watinne L, Remy J (1991) Transcatheter occlusion of pulmonary arterial circulation and collateral supply: failures, incidence and complications. Radiology 180:699–705

56. Remy J, Remy-Jardin M, Watinne L, Deffontaines C (1992) Pulmonary arteriovenous malformations: evaluation with CT of the chest before and after treatment. Radiology 182:809–816

57. Remy J, Remy-Jardin M, Giraud F, Wattine L (1994) Angioarchitecture of pulmonary arteriovenous malformations: clinical utility of three-dimensional helical CT. Radiology 191:657–664

58. Rotondo A, Scialpi M, Scapati C (1997) Pulmonary arteriovenous malformations: evaluation by MR angiography. Am J Roentgenol 167:452–454

59. Sagara K, Miyazono N, Inoue H, Ueno K, Nishida H, Nakajo M (1998) Recanalization after coil embolotherapy of pulmonary arteriovenous malformations: study of long-term outcome and mechanism for recanalization. Am J Roentgenol 171:1704

60. Saluja S, Sitko I, Lee DW, Pollak J, White RI Jr (1999) Embolotherapy of pulmonary arteriovenous malformations with detachable balloons: long-term durability and efficacy. J Vasc Interv Radiol 10:883–889

61. Seward JB, Tajik AJ, Spangler JG, Ritter DG (1975) Echocardiographic contrast studies: initial experience. Mayo Clin Proc 50:163–169

62. Shannon T, Pollak J, White RI Jr (1992) Redistribution of pulmonary blood flow by embolotherapy: a new method for improving oxygenation in patients with diffuse pulmonary arteriovenous malformations (abstract). Am Rev Respir Dis 145:600A

63. Shovlin CL, Hugues JM (1996) Hereditary hemorrhagic telangiectasia. N Engl J Med 334:330–332

64. Shovlin CL, Guttmacher AE, Buscarini E, Faughnan ME, Hyland RH, Westermann CJJ, Kjeldsen AD, Plauchu H (2000) Diagnostic criteria for hereditary hemorrhagic telangiectasia (Rendu-Osler-Weber syndrome). Am J Med Genet 91:65–67

65. Sluiter-Eringa H, Orie NG, Sluiter HJ (1969) Pulmonary arteriovenous fistula: diagnosis and prognosis in noncompliant patients. Am Rev Respir Dis 100:177–188

66. Stringer CJ, Stanley AL, Bates RC, Summers JE (1955) Pulmonary arteriovenous fistulas. Am J Surg 89:1054–1080

67. Swanson KL, Prakash UBS, Stanson AW (1999) Pulmonary arteriovenous fistulas: Mayo Clinic experience. Mayo Clin Proc 74:671–680

68. Takahashi K, Tanimura K, Honda M, Kikuno M, Toei H, Hyodoh H, Furuse M, Yamada T, Aburano T (1999) Venous sac embolization of pulmonary arteriovenous malforma-

tion: preliminary experience using interlocking detachable coils. CardioVasc Intervent Radiol 22:210–213

69. Tal MG, Saluja S, Henderson KJ, White RI Jr (2002) Vein of Galen technique for occluding the aneurysmal sac of pulmonary arteriovenous malformations. J Vasc Interv Radiol 13:1261–1264

70. Taxman RM, Halloran MJ, Parker BM (1973) Multiple pulmonary arteriovenous malformations in association with Fanconi's syndrome. Chest 64:118–120

71. Terry PB, White RI Jr, Barth KH, Kaufman SL, Mitchell SE (1983) Pulmonary arteriovenous malformations: physiologic observations and results of therapeutic balloon embolization. N Engl J Med 308:1197–1200

72. Todo K, Moriwaki H, Higashi M, Kimura K, Naritomi H (2004) Am J Neuroradiol 25:428–430

73. White RI Jr (1992) Pulmonary arteriovenous malformations: how do we diagnose them and why is it important to do so? Radiology 182:633–635

74. White RI Jr (1998) Recanalization after embolotherapy of pulmonary arteriovenous malformations: significance? Outcome? (Letter.) Am J Roentgenol 170:727–730

75. White RI Jr, Barth KH, Kaufman SL, de Caprio V, Strandberg JD (1980) Therapeutic embolization with detachable balloons. CardioVasc Intervent Radiol 3:229–241

76. White RI Jr, Mitchell SE, Barth KH, Kaufman SL, Kadir S, Chang R, Terry PB (1983) Angioarchitecture of pulmonary arteriovenous malformations: an important consideration before embolotherapy. Am J Roentgenol 140:681–686

77. White RI Jr, Lynch-Nylan A, Terry P, Buescher PC, Farmlett EJ, Charnas L, Shuman K, Kim W, Kinnison M, Mitchell SE (1988) Pulmonary arteriovenous malformations: technique and long-term outcome of embolotherapy. Radiology 169:663–669

78. White RI Jr, Pollak JS, Wirth JA (1996) Pulmonary arteriovenous malformations: diagnosis and transcatheter embolotherapy. J Vasc Interv Radiol 7:787–804

79. White RI Jr, Pollak JS, Picus D (2003) Are Guglielmi detachable coils necessary for treating pulmonary arteriovenous malformations? (Letter.) Radiology 226:599–600

Subject Index

List of Contributors

Volume 1

HICHAM T. ABADA, MD
Department of Imaging and Interventional Radiology
Centre Hospitalier René Dubos
6, Avenue de L'lle-de-France
95303 Cergy Pontoise Cedex
France

DOUGLAS M. COLDWELL, MD
Professor of Radiology
University of Texas Southwestern Medical Center
5323 Harry Hines Blvd.
Dallas, TX 75390-8834
USA

MICHAEL D. DARCY, MD
Professor of Radiology and Surgery
Mallinckrodt Institute of Radiology
Washington University School of Medicine
510 South Kingshighway Boulevard
Saint Louis, MO 63110-1076
USA

LUC DEFREYNE, MD
Department of Vascular and
Interventional Radiology
Ghent University Hospital
De Pintelaan 185
9000 Ghent
Belgium

ARNAUD FAUCONNIER, MD, PhD
Department of Obstetrics and Gynecology,
Centre Hospitalier de Poissy,
10, rue du Champ Gaillard,
78300 Poissy Cedex,
France

JAFAR GOLZARIAN, MD
Professor of Radiology
Director, Vascular and Interventional Radiology
University of Iowa
Department of Radiology
200 Hawkins Drive, 3957 JPP
Iowa City, IA 52242
USA

DAVID W. HUNTER, MD
Department of Radiology
J2-447 Fairview-University Medical Center
University of Minnesota
500 Harvard Street S.E.
Minneapolis, MN 55455
USA

PASCAL LACOMBE, MD
Department of Radiology Hôpital Ambroise Pare
9, Avenue Charles De Gaulle
92104 Boulogne Cedex
France

ALEXANDRE LAURENT, MD, PhD
Assistant Professor
Center for Research in
Interventional Imaging (Cr2i APHP-INRA)
Jouy en Josas, 78352
France

LINDSAY MACHAN, MD
Department of Radiology
University of British Columbia Hospital
2211 Wesbrook Mall
Vancouver, BC V6T 2B5
Canada

HIDEFUMI MIMURA, MD
Professor of Radiology
University of Iowa Hospitals and Clinics
Department of Radiology
200 Hawkins Dr, 3957 JPP
Iowa City, IA 52242
USA

TONY A. NICHOLSON, BScM, Sc, MB, ChB, FRCR
Consultant Vascular Radiologist & Senior Lecturer
Leeds Teaching Hospitals NHS Trust
Great George Street
Leeds, LS13EX
UK

JEAN-PIERRE PELAGE, MD, PhD
Department of Radiology
Hôpital Ambroise Pare
9, Avenue Charles De Gaulle
92104 Boulogne Cedex
France

JEFFREY S. POLLAK, MD
Yale University School of Medicine
Department Diagnostic Radiology
PO Box 20842
New Haven, CT 06504-8042
USA

MAHMOOD K. RAZAVI, MD
Director
Center for Research and Clinical Trials
St. Joseph Vascular Institute
Orange, CA 92868
USA

JIM A. REEKERS, MD, PhD
Department of Radiology, G1-207
Academic Medical Center
University of Amsterdam
Meibergdreef 9
AZ 1105 Amsterdam
The Netherlands

ANNE C. ROBERTS, MD
University of California, San Diego Medical Center
Division of Vascular and
Interventional Radiology
200 West Arbor Drive
San Diego, CA 92103-8756
USA

GALIA T. ROSEN, MD
Department of Radiology
J2-447 Fairview-University Medical Center
University of Minnesota
500 Harvard Street S.E.
Minneapolis, MN 55455
USA

MELHEM J. SHARAFUDDIN, MD
Departments of Radiology and Surgery, 3JPP
University of Iowa Hospitals and Clinics
200 Hawkins Drive
Iowa City, IA 52242-1077
USA

GARY P. SISKIN, MD
Associate Professor of Radiology and
Obstetrics & Gynecology
Albany Medical College
47 New Scotland Avenue, MC-113
Albany, NY 12208-3479
USA

SHILIANG SUN, MD
Department of Radiology
University of Iowa Hospitals and Clinics
200 Hawkins Dr, 3955 JPP
Iowa City, IA 52242
USA

KOJI TAKAHASHI, MD
Department of Radiology
Asahikawa Medical College
2-1-1-1 Midorigaoka
Asahikawa, 078-8510
Japan

JOS C. VAN DEN BERG, MD, PhD
Head of Service of Interventional Radiology
Ospedale Regionale di Lugano, sede Civico
Via Tesserete 46
6900 Lugano
Switzerland

DAVID A. VALENTI, MD
Royal Victoria Hospital
McGill University Health Centre
McGill University
687 Pine Avenue West, Suite A451
Montreal, Quebec H3A 1A1
Canada

ROBERT I. WHITE, Jr., MD
Yale University School of Medicine
Department of Diagnostic Radiology
333 Cedar Street, Room 5039 LMP
New Haven, CT 06520
USA

JEFFREY J. WONG, MB ChB, BMedSc
Senior House Officer
Royal National Orthopaedic Hospital
London
UK

Contents – Volume 2

List of Contributors – Volume 2

KAMRAN AHRAR, MD
Section of Interventional Radiology
Division of Diagnostic Imaging
The University of Texas
MD Anderson Cancer Center
1515 Holcombe Boulevard, Unit 325
Houston, TX 77030-4009
USA

HORTENSIA ALVAREZ, MD
Service de Neuroradiologie Diagnostique
et Thérapeutique
Hôpital Bicêtre
78 rue due Général Leclerc
94275 Le Kremlin Bicêtre
France

JOHN C. CHALOUPKA, MD, FAHA, FACA
Director of Interventional Neuroradiology
Professor of Radiology and Neurosurgery
University of Iowa Hospitals and Clinics
University of Iowa Carver College of Medicine
200 Hawkins Dr, 3893 JPP
Iowa City, IA 52242
USA

MICHAEL D. DARCY, MD
Professor of Radiology and Surgery
Division of Diagnostic Radiology
Chief, Interventional Radiology Section
Washington University School of Medicine
Mallinckrodt Institute of Radiology
510 South Kingshighway, 6th Floor
St. Louis, MO 63110
USA

JOSÉE DUBOIS, MD
Professor of Radiology
Pediatric and Interventional Radiologist
Department of Medical Imaging
Hôpital Ste-Justine
3175 Côte Ste-Catherine Road
Montreal, Quebec H3T 1C5
Canada

JAMES R. DUNCAN, MD, PhD
Assistant Professor of Radioloy and Surgery
Mallinckrodt Institute of Radiology and
Washington University School of Medicince
510 S. Kingshighway Blvd
St. Louis, MO 63110
USA

DOMINIQUE ELIAS, MD
Head of Digestive Surgery Section
Institut Gustave Rousssy
39, Rue Camille Desmoulins
94800 Villejuif Cedex
France

LAURENT GAREL, MD
Professor of Radiology
Pediatric and Interventional Radiologist
Department of Medical Imaging
Hôpital Ste-Justine
3175 Côte Ste-Catherine Road
Montreal, Quebec H3T 1C5
Canada

CHRISTOS S. GEORGIADES, MD, PhD
Assistant Professor of Radiology and Surgery
Johns Hopkins Medical Institutions
Blalock 545, 600 North Wolfe Street,
Baltimore, MD 21287
USA

JEAN-FRANCOIS H. GESCHWIND, MD
Associate Professor of Radiology, Surgery and Oncology
Division of Vascular and Interventional Radiology
The Russell H. Morgan Department of Radiolgy
and Radiological Sciences
Johns Hopkins Medical Institutions
Blalock 545, 600 North Wolfe Street
Baltimore, MD 21287
USA

CRAIG B. GLAIBERMAN, MD
Instructor, Radiology
Division of Interventional Radiology
Washington University School of Medicine
Mallinckrodt Institute of Radiology
510 South Kingshighway, 6th Floor
St. Louis, MO 63110
USA

JAFAR GOLZARIAN, MD
Professor of Radiology
Director, Vascular and Interventional Radiology
University of Iowa
Department of Radiology
200 Hawkins Drive, 3957 JPP
Iowa City, IA 52242
USA

MINAKO HAYAKAWA, MD
Visiting Assistant Professor of Radiology
University of Iowa Hospitals and Clinics
University of Iowa Carver College of Medicine
200 Hawkins Dr, 3893 JPP
Iowa City, IA 52242
USA

SAM HEYE, MD
Department of Radiology
University Hospitals Gasthuisberg
Herestraat 49
3000 Leuven
Belgium

SHIH-WEI HSU, MD
Visiting Scholar, University of Iowa Hospitals
and Clinics
University of Iowa Carver College of Medicine
200 Hawkins Dr, 3893 JPP
Iowa City, IA 52242
USA

and

Assistant Professor, Department of Diagnostic
Radiology
Chang Gung Memorial Hospital
Kaohsiung
Taiwan

MATTHEW S. JOHNSON, MD
Associate Professor of Radiology
Diector, Section of Interventional Radiology
Indiana University Hospital, UH0279
Department of Radiology
550 University Boulevard
Indianapolis, IN 46202-5253
USA

JOHN R. KACHURA, MD, FRCPC
Division of Vascular and Interventional Radiology
Department of Medical Imaging
Toronto General Hospital
200 Elizabeth Street, Eaton South 1-454d
Toronto, ON M5G 2C4
Canada

NEIL M. KHILNANI, MD
Cornell Vascular
Weill Medical College of Cornell University
416 East 55th Street
New York, NY 10022
USA

PAULA KLURFAN, MD
Interventional Neuroradioly Clinical Fellow
Department of Medical Imaging
University of Toronto
Toronto Western Hospital
399 Bathurst Street
Toronto, Ontario M5T 2S8
Canada

PIERRE LASJAUNIAS, MD, PhD
Service de Neuroradiologie Diagnostique et Thérapeutique
Hôpital Bicêtre
78 rue due Général Leclerc
94275 Le Kremlin Bicêtre
France

SEON KYU LEE, MD, PhD
Assistant Professor and Staff Neuroradiologist
Department of Medical Imaging
University of Toronto
Toronto Western Hospital
#399 Bathurst Street
Toronto, Ontario M5T 2S8
Canada

WALTER S. LESLEY, MD
Chief, Section of Surgical Neuroradiology
Assistant Professor of Radiology
The Texas A&M University Health Science Center
USA

ELENI LIAPI, MD
The Russell H. Morgan Department of Radiolgy
and Radiological Sciences
Johns Hopkins Medical Institutions
Baltimore, MD
USA

DAVID C. MADOFF, MD
Section of Interventional Radiology
Division of Diagnostic Imaging
The University of Texas
MD Anderson Cancer Center
1515 Holcombe Boulevard, Unit 325
Houston, TX 77030-4009
USA

GEERT MALEUX, MD
Department of Radiology
University Hospitals Gasthuisberg
Herestraat 49
3000 Leuven
Belgium

FRANCIS MARSHALLECK, MD
Assistant Professor of Radiology
Indiana University School of Medicine
Indiana University Hospital
Room 0279, 550 North University Boulevard
Indianapolis, IN 26202
USA

ROBERT J. MIN, MD
Cornell Vascular
Weill Medical College of Cornell University
416 East 55th Street
New York, NY 10022
USA

ANNE C. ROBERTS, MD
University of California, San Diego Medical Center
Division of Vascular and Interventional Radiology
200 West Arbor Drive
San Diego, CA 92103-8756
USA

ALAIN J. ROCHE, MD
Head of Interventional Radiology Section
Professor, Institut Gustave Rousssy
39, Rue Camille Desmoulins
94800 Villejuif Cedex
France

GEORGES RODESCH, MD
Service de Neuroradioloie Diagnostique et Thérapeutique
Hôpital Foch
40 rue Worth
B.P. 36
92150 Suresnes
France

RIAD SALEM, MD, MBA
Assistant Professor of Radiology and Oncology
Northwestern Memorial Hospital
Department of Radiology
676 North St. Claire, Suite 800
Chicago, IL 60611
USA

MELHEM J. SHARAFUDDIN, MD
University of Iowa Hospitals and Clinics
Department of Radiology
200 Hawkins Dr, 3957 JPP
Iowa City, IA 52242
USA

GARY SISKIN, MD
Albany Medical College
Vascular Radiology, A113
47 New Scotland Avenue
Albany, NY 12208-3479
USA

SHILIANG SUN, MD
Associate Professor of Radiology
Department of Radiology
University of Iowa, College of Medicine
200 Hawkins Dr., 3955 JPP
Iowa City, IA 52242
USA

KONG TENG TAN, MB, BCh, FRCS, FRCR
Division of Vascular and Interventional Radiology
Department of Medical Imaging
Toronto General Hospital
585 University Avenue, NCSB 1C-563
Toronto, ON M5G 2N2
Canada

MARIA THIJS, MD
Department of Radiology
University Hospitals Gasthuisberg
Herestraat 49
3000 Leuven
Belgium

KENNETH G. THURSTON, Ma
17 Bramble Lane
West Grove, PA 19390
USA

RAJIV VERMA, MD
Section of Interventional Radiology
Division of Diagnostic Imaging
The University of Texas
MD Anderson Cancer Center
1515 Holcombe Boulevard, Unit 325
Houston, TX 77030-4009
USA

LUCY A. WIBBENMEYER, MD
University of Iowa Hospitals and Clinics
Department of Radiology
200 Hawkins Dr.
Iowa City, IA 52242
USA

JEFFREY J. WONG, MB ChB, BMedSc
University of California, San Diego Medical Center
Division of Vascular and Interventional Radiology
200 West Arbor Drive
San Diego, CA 92103-8756
USA

DIAGNOSTIC IMAGING

Innovations in Diagnostic Imaging
Edited by J. H. Anderson

Radiology of the Upper Urinary Tract
Edited by E. K. Lang

**The Thymus - Diagnostic Imaging,
Functions, and Pathologic Anatomy**
Edited by E. Walter, E. Willich,
and W. R. Webb

Interventional Neuroradiology
Edited by A. Valavanis

Radiology of the Pancreas
Edited by A. L. Baert,
co-edited by G. Delorme

Radiology of the Lower Urinary Tract
Edited by E. K. Lang

Magnetic Resonance Angiography
Edited by I. P. Arlart, G. M. Bongartz,
and G. Marchal

Contrast-Enhanced MRI of the Breast
S. Heywang-Köbrunner and R. Beck

Spiral CT of the Chest
Edited by M. Rémy-Jardin and J. Rémy

Radiological Diagnosis of Breast Diseases
Edited by M. Friedrich and E.A. Sickles

Radiology of the Trauma
Edited by M. Heller and A. Fink

Biliary Tract Radiology
Edited by P. Rossi,
co-edited by M. Brezi

Radiological Imaging of Sports Injuries
Edited by C. Masciocchi

Modern Imaging of the Alimentary Tube
Edited by A. R. Margulis

Diagnosis and Therapy of Spinal Tumors
Edited by P. R. Algra, J. Valk,
and J. J. Heimans

**Interventional Magnetic
Resonance Imaging**
Edited by J.F. Debatin and G. Adam

Abdominal and Pelvic MRI
Edited by A. Heuck and M. Reiser

Orthopedic Imaging
Techniques and Applications
Edited by A. M. Davies
and H. Pettersson

Radiology of the Female Pelvic Organs
Edited by E. K.Lang

**Magnetic Resonance of the Heart
and Great Vessels**
Clinical Applications
Edited by J. Bogaert, A.J. Duerinckx,
and F. E. Rademakers

Modern Head and Neck Imaging
Edited by S. K. Mukherji
and J. A. Castelijns

**Radiological Imaging
of Endocrine Diseases**
Edited by J. N. Bruneton
in collaboration with B. Padovani
and M.-Y. Mourou

Trends in Contrast Media
Edited by H. S. Thomsen,
R. N. Muller, and R. F. Mattrey

Functional MRI
Edited by C. T. W. Moonen
and P. A. Bandettini

Radiology of the Pancreas
2nd Revised Edition
Edited by A. L. Baert. Co-edited by
G. Delorme and L. Van Hoe

Emergency Pediatric Radiology
Edited by H. Carty

Spiral CT of the Abdomen
Edited by F. Terrier, M. Grossholz,
and C. D. Becker

Liver Malignancies
Diagnostic and
Interventional Radiology
Edited by C. Bartolozzi
and R. Lencioni

Medical Imaging of the Spleen
Edited by A. M. De Schepper
and F. Vanhoenacker

Radiology of Peripheral Vascular Diseases
Edited by E. Zeitler

Diagnostic Nuclear Medicine
Edited by C. Schiepers

Radiology of Blunt Trauma of the Chest
P. Schnyder and M. Wintermark

Portal Hypertension
Diagnostic Imaging-Guided Therapy
Edited by P. Rossi
Co-edited by P. Ricci and L. Broglia

**Recent Advances in
Diagnostic Neuroradiology**
Edited by Ph. Demaerel

**Virtual Endoscopy
and Related   3D Techniques**
Edited by P. Rogalla, J. Terwisscha
Van Scheltinga, and B. Hamm

Multislice CT
Edited by M. F. Reiser, M. Takahashi,
M. Modic, and R. Bruening

Pediatric Uroradiology
Edited by R. Fotter

**Transfontanellar Doppler Imaging
in Neonates**
A. Couture and C. Veyrac

Radiology of AIDS
A Practical Approach
Edited by J.W.A.J. Reeders
and P.C. Goodman

CT of the Peritoneum
Armando Rossi and Giorgio Rossi

Magnetic Resonance Angiography
2nd Revised Edition
Edited by I. P. Arlart,
G. M. Bongratz, and G. Marchal

Pediatric Chest Imaging
Edited by Javier Lucaya
and Janet L. Strife

**Applications of Sonography
in Head and Neck Pathology**
Edited by J. N. Bruneton
in collaboration with C. Raffaelli
and O. Dassonville

Imaging of the Larynx
Edited by R. Hermans

3D Image Processing
Techniques and Clinical Applications
Edited by D. Caramella
and C. Bartolozzi

**Imaging of Orbital and
Visual Pathway Pathology**
Edited by W. S. Müller-Forell

Pediatric ENT Radiology
Edited by S. J. King
and A. E. Boothroyd

Radiological Imaging of the Small Intestine
Edited by N. C. Gourtsoyiannis

MEDICAL RADIOLOGY Diagnostic Imaging and Radiation Oncology

Titles in the series already published

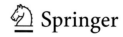

MEDICAL RADIOLOGY Diagnostic Imaging and Radiation Oncology

Titles in the series already published

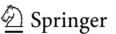 Springer